Neural Modeling of Brain and Cognitive Disorders

PROGRESS IN NEURAL PROCESSING

Series Advisors

Alan Murray *(University of Edinburgh)*
Lionel Tarassenko *(University of Oxford)*
John Taylor *(King's College, London)*
Andreas Weigend *(University of Colorado)*

Neural Modeling of Brain and Cognitive Disorders

Editors

James A Reggia
University Maryland, USA

Eytan Ruppin
Tel Aviv University, Israel

Rita Sloan Berndt
University Maryland, USA

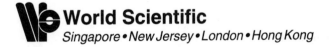

World Scientific
Singapore • New Jersey • London • Hong Kong

Published by

World Scientific Publishing Co. Pte. Ltd.

P O Box 128, Farrer Road, Singapore 912805

USA office: Suite 1B, 1060 Main Street, River Edge, NJ 07661

UK office: 57 Shelton Street, Covent Garden, London WC2H 9HE

Library of Congress Cataloging-in-Publication Data
Neural modeling of brain and cognitive disorders / [edited by] James
    A. Reggia, Eytan Ruppin, & Rita Sloan Berndt.
       p.   cm.
    Consists of presentations made at the Workshop on Neural Modeling
of Cognitive and Brain Disorders, held at the University of Maryland, June 1995.
    Includes bibliographical references.
    ISBN 9810228791
    1. Cognition disorders -- Computer simulation -- Congresses.
2. Brain -- Diseases -- Computer simulation -- Congresses.   3. Psychoses -
- Computer simulation -- Congresses.   4. Neural networks
(Neurobiology) -- Congresses.   I. Reggia, James A.   II. Ruppin, Eytan.
III. Berndt, Rita Sloan.   IV. Workshop on Neural Modeling of
Cognitive and Brain Disorders (1995 : University of Maryland)
    [DNLM: 1. Nervous System Diseases -- Congresses.   2. Cognition
Disorders -- Congresses.   3. Mental Disorders -- Congresses.   4. Models,
Neurological -- Congresses.   WL 140 N4905 1996]
RC553.C64N47   1996
616.8--dc20
DNLM/DLC
for Library of Congress   96-35593
                                          CIP

British Library Cataloguing-in-Publication Data
A catalogue record for this book is available from the British Library.

This book is printed on acid-free paper.

Printed in Singapore by Uto-Print

PREFACE

Neural modeling, the study of networks of artificial neurons, has had its ups and downs. In the 1960's, neural modeling research was a very dynamic and exciting part of the field known today as artificial intelligence. However, it is fair to say that during the subsequent 15 years very little interest was exhibited in neural networks. Only a relatively few individuals worked in this area during the 1970's, and the work that was done, which was often primarily theoretical analysis, did not receive the attention it deserved.

Times have changed. Since the mid 1980's there has been a tremendous surge of interest in and applications involving neural models. Today not only mathematicians, physicists, computer scientists and engineers regularly study neural models, but so do neuroscientists and cognitive psychologists. Individuals in both these latter fields view computational modeling with neural networks (or connectionist networks, as they are often called in cognitive science) as a major theoretical tool.

To date, the vast majority of work using neural networks in neuroscience and cognitive psychology has focused on modeling *normal* functions. There are now numerous neural models of intact memory, language, perception and related functions. The earliest models we know of addressing *abnormal* functionality in these areas appeared around 1980. It is these models of brain and cognitive disorders that are the focus of this book, which was prompted by the growing interest in applying neural modeling to the understanding of clinical disorders. In June 1995 about 150 individuals from around the world met at a workshop we organized at the University of Maryland to discuss and debate issues in this area. The shared enthusiasm for this new approach to studying clinical disorders was very encouraging. The multidisciplinary background of participants led to exciting discussions and exchanges of views.

The contributions in this book represent only a subset of the presentations made at the Workshop. Space limitations prevented inclusion of all of the presentations made; many of those not included here also described very interesting results.[1] The contributions that are included are representative of the challenging and productive work currently under way.

The Workshop, and this book, would never have happened without contributions from many individuals and institutions. The meeting itself was supported by NIH Grant MH-54266, with financial contributions from the National Institute of Mental Health, National Institute of Neurological Disorders

---

[1] An informal "Proceedings" of all 45 presentations made at the 1995 Workshop on Neural Modeling of Cognitive and Brain Disorders can be obtained by contacting the Publications Officer, UMIACS, University of Maryland, College Park MD 20742, USA.

and Stroke, National Institute on Deafness and Other Communication Disorders, and National Institute on Aging. Just as importantly, individuals like Dennis Glanzman, John Marler and Judith Cooper at NIH provided crucial encouragement, as did Joseph JaJa, Director of the Institute for Advanced Computer Studies at the University of Maryland. The Institute for Advanced Computer Studies also provided a substantial financial contribution to support the meeting. Other sponsors include the Department of Neurology, University of Maryland School of Medicine; the Center for the Neural Basis of Cognition, Carnegie Mellon & Pittsburgh Universities; the Adams Super Center for Brain Studies, Tel Aviv University; the Upjohn Company; and the Center for Neural and Cognitive Sciences, University of Maryland. Johanna Weinstein and Cecilia Kullman provided invaluable assistance in organizing and administering the workshop. Finally, Richard Lim, Connie Liu and others at World Scientific provided a great deal of assistance in preparing this book.

James A. Reggia
Eytan Ruppin
Rita Sloan Berndt

June 1996

TABLE OF CONTENTS

PSYCHIATRIC DISORDERS

INTRODUCTION

MODELING BRAIN AND COGNITIVE DISORDERS

James A. Reggia

Depts. of Computer Science & Neurology, Inst. Advanced Computer Studies
A.V. Williams Bldg., University of Maryland, College Park, MD 20742, USA
Email: reggia@cs.umd.edu

Eytan Ruppin

Depts. of Computer Science & Physiology, Tel Aviv University,
Tel Aviv 69978, Israel
Email: ruppin@math.tau.ac.il

Rita Sloan Berndt

Dept. of Neurology, University of Maryland School of Medicine
Baltimore, MD 21201, USA
Email: rberndt@umabnet.ab.umd.edu

Abstract

During the last several years there has been a growing interest in developing computational models of phenomena associated with brain and cognitive disorders. Work in this area has included studies of Alzheimer's disease, aphasia and dyslexia, epilepsy, stroke, Parkinson's disease, schizophrenia, depression, and related problems. In this chapter, we give a broad overview of past work in this area as background for the specific topics addressed in the rest of this book.

1. Introduction

Neural modeling research is currently a very active scientific field involving substantial multidisciplinary work. The main emphasis in the past has been on the investigation of cognitive and neural functions in normal, healthy subjects. Recently, a new direction has emerged, that of using "lesioned" neural models to study various brain and cognitive disorders from a computational point of view. The term "lesioned" is interpreted broadly here to mean that an intact model's structural or functional mechanisms are disrupted in some fashion. The goals of this research have been to construct computational models that can explain how specific neuroanatomical and neurophysiological pathological changes can result in various clinical manifestations, and to investigate the functional organization of the symptoms that result from specific brain pathologies.

Neural models necessarily simplify the biological phenomena occurring in the nervous system and are generally constrained in size. The simulated lesions in such models are also substantial simplifications of pathophysiological events occurring within

3

the brain and/or in cognitive processes. Nevertheless, such computer-based models complement traditional methods of studying brain disorders in substantial and important ways. Lesion size and location can be controlled precisely and can be systematically varied over arbitrarily large numbers of experimental 'subjects' and information processing tasks. Further, computational experiments are open to detailed inspection in ways that biological systems are not, permitting one to determine the underlying mechanisms and trace the behavioral changes following a lesion.

In this chapter, we give a broad overview of representative past efforts to model brain and cognitive disorders computationally. We divide this past work into four categories:

- Memory Disorders
- Language Disorders
- Neurological Disorders
- Psychiatric Disorders

This division[a], which parallels that of the rest of this book, is somewhat arbitrary in that some studies fall into more than one of these categories. For example, simulations of memory impairments in Alzheimer's disease might be grouped with neurological disorders or models of memory impairment. Nevertheless, it provides a useful starting orientation for someone previously unfamiliar with this work.

2. Memory Disorders

Simulating various aspects of memory has been of central importance in neural modeling. Because of this, it is not surprising that substantial efforts have also gone into developing models of memory disorders, and that some of the earliest modeling of disorders was in this area. Representative examples are listed in Table 1.

---

[a]Another category of clinical applications of neural models involves their use as decision aids in clinical practice. What is being modeled with these systems is not a neurological or cognitive disorder, but the clinical decision making that goes into analysis of data about a patient with such a disorder. For this reason, we do not consider such models in this book.

Table 1: Example Neural Models of Memory Disorders

Abnormality	Investigators	Year
random network lesions	Wood	1978
	Anderson	1983
disconnection syndromes	Gordon	1982
amnesia	McClelland & Rumelhart	1986
Alzheimer's disease	Horn et al	1993, 1995
	Hasselmo	1994
	Ruppin & Reggia	1995a
agnosia	Farah & McClelland	1991
consolidation and catastrophic forgetting	McClelland et al	1995
semantic memory impairments	Small et al 1995	1995
structural vs. functional damage	Ruppin & Reggia	1995b

2.1 Early Associative Memories

Some of the earliest neural models that were systematically studied and analyzed were simple linear associative memories. Anderson (1983) and Kohonen (1989) summarize some of this early work. Lesion studies with these models can be viewed as precursors of both the contemporary models of Alzheimer's disease to be discussed in this section and the focal cortical lesions described later in this chapter. In a neural model of this kind, there is a set of input neurons and a set of output neurons. Each input neuron sends a one-way connection to every output neuron, so this is a fully-connected, feedforward architecture. Output neurons compute their activation level as a linear sum of their inputs where the coefficients in this sum are the weights on the respective connections. It is this linearity that makes such models readily analyzable and thus encouraged their early development. These models typically used a distributed representation of information and learned using Hebb's rule. They are generally said to be associative memories because they are trained to produce a specific output pattern in response to each input pattern they are given.

Perhaps the earliest systematic lesioning study of brain models was done with linear associative memories (Wood, 1978). In this study there were only eight input neurons and eight output neurons, and the model was trained with four pairs of input-output patterns. A very large number of simulations were run in which a set of cells and all of their connections were deleted from the network. All possible lesions involving combinations of one to seven input neurons, one to seven output neurons, and one to fourteen input and output neurons were tested. Performance of a lesioned model was measured based on how well it generated the correct output pattern for each of the input patterns it was given.

The lesioned models in this study exhibited a number of interesting properties. They were fault tolerant in that small lesions tended to have little effect. As lesion size increased, performance decreased. On the other hand, removal of any neuron produced a roughly similar deficit as removal of any other neuron in terms of its effect on performance. These results led to the conclusion that lesioning of associative networks of linear neurons produced effects resembling Lashley's "mass action" and "equipotentiality" (Wood, 1978). While this is true, the situation is more complex than such statistical measures might suggest, e.g., removing some neurons may be more harmful for specific associations than for others (see Dean (1980) and Wood (1980) for further discussion).

Subsequent work with similar but more sophisticated networks of neurons largely confirmed the above results and demonstrated new phenomena. One well-known related model that has been lesioned is the autoassociative memory sometimes called the "brain-state-in-a-box" (Anderson, 1983). This model consists of a single set of neurons fully-connected to one-another. It is "autoassociative" in that activity patterns became associated with themselves during Hebbian learning. The network thus serves as an associative memory: complete patterns "stored" in the network are retrieved by presenting the network with part of the pattern or a noisy version of the pattern.

A fifty neuron autoassociative memory trained on images representing the twenty-six letters of the alphabet was systematically lesioned, and its degradation in performance was assessed as a function of lesion size (Anderson, 1983). Lesions consisted of randomly removing a specific percentage of the synapses (connections) rather than neurons as was done in (Wood, 1978). In spite of this difference and the different network structures, the same pattern of results was obtained. In addition, it was observed that if lesions were made incrementally rather than all at once while synaptic modifiability was allowed to continue, then there was much less deterioration in performance for a given lesion size. This latter result is intriguing because it is consistent with observations that slow damage is less harmful than rapid damage in animal ablation studies (Anderson, 1983) and in clinical experience (Brain & Walton, 1969; Walsh, 1978; Heilman & Valenstein, 1979).

A more complex architecture has been used to simulate various disconnection syndromes manifested by deficits in confrontation naming (Gordon, 1982). The network in this study was composed of four sets of 32 neurons, each set combining features of the simple associative and autoassociative memories described above. The four sets of neurons represented visual input, tactile input, "semantics", and motor output brain regions. Lesions were induced by partially or completely removing the connections between these sets. The resulting degraded performance in the network was interpreted as being consistent with optic aphasia, tactile aphasia, and other clinical syndromes.

These early lesioning studies of neural models were intended, at least loosely, as models of cerebral cortex and its connections. They showed how lesions of highly parallel information processing systems could account for various neuropsychological phenomena. However, their small size and abstract nature make it difficult to relate them directly to real biophysical neural circuitry. For example, the neurons in these models generally do not have a spatial relationship to one another as occurs in the brain. All neurons in a set of neurons in these models are "equidistant" from one another so that there cannot be a concept of topographic map formation or of a "focal lesion" in the physical sense that a neuropsychologist or neurologist would mean.

2.2 Alzheimer's Disease

Alzheimer's disease is the most common dementing illness. Because of its clinical importance, we focus on this topic in the rest of this section. The essential feature of Alzheimer's is broad-based intellectual decline from previous levels of functioning. Although Alzheimer's disease is characterized by the development of multiple cognitive deficits manifested by disturbances in language, motor and executive functions, a major clinical hallmark of the disease is memory impairment, which manifests itself as an inability both to recall previously learned knowledge and to learn new information.

The clinical course of Alzheimer's disease is usually characterized by gradual deterioration, although both slow and rapidly progressive forms have been reported, exhibiting a large variation in the rate of progression. The diagnosis of Alzheimer's disease is traditionally based on the presence of specific microscopic abnormalities such as neurofibrillary tangles and senile plaques in brain tissue (which in small numbers are found also in the normal aging brain). A confirmed diagnosis of Alzheimer's disease is usually made only after autopsy, or, less frequently, after brain biopsy. Although considerable progress has been made recently in understanding some neurobiological features of Alzheimer's disease, its causes and pathogenesis are still generally unknown (the interested reader is referred to (Katzman 1986) for a review of Alzheimer's disease).

In the following we summarize two previous neural models of the pathogenesis of Alzheimer's disease. The first concentrates on studying the possible role of synaptic deletion and compensation, while the second investigates the role of synaptic runaway.

2.3. Synaptic Deletion and Compensation

Recent neuroanatomical investigations have repeatedly demonstrated that the progress of Alzheimer's disease is accompanied by considerable synaptic changes, including synaptic deletion and compensation. While *synaptic deletion* is manifested in a reduction of the number of synapses per unit of cortical volume, a concomitant increase in the size of the remaining synapses has also been observed and is referred to as *synaptic compensation.*

In light of the major place that memory impairment occupies among the clinical manifestations of Alzheimer's disease, the neuronal and synaptic degenerative changes that occur as the disease progresses are an ideal candidate for neural modeling. This approach was taken by (Horn et al., 1993) in studying how the interplay between synaptic deletion and compensation determines the observed patterns of memory deterioration, and what strategies of increased synaptic efficacy could best maintain memory capacities in face of synaptic deletion.

Investigating these synaptic changes in a Hopfield-like attractor neural network model of associative memory, (Horn et al., 1993) have shown that the deterioration of memory retrieval due to synaptic deletion can be much delayed by strengthening the remaining synaptic weights by a uniform compensatory factor. Variations on the rate and exact functional form of synaptic compensation were used to define various compensation strategies, and these could account for the observed variation in the severity and progression rate of Alzheimer's disease. These results explain the specific patterns of cognitive decline observed in various clinically-defined subgroups of patients with Alzheimer's disease, and have led to the formulation of a new hypothesis accounting for the appearance of parkinsonian symptoms in Alzheimer's disease patients (Horn & Ruppin 1992). This work is however limited in two important ways. First, since a prescribed synaptic memory matrix was used, only memory retrieval and not storage could be addressed. Second, the synaptic compensation dependencies employed were realized in a 'global' manner which is biologically unrealistic.

The first limitation was addressed in (Ruppin & Reggia, 1995a), using a simple, activity-dependent Hebbian synaptic storage scheme to simulate memory acquisition in the framework of an attractor neural network model. This work countered a recent claim that neural models cannot account for more detailed aspects of memory impairment, such as the relative sparing of remote versus recent memories observed in Alzheimer's patients (Carrie 1993). The model exhibits differential sparing of remote versus recent memories, accounts for the experimentally observed temporal gradient of memory decline, and shows that neural models can account for a large variety of experimental phenomena characterizing memory degradation in Alzheimer patients. Specific testable predictions were generated concerning the relation between the neuroanatomical degenerative findings and the clinical manifestations of Alzheimer's disease.

The biological appeal of the uniform synaptic compensatory regimes studied by (Horn et al., 1993) hinges upon the ability to show that they can actually be realized in a 'local' manner, where each neuron readjusts its synaptic weights only as a function of local information such as its post-synaptic potential. A recent study of such local compensatory mechanisms demonstrates that this is a non-trivial but feasible task (Horn et al., 1995). This study has revealed a new dependency between the extent of synaptic changes and the retrieval properties of the network. In contradistinction to the case of global compensatory strategies, the network's performance not only depends on the current magnitudes of deletion and compensation, but also on the precise rates at which these processes progress. That is, the performance of the network is history-dependent. This dependency provides a new explanation for the rather puzzling broad variability in structural indicators of damage observed in Alzheimer's disease patients having approximately similar levels of cognitive function. Further details about modeling synaptic deletion and compensation are given in (Ruppin et al., this volume).

2.4. *Synaptic Runaway*

While the studies reviewed above have sought to explain memory degradation in Alzheimer's disease as a failure of synaptic compensatory responses to account for ongoing accelerated synaptic deletion, a different approach, *runaway synaptic modification*, has been studied in both attractor and feed-forward networks (Hasselmo et al., 1992, 1993, 1994). Runaway synaptic modification denotes a pathological exponential growth of synaptic connections that may occur due to interference by previously stored patterns during the storage of new patterns. This interference occurs because, when a new memory pattern is being stored in the network, the resulting network activity is not only guided by the new pattern but also by all the previous memory patterns which are engraved in the synaptic matrix. Thus, previously memorized patterns tend to bias the activation in 'their direction' during new storage. This inherent reinforcement may lead to exponential synaptic growth and to a pathological increase in the number of synapses.

One possible way to prevent synaptic runaway is to assume that the strength of the external projections by which new patterns are stored in the network is sufficiently strong to overcome the interference of other memories (this assumption does not necessarily imply the use of strong external fields that 'clamp' the activation in the network; see (Ruppin & Reggia 1995a)). Another alternative is that runaway synaptic modification can be inhibited by suppression of internal synaptic connections (synapses between neurons belonging to the same cortical module) during learning.

What is the hypothesized role of synaptic runaway in the pathogenesis of Alzheimer's disease? Analysis shows that there is a critical storage capacity beyond which interference during learning cannot be prevented and synaptic runaway is unavoidable (Hasselmo et al., 1992, 1993, 1994). Several factors can lead to the initiation of synaptic runaway, such as a decrease in the level of cortical inhibition, reduced synaptic decay, and excess memory storage. Once synaptic runaway occurs, it is claimed that its increased metabolic demands or excitotoxic effects could be sufficiently severe to cause neuronal degeneration, parallel to that found in Alzheimer's disease. Furthermore, this work provides a theoretical framework for describing the specific distribution of neuronal degeneration observed in Alzheimer's disease, where entorhinal regions lacking suppression of internal synaptic transmission are more markedly damaged than other cortical regions.

The synaptic runaway theory has been inspired by experimental work (Hasselmo and Bower 1992; Hasselmo and Barkai 1992) that provides evidence that acetylcholine selectively suppresses excitatory synaptic transmission at the internal synapses, while allowing external afferent synaptic transmission (i.e., projections from neurons belonging to other modules) to operate at full strength. Accordingly, it is claimed that the loss of cholinergic innervation in Alzheimer's disease may underlie the initiation of runaway synaptic modification, and that sprouting of cholinergic innervation observed in the dentate gyrus during Alzheimer's disease reflects attempts to arrest the progress of synaptic runaway.

This work on synaptic runaway is an excellent example of research that combines experimental physiological studies with computational modeling. It demonstrates how a computational model can raise a quandary (how are patterns actually stored without being accompanied by synaptic runaway?) which motivates an experimental study (the differential effects of acetylcholine on internal and external synapses). Moreover, the theoretical solution to this question gives rise to further hypotheses concerning the possible consequences of a disruption of the newly revealed computational mechanism (i.e., the role of synaptic runaway in the pathogenesis of Alzheimer's disease). Further details on these issues can be found in (Hasselmo & Wyble, this volume).

3. Language Disorders

Many different types of brain pathologies can have devastating effects on the human cognitive system. Neurologists and neuropsychologists have identified a wide variety of cognitive and language disorders that are associated with both focal and diffuse brain lesions. Connectionist models have been developed to simulate normal cognitive function and the ways in which normal cognition is affected by brain injury. Although these cognitively-oriented connectionist models often use a neuron-like processing structure, they are *not* brain models in the sense that they model neuroanatomic and neurophysiological function. They are best viewed as simulations of cognitive functions and related phenomena that emanate from brain function, in contrast to the neural models described elsewhere in this volume that attempt to simulate specific aspects of brain anatomy and physiology.

Networks in cognitive connectionist models often represent concepts and associations, entities in the cognitive domain rather than biological structures. Such models often adopt a *local representation* of information, with nodes representing a complex psychological construct (e.g., words or morphemes) and connections representing associations between such constructs. Models with this local representation of information are sometimes referred to as "symbolic" models, and they may assume the existence of relatively complex cognitive units as part of the normal cognitive architecture. Many of these models use a neuron-like activation rule borrowed from the neural modeling literature, although others do not. In either case, these spreading activation networks can be regarded as viable models of mental functional processes independently of the extent to which they are intended as models of brain activity.

Other connectionist models studied in cognitive science use a *distributed represen-*

tation of information. In these "subsymbolic" models cognitive constructs are typically represented as patterns of activity across a population of primitive nodes that develop from repeated pairings of information from different sources. Such models do not represent symbolic cognitive constructs explicitly, although patterns of activity that develop over time may function much like such a representation (Forster, 1994).

Fully distributed connectionist models simulating cognitive mechanisms, just as models with local representations of information, must be distinguished from neural models of brain function. However, since biologically-based neural models generally use distributed representations of information that appear to be very similar to the distributed representations of the cognitive models, there is a tendency to blur this distinction and to regard distributed cognitive models as direct representations of some level of brain activity. In fact, the details of how connectionist cognitive models map onto a neural substrate is an open research question. Table 2 presents a selective list of some connectionist models of neurogenic language dysfunction.

Table 2: Example Neural Models of Language Disorders

Abnormality	Investigators	Year
symptoms of aphasia	Gigley	1983
	Cottrell	1985
	Martin et al.	1994, 1996
	Harley	1995
symptoms of acquired dyslexia	Reggia, Marsland & Berndt	1988
	Patterson et al.	1989
	Mozer & Behrmann	1990
	Hinton & Shallice	1991
	Plaut & Shallice	1993
	Coltheart et al.	1993
	Plaut	1996
	Plaut et al.	1996
symptoms of acquired dysgraphia	Olson & Caramazza	1994
	Shallice et al.	1995

3.1 Structural vs. emergent cognitive components

The distinction between completely distributed connectionist models and those employing a local representation is more than a minor detail of the model's implementation, and can imply quite different views of the principles underlying cognitive processing. Several chapters in this volume report investigations of the behavior of lesioned distributed connectionist models that question the necessity of components within symbolic cognitive models that are assumed to be necessary structural requirements of the normal cognitive architecture. Although each of these chapters focuses on a specific type of cognitive disorder arising from brain lesions, their goal is to demonstrate that, in principle, specific symptoms can arise from very general degradations of activation across fully distributed representations. For example, Farah and Tippett (this volume) consider symptoms shown by patients with Alzheimer's Disease that have been interpreted as evidence for multiple cognitive deficits arising from disruption to distinct levels of processing (i.e., visual, lexical, semantic) within a symbolic framework. Farah and Tippett show that these distinct symptoms may arise from degradation of information flow within a single, putatively semantic, information layer that mediates between visual and lexical information (e.g., between pictures of objects and their names). This chapter also questions the need for an explicit level of knowledge representation that distinguishes among semantic categories. Rather, it is argued that category knowledge (which is frequently retained in Alzheimer's Disease) and knowledge about the identity of category exemplars (which is subject to earlier deterioration) emerges naturally from frequency-sensitive graded processing of distributed representations of exemplar attributes. A similar conclusion is reached by Small and colleagues (this volume), who demonstrate the emergence of semantic category structure from feature representations of objects. This finding is used as a basis to account for cases of selective semantic category impairment that have been reported in patients with a variety of brain pathologies.

In a similar vein, Mayall and Humphreys (this volume) consider the topic of "covert recognition" following brain damage–the finding that patients may have information that they are not aware of about characteristics of stimuli. Interpretations of covert recognition have relied on structural distinctions between qualitatively different types of information. These accounts have postulated either separate processors for consciously perceived vs. unconscious knowledge, or have speculated about possible "disconnections" between intact processing components and a separate component of conscious awareness. Mayall and Humphreys describe a simple, distributed word recognition system that, when damaged in a variety of ways, simulates performance found among patients with a specific type of acquired dyslexia ("pure alexia"). The symptoms demonstrated include the ability to report information about words that are not recognized and cannot be pronounced. Thus, as in the examples described above, it is argued that dissociations of symptoms (conscious vs. unconscious "recognition") do not necessarily signal the selective disruption of discrete components in a complex, symbolic architecture. The contrast between completely distributed cognitive models and those with local representation of symbolic information are most evident in studies of language disorders involving focal brain injury, where both types of models have found some support.

3.2 Focal language disorders: aphasia

Although some of the earliest attempts to model aphasic disturbances focused on disturbances of sentence processing (Gigley, 1983; Cottrell, 1985), and despite the fact that non-connectionist, computational models have been developed to simulate sentence comprehension (Haarman & Kolk, 1991; Haarman, Just & Carpenter, 1996), recent connectionist studies of language have been concerned not with sentence processing but with simple transcoding of information at the single word level. Many of these efforts have been concerned with the issue of how information of different types (e.g., phonological, semantic) serves to trigger word responses under different conditions of stimulation: picture naming, word repetition, or written word naming.

In the auditory-verbal domain, a single-word model with local representation of information has been used to simulate the performance of individual patients with impaired picture naming and word repetition. Martin, Dell, Saffran and Schwartz (1994) used Dell's (1986) interactive activation model of sentence production to simulate the performance of a patient with "deep dysphasia". This type of aphasia is defined by a high rate of semantic substitutions ("semantic paraphasias") in repetition tasks and an inability to repeat nonsense words. The patient also produced many errors when naming pictures, but these errors were primarily substitutions of words with a phonological, rather than semantic, relationship to the target ("formal paraphasias"). With recovery, these characteristic error patterns in the two tasks changed to a more "normal" pattern: more semantic than formal paraphasias in picture naming, and more formal than semantic paraphasias in repetition.

The model used for the simulations combined three levels of linguistic representation (semantic, lexical and phonological) with a spreading activation retrieval mechanism with feedforward and feedback connections that carry priming activation to target and related nodes in a small lexical network (Dell, 1986). In naming tasks, a target lexical node is activated by semantic processes (as if stimulated by the presence of a picture), and successively activates its corresponding phonemes. Feedback from all activated nodes reinforces activation of the target node, but also activates phonologically related nodes. If this feedback raises activation of a non-target node to a level higher than that of the target, a phonological error (formal paraphasia) will occur. In repetition tasks, the order of information flow is altered, with phonological activation occurring before semantic activation (as if from an aural stimulus presented for repetition).

Two parameters of the model, connection strength and decay rate, regulate the flow of information through the network, and these parameters were manipulated in the "lesion" simulations. Increasing the decay rate produced the specific effects that were found in the patient's data: a higher percentage of formal paraphasias in naming and of semantic errors in repetition. Further, reduction of the decay rate "impairment" toward normal successfully reproduced the patient's error patterns as he recovered. These results suggest that a single impairment in a dynamic processing parameter within the language system can produce a variety of error patterns across different tasks.

In the most recent simulations of aphasic naming errors using this approach, Dell and colleagues (this volume) simulated the individual error type distributions of 21 fluent aphasic patients by altering the model's parameters of connection weight and/or decay rate. Once the model was individually fitted to each aphasic patient's data, predictions were made about a number of other aspects of patient performance. The work described in this chapter contrasts markedly with the studies of completely distributed networks in the specificity of what the computational "lesion" represents. For Dell and colleagues, the nature and extent of information degradation is critical to interpreting the outcome; for many simulations with completely distributed models lesion severity is the only lesion parameter of interest.

3.3 Single and multiple "routes" to reading: acquired alexia

Many of the connectionist models of cognitive dysfunction that have been developed to date are concerned with disorders of the ability to transcode between print and pronunciation - to read aloud and to write to dictation (see Table 2). Symptoms involving reading and writing disorders have been a favored research topic among cognitive neuropsychologists and have generated considerable interest among connectionists. This attention has in large measure been engendered by the interesting and distinct patterns of impairment that can occur in these disorders. Patient performance has been shown to reflect characteristics of stimulus words such as lexical status, grammatical class and imageability. The errors produced can bear different types of relations to the target (e.g., semantic, visual), and may reflect aspects of the spatial configuration of the word. These disorders thus provide a rich source of information about the relative importance of a variety of factors in the reading and writing of words.

Four distinct types of acquired alexia (or dyslexia) that have been simulated using connectionist models are discussed in chapters in this volume. Two of these types are characterized by special difficulty reading unfamiliar or "made-up" words; when such "non-words" are misread, patients frequently produce a visually similar real word (a "lexicalization") that overlaps orthographically with the target. Among these patients with non-word reading impairment, *deep dyslexics* also demonstrate a variety of problems reading aloud real words, particularly abstract words, and they often produce errors that are either semantically or visually related to the target (Coltheart, Patterson & Marshall, 1980). *Phonological dyslexics*, who are also impaired in non-word reading, do not produce semantic errors when reading words, and in fact may read real words very well (Beauvois & Derouesne, 1979; Funnel, 1983). These two patient types, sharing the symptom of non-word reading impairment, have been described as falling at different points of severity along a single continuum of disorder (Glosser & Friedman, 1990). In contrast to these patterns of reading symptoms, *surface dyslexic* patients can read aloud non-words and many real words, but have difficulty reading words with irregular spelling/sound correspondences (Patterson, Marshall, & Coltheart, 1985).

These generalizations about the performance of patients of different types obscure considerable individual variability among patients within a type, and fail to consider numerous aspects of their performance (e.g., in lexical decision and comprehension tasks) that might well influence the interpretation of the impairment. Nonetheless, the occurrence of the dissociation between the ability to read words and non-words has been used as a primary piece of data supporting the necessity of a distinction between lexical and non-lexical reading procedures or *routes* from print to sound (e.g., Coltheart, 1985). The *dual route model* postulates different procedures for achieving a pronunciation for a letter string when reading words and non-words; thus, this view easily accommodates the occurrence of these different patient types by postulating selective impairments to one of the two routes. Challenges to the dual route model have mounted numerous different types of arguments that the operation of a single routine can explain the relevant data, (e.g., Glushko, 1979; Kay & Marcel, 1981; Shallice & McCarthy, 1985), but those models have had difficulty accounting for the distinct patterns found in patients with acquired dyslexia.

Several of the characteristics of deep dyslexia have been simulated in a connectionist model that links orthography (word form) and meaning (semantic features)(Hinton & Shallice, 1991; Plaut & Shallice, 1993). In the initial implementation, a "direct" pathway generated initial semantic activity from visual input, and a "clean-up" pathway refined this activity into the appropriate semantic activation for the target word. Although the model uses two pathways, it does not constitute a dual route model since both pathways must be considered to support lexical reading only; Hinton and Shallice (1991) did not attempt to simulate non-word reading (or its impairment), but did perform lesion simulations that succeeded in producing errors that were semantically related to the targets. The lesioned model also produced other interpretable error patterns that have been argued to occur in deep dyslexia, including errors visually related to the target and a higher proportion of "mixed" (semantic/visual) errors than would be expected by chance.

A summary of these simulations of Deep Dyslexia, and a discussion of recent development of the model, are provided in this volume by Plaut. This new work includes the addition of abstract words (and representations of their meaning) to the model, which allows the simulation of the finding that Deep Dyslexic patients read concrete words better than abstract. The recent work also includes some initial investigations of the utility of modeling rehabilitation and recovery of function using connectionist models.

The model described above concerns the mapping from orthography to semantics and does not consider the processes necessary to achieve a pronunciation. Thus, although it was able to simulate some aspects of Deep Dyslexia - a disorder that arguably involves a disruption within the semantic system as well as other impairments - it did not consider symptoms involving word regularity or non-word reading. Several other connectionist models have been proposed that focus on conversion of orthography to phonology, with or without a consideration of semantics, and thus provide a means for modeling the phonological and surface forms of dyslexia.

Seidenberg and McClelland (1989) developed a model of normal word recognition and pronunciation that simulates a variety of empirical findings from normal subjects. It was also claimed that the model could be lesioned to simulate some of the characteristics of surface dyslexia (Patterson, Seidenberg & McClelland, 1989). The fact that the model contained no explicit representations of morphemic or lexical information, nor of specific rules for conversion of orthography to phonology, lent considerable theoretical interest to the model's performance. If a model with this completely "sub-symbolic" architecture could successfully reproduce phenomena such as normal subjects' ability to pronounce unfamiliar letter strings, and at the same time could succeed in pronouncing words with exceptional spelling/sound correspondences, dual route reading models would face a formidable challenge. Moreover, some fundamental assumptions about the organization and processing of language would need to be re-evaluated, with the need for explicit components dedicated to specific linguistic functions being supplanted by more general principles based on patterns of associations across domains.

These theoretical implications fueled interest in the model's performance, and led to serious challenges of the strong claims that have been made for this and related models with completely distributed architectures (e.g., Fodor & Pylyshyn, 1988; Forster, 1994; McCloskey, 1991; Pinker & Prince, 1988). Some of the specific critiques that were leveled at the initial version of the model led to revision of how information was represented in the model. For example, Besner, Twilley, McCann and Seergobin (1990) challenged the model's ability to pronounce non-words and to perform lexical decisions. Changes were made to the way orthographic input and phonological output were represented, and the model's ability to "pronounce" non-words improved markedly (Seidenberg, Plaut, Petersen, McClelland & McRae, 1994).

For present purposes, the most important critiques of the original Seidenberg and McClelland model are those directed at its limited ability to simulate the performance patterns of the acquired dyslexias. Coltheart, Curtis and Atkins (1993) offered a particularly detailed critique of the model's potential to achieve a reasonable simulation of acquired reading disorders without the provision of separate mechanisms for the reading of words and non-words. With regard to Surface Dyslexia, the initial lesion simulation succeeded in producing better performance with regular than irregular words, but failed to reproduce the preserved non-word reading and regularization errors that are characteristic of surface dyslexic reading. Again, modifications of the original model, this time involving the addition of semantic activation (described by Patterson and colleagues in this volume), led to much improved simulation of these and other characteristics of Surface Dyslexia (Plaut, McClelland, Seidenberg & Patterson, 1996). The chapter in this volume also describes the simulation of data from specific dyslexic patients, including changes in the performance of patients with progressive Surface Dyslexia.

In addition to providing a critique of the Seidenberg and McClelland model, Colt-heart and colleagues (1993) advanced strong arguments that the basic architecture required for any model of written word pronunciation to simulate patterns of acquired dyslexia must incorporate separate mechanisms for reading words and non-words. These authors argued that this requirement is not inconsistent with connectionist models, and they outlined the elements of a dual-route model that would be likely to perform better than the fully distributed model in a wide range of oral reading tasks. The non-lexical pathway of their model translates input letter strings into strings of phonemes using explicit grapheme-to-phoneme translation rules. The system learns these rules through recurrent pairings of spellings and phonetic transcriptions.

This implemented non-lexical portion of the Coltheart et al. model is fully com-putational, although not connectionist, in its design. The lexical pathway is a local connectionist model with separate architectures for input (essentially reproducing McClelland and Rumelhart's (1981) interactive activation model of word recogni-tion) and for output (using Dell's (1986) model of spoken word production, discussed above). Coltheart and colleagues motivate the borrowing of these elements from other models by their strong assumption of modularity; word recognition and production are separate components of lexical processing and should be implemented separately. This approach to connectionist modeling of cognitive function stands in sharp con-trast to that of proponents of completely distributed systems, in which the structure of the system emerges from recurrent association of input and output.

A different approach to a dual-route reading model was taken by Reggia, Marsland and Berndt (1988; see also Goodall, Reggia, Peng & Berndt, 1990). This model takes input in the form of pre-segmented "grapheme" units - one or more printed charac-ters that serve as the written representation of a single phoneme. The non-lexical route provides for the mapping of graphemes onto their corresponding phonemes by weighted links based of the probability of association between specific graphemes and phonemes. These probabilities were not derived by rules such as those used in the model of Coltheart and colleagues (1993), or from linguistic principles (Venezky, 1970), but are based on empirical observation of correspondences in a large corpus of English words (Berndt, Reggia & Mitchum, 1987). This representation of how pro-nunciations are derived from print non-lexically carves out a middle ground between the completely distributed models (e.g., Seidenberg & McClelland, 1989), in which association strength is derived through learning from repeated pairings of written and spoken words, and the rule-based approach taken by Coltheart and colleagues (1993). The lexical route in this model consists of connections from the same grapheme nodes to a set of word nodes, and connections from the word nodes to phoneme nodes. One unusual feature of this model is that it does not implement inhibitory connections between nodes as a means of controlling competition among elements. Rather, nodes compete directly for activation within each of the two routes.

The early implementations of this network succeeded in simulating several important characteristics of normal word pronunciation, including the frequency-by-regularity interaction in reading words; the model also achieved a high degree of success in pronouncing non-words. Most importantly, performance patterns characteristic of both Surface and Phonological Dyslexia were produced when the lexical and non-lexical routes, respectively, were degraded. This model has undergone a number of modifications, including the provision of competition between the two routes to allow for the simulation of behaviors that appear to reflect route interactions. The most recent version of the model, described by Whitney, Berndt and Reggia in this volume, has also been used to simulate distinct performance patterns produced by individual patients with Phonological Dyslexia. As noted above with regard to the model of Dell and colleagues, models with local information representation allow the study of specific sites, types and severities of lesions, with different lesions showing distinct effects. Whitney and colleagues describe simulation of qualitatively different patterns of patient performance with lesions of different type and severity.

4. Neurological Disorders

We now turn to models of neurological disorders such as stroke, epilepsy, migraine and parkinsonism. In contrast to the more abstract "cognitive models" of the preceding section, this class of models is more closely related to anatomical structure and physiological processes occurring in the brain. Typically, each node represents a neuron or population of neurons, and its connections represent synapses or groups of synapses with other neurons. A weight on a connection represents a measure of synaptic strength or effectiveness (positive = excitatory; negative = inhibitory). The input to a node often represents the corresponding neuron's membrane potential, and the node's activation level or output often represents its firing rate. While there are numerous models that fit this description, relatively few of these models have been used to study the effects of brain damage or dysfunction. Representative examples of these latter models are summarized in Table 3.

Table 3: Example Neural Models of Neurological Disorders

Abnormality	Investigators	Year
focal cortical deafferentation	Pearson et al.	1987
	Sklar	1990
	Spitzer et al.	1995
focal cortical lesions/stroke	Grajski & Merzenich	1990
	Sutton et al.	1993
	Weinrich et al.	1993
	Armentrout et al.	1994
	Ruppin & Reggia	1995b
	Xing & Gerstein	1996
seizures/epilepsy	Wong et al.	1986
	Barth et al.	1989
	Zepka & Sabbatini	1991
	Mehta et al.	1993
	Traub	1995
movement disorders	Borrett et al.	1993
	Contreras-Vidal & Stelmach	1995
migraine aura	Reggia & Montgomery	1996

Memory and language disorders are, of course, of great importance in clinical neurology. They have been the subject of several modeling efforts, as has already been described in the preceding sections of this chapter. In this section we review simulations related to cortical effects of peripheral nerve lesions, stroke, epilepsy, extrapyramidal disorders and migraine. Further discussion of issues involved in modeling neurological disorders can be found in (Crystal & Finkel, this volume).

4.1 Focal Deafferentation of Cortical Maps

During the last several years there have been numerous efforts to develop computational models of cortex that, unlike many earlier models (e.g., simple associative memories; see section 2.1), incorporate more realistic spatial relationships (Kohonen, 1982; Obermayer et al., 1990; Pearson et al., 1987; Grajski & Merzenich, 1990; Sklar, 1990; von der Malsburg 1973; Ritter et al., 1989 Reggia et al., 1992). These models typically are concerned with simulating map formation in primary sensory cortex. It has long been known that each primary sensory region of the cerebral cortex has a "map" of relevant aspects of the external world (e.g., the homunculus in somatosensory cortex) (Knudsen et al., 1987; Udin & Fawcett, 1988). The term "map" here refers to the fact that stimuli in the sensory space (e.g., tactile stimuli on the surface of the hand) are projected in an order-preserving fashion onto the cortex so that similar stimuli generally excite cortical elements close to one another (e.g., adjacent points on the hand's surface are represented close to one another in the cortex). Perhaps most intriguing has been the repeated experimental demonstration that such maps are highly plastic in adult animals: they undergo a reorganization in response to deafferentation (Merzenich et al., 1983a&b; Pons et al., 1988; Kaas, 1991), de-efferentation (Sanes et al., 1988), localized repetitive stimuli (Jenkins et al., 1990), and focal cortical lesions (Jenkins & Merzenich, 1987). For example, following a peripheral nerve lesion that deprives part of the somatosensory cortex of its input, the somatosensory map reorganizes to reuse the area of cortex that has lost its primary input. The map shifts so that the deafferented part of the cortex comes to represent other parts of the body surface. Recent noninvasive studies have suggested that such plasticity is also found in human cortical maps (Pascual-Leone et al., 1995).

Models of normal cortical map formation typically take the form of a two or three layer network, and use an unsupervised learning method (often a variant of Hebbian learning called competitive learning). For example, computational models of the hand region of primary somatosensory cortex have demonstrated map refinement (transformation from an initially coarse, poorly organized map to a sharply-defined and highly organized one) and map reorganization in response to localized repetitive stimulation (Pearson et al, 1987; Grajski & Merzenich, 1990; Sklar, 1990). These models have been partially deafferented by removing a portion of their input connections to cortex, e.g., by removing input from the palm surface of the first two fingers to simulate a median nerve lesion. When such deafferentation is done the cortical map spontaneously reorganizes in a fashion reminiscent of experimental studies (Pearson et al, 1987; Sklar, 1990); the map shifts so that the part of cortex originally representing the deafferented region of the sensory surface is reused to represent other nearby sensory surface areas. Receptive field changes consistent with an inverse magnification rule have been demonstrated (Grajski & Merzenich, 1990). See (Crystal & Finkel, this volume) for further discussion of these models.

Similar models of cortical deafferentation have been used more recently to support a theory of phantom limb experiences (Spitzer et al, 1995). *Phantom limbs* are the sensation that an extremity is still present after it has been lost (e.g., by traumatic amputation). Spitzer and colleagues combine a model of focal cortical deafferentation with input noise to account for various observations related to phantom limbs. Their model is summarized and its implications discussed in detail in (Spitzer, this volume).

4.2 Focal Cortical Lesions and Stroke

The above computational studies of cortical maps provide an impressive demonstration that fairly simple assumptions about network architecture and synaptic modifiability can qualitatively account for several fundamental facts about map self-organization and reorganization following deafferentation. However, they have been less successful in accounting for some other effects. For example, it is known from limited animal experiments that focal cortical lesions also produce spontaneous map reorganization (Jenkins & Merzenich, 1987). In the first computational model we know of that simulated a focal cortical lesion, map reorganization would not occur unless implausible steps were taken (complete re-randomization of weights) (Grajski & Merzenich, 1990). Map reorganization following a cortical lesion is fundamentally different from that involving deafferentation or focal repetitive stimulation described above. In both of the latter situations there is a change in the probability distribution of input patterns seen by the cortex. Such a change has long been recognized to result in map alterations (Kohonen, 1987). In contrast, with a focal cortical lesion there is no change in the probability distribution of input patterns, so some other factor must be responsible for map reorganization.

Motivated primarily by a desire to better understand the events occurring in stroke, recent work has developed successful computational models of acute focal lesions in cortex. A *stroke* is acute, focal brain damage due to altered blood supply to the brain. When there is sudden loss of blood flow to an area of the brain due to occlusion of an artery, the resultant brain damage is referred to as an *ischemic stroke*. Stroke is a common neurological disease; for example, it is the third leading cause of death in the United States. Because it often causes partial paralysis and/or language and memory problems, it is also a major cause of chronic disability.

The complexity of brain changes during a stroke suggests that computational models can be powerful tools for its investigation. Ultimately, one seeks a sufficiently powerful model that can be used to understand better the acute post-stroke changes in the ischemic penumbra, to determine which factors lead to worsening or recovery from stroke, and to suggest new pharmacologic interventions and rehabilitative actions that could improve stroke outcome. However, the complexity of stroke pathophysiology, and the limitations of current neural modeling technology and neuroscientific knowledge, make it impractical to create immediately a detailed, large scale model of the brain and all of the effects of a major stroke. The computational models done so far have involved simulating the effects of small ischemic cortical strokes.

Several modeling studies of acute focal cortical lesions have focused primarily on topographic somatosensory maps (Sutton et al., 1993; Armentrout et al., 1994). In such maps, points close to one another on the body surface are represented close to each other in the cortical map. This work again involved the region of somatosensory maps representing the surface of the hand. When a focal lesion was introduced into the topographic map, the model reorganized such that the sensory surface originally represented by the lesioned area spontaneously reappeared in adjacent cortical areas, as has been seen experimentally in animal studies (Jenkins & Merzenich, 1987). Perilesion receptive field sizes increased too, consistent with an inverse magnification rule. A more recently developed model of somatosensory cortex differing substantially in details (e.g., use of spiking neurons) has essentially duplicated these post-lesion findings (Xing & Gerstein, 1996). Two key hypotheses emerged from this modeling work. First, post-lesion map reorganization is a two-phase process, consisting of a rapid phase due to the dynamics of neural activity and a longer-term phase due to synaptic plasticity. Second, increased perilesion excitability is necessary for useful map reorganization to occur.

Work in this area has subsequently evolved in a number of different ways. The initial cortical lesion studies, as well as other work with more abstract computational models of cortex not involving map organization, indicated the important role of intracortical interactions in post-lesion brain reorganization. Specifically, following a *structural lesion* that simulates a region of damage and neuronal death, a secondary *functional lesion* can arise in nearby cortex due to loss of synaptic connections from the damaged area to surrounding intact cortex (we use the term "functional lesion" in this limited sense and not to indicate the ischemic penumbra). This issue is considered in detail in (Ruppin & Reggia, this volume).

Recent work has also examined the effects of focal damage in a computational model of primary sensorimotor cortex that controls the positioning of a simulated arm in three-dimensional space (Chen & Reggia, 1996). This model involves both proprioceptive input as well as motor output in a "closed-loop" network. Maps initially form in the two cortical regions represented in the model: proprioceptive sensory cortex and primary motor cortex (MI). Unlike the previous computational models of cortex described above that were subjected to simulated focal lesions, the maps involved here are non-topographic feature maps and involve motor output as well as sensory input information. In simulations with this model, both perilesion excitability and cortical map reorganization have been examined, immediately after a lesion and over the long term. As described in (Reggia et al, this volume), the results obtained are consistent with the two hypotheses given above.

4.3. Epilepsy

Epilepsy is another very common and important disorder in clinical neurology. It is characterized by sudden, excessive electrical discharges in the cerebral cortex. Patients with epilepsy typically have recurrent convulsions, loss of consciousness, disturbances of sensation, impaired mentation, and related symptoms. These episodes are caused by paroxysmal high-frequency or synchronous low-frequency, high-voltage electrical disturbances observable in the EEG. While many biochemical and physiological abnormalities have been described in epileptic brain tissue, at present the precise pathophysiology of these abnormalities is only partially understood. Contemporary research on the mechanisms underlying seizures and on pharmacological treatments is very active, involving both human subjects and animal models.

Some of the most detailed and well known neural models of epileptic abnormalities have been developed by Traub and colleagues over a period of several years (Wong et al, 1986; Traub, 1995). They have primarily investigated a complex, multicompartmental model of area CA3 of the hippocampus, a brain region in which highly synchronized electrical activity and EEG spikes and sharp waves occur with certain types of epileptiform activity. By manipulating their models in ways corresponding to experimental procedures (e.g., simulating blockage of the inhibitory neurotransmitter

GABA$_A$ caused by picrotoxin), they were able to gain insight into the mechanisms underlying abnormal neuronal bursting and afterdischarges. More recently it has been shown that a much simplified model of hippocampal pyramidal neurons is still able to account for many of the same sorts of abnormal neuronal firing (Pinsky & Rinzel, 1994); such "reduced" or "minimal" models are discussed further in (Golomb & Rinzel, this volume).

Another very interesting phenomenon related to epilepsy is *kindling*. Kindling occurs when repeated electrical or chemical stimulation of a cortical region leads to generation of a new focus of abnormal, epileptogenic activity. Mehta and colleagues have developed and studied a neural model in which repeated simulated electrical stimuli produce kindling due to synaptic changes (Mehta et al, 1993). Their results are consistent with the hypothesis that kindling is due to the formation of a large number of excitatory synapses arising in the context of operation of Hebb's rule. This work and recent extensions of it are described in (Mehta et al, this volume).

4.4 Other Neurological Disorders

A number of neural models have recently been developed of movement disorders associated with dysfunction of the basal ganglia. Most attention has been paid to *Parkinson's disease* in which there is a loss of dopaminergic neurons in the substantia nigra. Patient's have rigidity, tremor, slow movements and poor balance. As discussed further in (Crystal & Finkel, this volume), it has been possible to simulate the emergence of tremor as an oscillatory state in a recurrent neural network (Borrett et al, 1993). More recently, a neural model of the opponent process occurring in basal ganglia and thalamocortical circuitry has been developed and used to simulate movement abnormalities in both Parkinsonism and Huntington's disease (Contreras-Vidal & Stelmach, 1995). As discussed further in (Contreras-Vidal et al, this volume), their model provides a unified and detailed theory of both of these disorders.

Migraine is another common neurological disorder that has recently been studied computationally. Migraine is an inherited disorder characterized by recurrent, usually unilateral throbbing headaches. In the "classic" form of migraine, pain is often preceded by an aura involving sudden, bright visual hallucinations in a crescent-shaped region which move across the visual field. The specific visual patterns that occur in migraine aura have never been definitively explained, although they are generally accepted to have a cortical origin. For many years, it has been hypothesized that they arise due to a wave of cortical spreading depression, but this is difficult to test in humans or animals. For this reason, a neural model of visual cortex incorporating spreading depression was developed and examined (Reggia & Montgomery, 1996). It was found that during the wave of cortical spreading depression, the spatial pattern of neural activity broke up into irregular patterns of lines and small patches of highly activated elements. The corresponding visual disturbances that would be produced by these patterns of neural activity resemble the hallucinations reported during the migraine aura, providing strong support for the cortical spreading depression hypothesis of migraine. This model also makes the testable prediction that these hallucinations move at an increasing speed as they cross the visual fields.

There are many other neurological disorders in which computational models might be fruitful in understanding pathophysiology, making testable predictions, or suggesting innovative therapy. As work emerges in these areas, and further work appears in modeling the disorders described above, a recurring issue is going to be the level of detail at which the modeling should be done. The models of neurological disorders described in this section have spanned a range from complex, multicompartmental biophysical models of individual neurons to much more abstract simulations where the atomic elements were abstract representations of sizable populations of neurons. Very few models to date have tried to model across these different scales of neural organization. In (Sutton, this volume), a general framework is described for modeling "nested" neural networks of cortex spanning multiple levels of representation. The successful use of this approach to simulate various aspects of memory impairment in Alzheimer's disease is also described.

5. Psychiatric Disorders

Neural models have also been created for a wide range of psychiatric disorders. Representative examples are given in Table 4. We consider primarily schizophrenia, paranoid processes, delirium, and affective disorders.

Table 4: Example Neural Models of Psychiatric Disorders

Abnormality	Investigators	Year
schizophrenic vs. manic thought disorders	Hoffman	1987
schizophrenia (negative symptoms)	Cohen & Servan-Schreiber	1992a,b
schizophrenia (positive symptoms)	Hoffman & Dobscha	1989
	Hoffman & McGlashan	1993
	Hoffman et al.	1994
	Horn & Ruppin	1995
	Ruppin et al.	1995
depression	Webster et al.	1988
	Leven et al.	1992
	Luciano et al.	1994
paranoid disorder	Vinograd et al.	1992
delirium	Avni et al.	1995
drug effects	Callaway et al.	1994

5.1 Schizophrenia

Schizophrenia is a clinically heterogeneous disorder with a broad spectrum of manifestations. Its symptoms are diverse, and include both "positive symptoms" such as hallucinations, delusions, disorganized speech and behavior, and "negative symptoms" such as loss of fluency of thought and speech, impaired attention, abnormalities in the expression and observation of emotion, and loss of volition and drive. The course of the illness tends to be marked by exacerbations and remissions, but the persistence of the impairment gives the disease a 'dementia-like' quality. It differs from classic dementia in that most schizophrenic patients stabilize at moderate levels of cognitive impairment, and the disease does not have a progressive downhill course leading eventually to death. The interested reader is referred to (Roberts 1990; Waddington 1993; Carpenter & Buchanan 1994; Andreasen 1994) for recent reviews of schizophrenia.

The pathogenesis of schizophrenia is unknown. A few theories have been raised, based on neuropathological observations, the actions of anti-psychotic medications, and ideas about the relation between brain and behavior. Perhaps the most enduring biochemical explanation of the pathophysiology of schizophrenia is the dopamine hypothesis, which postulates the coexistence of hypodopaminergic activity in the mesocortical system, resulting in negative symptoms, and hyper-dopaminergic activity in the mesolimbic system, resulting in positive symptoms. Structural and functional imaging and neuroanatomical postmortem studies are providing converging evidence of the involvement of specific brain regions in schizophrenia, such as the prefrontal areas, temporal lobes and the temporo-limbic circuitry, and subcortical and midline circuitry. Integrative pathophysiological hypotheses have attempted to explain schizophrenic symptoms in terms of biochemical and neuroanatomical alterations in specific brain circuits, but at present no single explanatory mechanism has prevailed (a few of the most prominent of these theories were presented in (Stevens 1973; Weinberger 1987; Carlsson & Carlsson 1990; Stevens 1992).

Neural modeling of schizophrenia has also taken two main paths, perhaps reflecting the view of schizophrenia as composed of positive symptoms that arise due to temporo-frontal pathology, and negative symptoms that are a result of prefrontal abnormalities. This is true both with regard to the symptoms modeled and to the models employed. The first avenue, pioneered by Hoffman, has concentrated on modeling schizophrenic positive symptoms in the framework of an associative memory attractor network (Hoffman 1987; Hoffman & Dobscha 1989). This work has pointed to a possible link between the appearance of specific neurodegenerative changes and the emergence of 'parasitic foci', states in which a neural network's normal processing is disrupted and locked in dysfunctional patterns of activity. In another framework, that of feed-forward layered networks employing back-propagation learning, Cohen and Servan-Schreiber have provided a detailed computational account of how schizophrenic functional deficits can arise from neuromodulatory effects of dopamine

(Servan-Schreiber et al. 1990; Cohen & Servan-Schreiber 1992a,b,c).

5.2 Modeling Positive Symptoms of Schizophrenia with Attractor Networks

While a few formal models of information processing breakdown were presented earlier (e.g., Callaway 1970; Broadbent 1971; Joseph et al. 1979; Callaway & Naghdi 1982), the publication of Hoffman's (1987) paper probably marks the beginning of 'the era of neural modeling' of schizophrenia. In this paper, Hoffman describes how pathological alterations in a Hopfield attractor neural network can lead to the formation of *parasitic attractors*, whose cognitive and perceptual manifestations may play an important role in the emergence of schizophrenic delusions and hallucinations. These parasitic states are spurious states that are generated when the network becomes 'overloaded', i.e., its memory capacity is exceeded and catastrophic breakdown occurs (Amit 1989). Such memory overload presumably occurs in the brain of schizophrenics as a result of neurodegenerative changes, or as a result of selective attention deficits.

Delusions (false beliefs) are common abnormalities of thought among schizophrenics. Typical delusional themes of schizophrenic patients consist of externally imposed influences (thought insertion and thought broadcasting), grandiose delusions (a belief that one has unusual talents or an identity of a famous person), erotomania (in which the patient believes that a famous person is in love with him), and persecutory delusions (being a target of malevolent action). The inescapability of delusions, and their being spontaneously invoked at times by seemingly irrelevant experiences, led Hoffman to the idea that they can be conceived as parasitic attractor states which have broad and 'deep' basins of attraction. Hoffman also proposed that hallucinations have a similar linkage to parasitic states.

The linkage between parasitic states and delusions and hallucinations stems from the alien nature of the latter and their tendency to be repetitive. Building upon the basic linkage between parasitic states and positive symptoms, Hoffman & Dobscha (1989) presented a detailed simulation study that examined the hypothesis that the onset of schizophrenia (usually marked by a psychotic crisis and positive symptoms) is triggered by progressive elimination of synapses in the prefrontal cortex. In accordance with this hypothesis, the pathological excess of synaptic pruning reflects a normal developmental synaptic elimination process that fails to arrest in time and proceeds too far (interestingly, the typical onset period of schizophrenia is during late adolescence, when synaptic pruning supposedly reaches it peak). Studying this hypothesis in a 2-D associative memory attractor neural network, prefrontal synaptic pruning is modeled as a process of random synaptic deletion that tends to damage weak and distal synaptic connections more than strong and proximal ones. This type of spatial-selective damage was found to lead to two kinds of behavior in the network that may have interesting parallels in schizophrenic symptomatology: 1. 'Functional fragmentation' - denoting patches of convergence to different memories in distinct regions of the network. 2. Spatially organized 'parasitic foci' - denoting patches of the network that tend to lock into some non-memory activation patterns regardless of initial input cues applied to the network. Hoffman & Dobscha (1989) suggest that the observed functional fragmentation models the 'contamination response' that is specific to schizophrenics, i.e., the fusion of multiple distinct gestalts presented in each image of the Rorschach personality test.

In addition to the intuitive notion that schizophrenic delusions and hallucinations typically arise in a spontaneous and repetitive manner, what other characteristics of ill-formed attractor states can be thought of as linked to the pathogenesis and manifestations of schizophrenic positive symptoms? Hoffman & McGlashan (1993) have recently provided a detailed account of the possible role of parasitic foci in the formation of schizophrenic positive symptoms, suggesting that parasitic foci produce their effects by altering speech perception and production processes. For example, suppose that cortical speech production regions become dominated by a parasitic attractor. This may result in an experience of inner speech, which, because of the parasitic focus, is stereotyped in nature. Due to the possible detachment of such inner mental events from corresponding motor actions, these events may be experienced as unintended. This, combined with their stereotyped nature, may induce the patient to conclude that a particular alien non-self force is inserting thoughts into his head. Hoffman's work is described further in detail in (Hoffman, this volume). In a closely related spirit, Globus & Arpia (1994) have recently proposed that due to pathological changes the brain tends to settle in certain attractors which obtain a psychotic 'attunement'.

Following the work of Hoffman and his colleagues, Horn & Ruppin (1995) have examined a recent theory of Stevens (1992) in the framework of an attractor neural network model. As summarized in (Stevens 1992), the wealth of data gathered concerning the pathophysiology of schizophrenia suggests that there are atrophic changes in temporal lobe regions in the brains of a significant number of schizophrenic patients, including neuronal loss and gliosis. On the other hand, neurochemical and morphometric studies testify to an expansion of various receptor binding sites and increased dendritic branching in the projection sites of temporal lobe neurons, including the frontal cortex. These findings have led Stevens to hypothesize that the onset of schizophrenia is associated with reactive anomalous sprouting and synaptic reorganization taking place in the projection sites of degenerating temporal neurons.

To study the functional implications of Stevens' hypothesis, Horn & Ruppin (1995) modeled a frontal module as an associative memory neural network receiving its inputs from degenerating temporal projections and undergoing reactive synaptic regeneration. In this model, it is shown that while preserving memory performance, compensatory synaptic regenerative changes modeling those proposed by Stevens may lead to adverse, spontaneous activation of stored patterns. When *spontaneous retrieval* emerges, the incorporation of Hebbian activity-dependent synaptic changes leads to a *biased* retrieval distribution that is strongly dominated by a single memory pattern (Ruppin et. al. 1996). The formation of biased, spontaneous retrieval is shown to require the concomitant occurrence of both degenerative changes in the external input (temporal) fibers and regenerative activity-dependent Hebbian changes in the intra-modular (frontal) synaptic connections.

A few important characteristics of positive symptoms are reflected in the behavior of the network: 1. The emergence of spontaneous, non-homogeneous retrieval is a self-limiting phenomenon; eventually, a global, spurious, attractor is formed. The formation of such a cognitively meaningless spurious attractor, accompanied by a decrease in the size of basins of attraction of the memory patterns, may lead to the emergence of deficit, negative symptoms. This parallels the clinical observation that as schizophrenia progresses positive symptoms tend to wane, while negative symptoms are enhanced. 2. When the network converges to a memory pattern that dominates the output in the spontaneous-retrieval scenario, it has increased tendency to remain in this state for a much longer time than in its normal functioning state, in accordance with the persistence of positive symptoms. 3. The model points to the possibility that maintenance therapy may have an important role not only in preventing the recurrence of positive symptoms, but also in slowing down the progression of the disease, by arresting the pathological evolution of the synaptic memory matrix. 4. In its spontaneous retrieval mode, the network may also converge to mixed retrieval states, which have some similarity to a few patterns concomitantly. Such retrieval of mixed patterns may play a part in explaining the generation of more complex forms of schizophrenic delusions and hallucinations, involving abnormal condensation of thoughts and imaginings. Interestingly, Ruppin and co-workers' account provides a neural 'correlate' of the widely held notion that delusions and hallucinations are adaptive responses to preexisting disorganization as part of a compensatory 'defense' mechanism. The model can be tested by quantitatively examining the correlation between a recent history of florid psychotic symptoms and postmortem neuropathological findings of synaptic compensation in schizophrenic subjects. The generation of spontaneous pattern activation following neural damage that alters the input/internal synaptic balance is a quite general phenomenon, as recently demonstrated in (Thaler 1995).

5.3 Modeling Cognitive Functions With Layered Networks

A different approach, both with regard to the phenomena studied and the models employed, has been taken by Cohen and Servan-Schreiber, whose work is reviewed in detail in (Servan-Schreiber & Cohen, this volume) Building upon their work on modeling the neuromodulatory effects of catecholamines on information processing (Servan-Schreiber et al., 1990; Servan-Schreiber & Cohen 1992), they have presented a comprehensive modeling study of the performance of normal subjects and schizophrenics in three attentional and language processing tasks (Cohen & Servan-Schreiber 1992b; Cohen et al., 1992). These tasks are important indices of cognitive dysfunction in schizophrenia, and are related to schizophrenic negative symptoms. Their modeling has enabled a detailed quantitative investigation, which is not confined to the qualitative realm of positive symptoms. In all the tasks modeled, a back propagation algorithm was used to train the networks to simulate normal performance. Although each task was modeled by a network designed specifically for that task, the networks used rely on similar information processing principles and share a common module for representing context, which is identified with the prefrontal cortex. Neuronal firing is governed by a sigmoidal function. The hypothesized neuromodulatory effects of dopamine on information processing (which may play a major role in the pathogenesis of schizophrenia, as described above) were modeled as a global change of the input gain. The simulations performed demonstrate that a change in the gain of neurons in the context module can quantitatively account for the differences between normal and schizophrenic performance in the tasks examined.

Cohen and Servan-Schreiber's work on modeling dopamine effects and schizophrenic deficits leaves many questions open, which has led to a vigorous discussion of their theory and its implications (primarily, the relation between the neuromodulatory 'gain' and dopamine) in the psychiatric literature (Jobe et al., 1994; Cohen & Servan-Schreiber 1995). Based on the work of (Servan-Schreiber 1990) on simulating human performance in a choice-reaction time task (Eriksen task), Callaway et al., (1994) have recently reanalyzed data from a similar task performed by subjects under the influence of various drugs. The authors maintain that patterns of performance observed in the data are in accordance with those predicted by Servan-Schreiber's model, when considering possible drug neuromodulatory effects on the gain and bias of units in different layers. They claim that "neural network models offer a better chance of rescuing the study of human psychologic responses to drugs than anything else currently available" (Callaway et al., 1994).

Although the model presented in (Cohen & Servan-Schreiber 1992a,b) has not addressed schizophrenic positive symptoms, the authors have pointed out that these may be studied in a similar modeling framework. This issue is precisely the goal of a recent study by Hoffman et al., (1994). Aiming to provide a quantitative description of the pathogenesis of auditory hallucinations, the authors have studied the hypothesis that hallucinated 'voices' arise from altered verbal working memory. The model consists of a recurrent layered neural network with a temporary storage layer and uses backpropagation to learn a speech perception task. In this task, sequences of randomly coded input words (referred to as 'phonetic') are translated into sequences of outputs (referred to as 'semantic') in a semantic feature space. In parallel to the simulation studies, an experimental study of speech perception in schizophrenics and normal controls was conducted. In accordance with the now 'standard' paradigm in these type of combined experimental/modeling studies, the network's architectural and dynamical parameters were first tuned to model the performance of normal subjects. Thereafter, various alterations of network connectivity and dynamics were systematically studied and the resulting network performance patterns were compared with the experimental findings. Several interesting insights and predictions have been generated: 1. Schizophrenics with auditory hallucinations should have significantly more severe speech perception abnormalities relative to non-hallucinating patients. 2. Several types of alterations can lead to auditory hallucinations, but the combined anatomical/modulatory model is the most likely one. 3. Drugs altering the response profile of neurons may be effective even when the primary pathology is neuroanatomical rather than neuromodulatory. 4. With severe neuroanatomical damage, perceptual function must be sacrificed in order to reduce hallucinations. Interestingly, this finding closely corresponds to that of Ruppin et al. (1995) in an entirely different framework.

5.4 Other Psychiatric disorders

Perhaps the topic most closely related to schizophrenia modeling is the study of paranoid processes. Paranoia is a tendency to develop suspicions and ambitions that gradually progress to 'systematized' delusions of persecution and grandeur. This chronic and unremitting system of delusions encompasses a broad set of false ideas that are connected by a common theme and are rigidly adhered to despite all contradictory evidence. Vinograd et al., (1992) have recently described a model of paranoid processes within the framework of spreading activation networks. Motivated by high-level psychological models of semantic memory and associations, each computational unit represents a distinct cognitive item, and the links between units represent associations. The authors propose that paranoia gradually forms in a process where initial suspicions consolidate into a delusional system. In this process, associations are constructed among temporally contiguous perceptions in an excessive manner, and are assigned an idiosyncratic meaning of malevolent motives or persecution by others. The authors suggest that this process can be modeled by a spreading activation network whose connectivity and dynamical parameters are altered, reflecting a 'hyper-associative' state. Relying on the work of Shrager et al. (1987), Vinograd et al. (1992) describe various phase transitions that the network undergoes when its structural and dynamical parameters are changed. There are three possible phases characterized by different sizes of activity clusters, where large and persistent clusters represent a delusional system. The work of Vinograd et al., (1992) concentrates more on the conceptual level and not on a neural network realization. As such, it does not suggest a link between specific neuropathological changes and paranoid symptoms, but presents a formal framework that may be relevant for studying the pertaining psychological data.

In addition to modeling memory deterioration and schizophrenic positive symptoms, attractor neural networks have been considered as a framework for modeling a few cognitive manifestations of manic-depressive disorder. Manic-depressive disorder is an affective disorder which includes patients with mania and depression or mania only. The manic bouts are characterized by a distinctly elevated, expansive or irritable mood, accompanied by 'hyperactivity' symptoms such as decreased need for sleep, pressure to keep talking, 'racing' of thoughts and inflated self-esteem. Hoffman (1987) has proposed that in contradistinction to schizophrenic positive symptoms, manic 'hyperactivity' arises not as a result of structural damage leading to the formation of pathological attractors, but due to an increase in the noise levels resulting in enhanced rate of transition between attractors. Hoffman's views were inspired by the lack of evidence for widespread neuroanatomic damage in manic-depressive disorder, by the success of lithium drugs which alter neural metabolic pathways and possibly their firing dynamics, and by discourse studies showing that the basic structure of manic discourse is intact. Obviously, the neural representation of a 'thread of thoughts' as a series of transitions between attractor states might be a gross simplification, but perhaps the principles of structural versus functional damage embodied in the metaphors described above would remain of relevance also in more developed descriptions.

The possible role of threshold variation in the pathogenesis of delirium has been recently explored in a neural modeling study by Avni et al. (1995). Delirium is characterized by a transient impairment of a wide range of cognitive functions due to a diffuse derangement in cerebral metabolism. Impairment of consciousness and reduced awareness of the environment are hallmarks of the disorder, together with cognitive dysfunction which may include poor memory, slowness of thinking, inconsistent responses and difficulty in concentrating. Almost any process that causes a diffuse disruption of brain homeostasis, such as fluid and electrolyte disturbances, drugs and infections, may cause delirium. Avni et al. (1995) have examined the hypothesis that variations in the neural threshold underlie some memory-related cognitive disturbances in delirium. The attractor neural network model they used incorporates two sets of connections: Hebbian connections storing memory patterns, and randomly-weighted connections. Depending on the values of the neuronal threshold and synaptic connectivity parameters, the network may either converge to a stable state or wander through its state space in a seemingly chaotic manner. The transition from the region of single stable states with near perfect retrieval to unstable end states is sharp, and is accompanied by a 'syndrome' of poor memory retrieval, slower retrieval time, instability and inconsistency of end states, and storage disturbances, all of which are typical characteristics of memory and cognitive functioning in delirium. Interestingly, similar unstable end states were found in the model at high and low levels of neuronal activity, offering some insight as to how both excitatory and inhibitory etiological factors (such as low or high levels of some electrolytes) can cause delirium.

Major depression has also been the focus of recent modeling work. Major depression, the most prevalent affective disorder, is characterized by depressed mood and symptoms like loss of interest, psychomotor retardation, fatigue, sleeplessness, impaired concentration and suicidal ideation. The difficulty of representing the symptoms above in neural network models has restricted current modeling attempts to some cognitive aspects of major depression. Past work related to major depression has concentrated primarily on modeling learned helplessness, an experimental psychological model of depression, in an adaptive resonance network (Levine et al., 1992). A similar modeling framework has been used by Hestenes (1992) to model the selection and execution of behavioral plans in manic-depressive patients. A new approach to studying major depression is described in (Luciano et al., this volume); see also (Luciano et al., 1994a,b). The goal of their investigation is to develop a neural model examining the possible role of the limbic system in depressive disorders, creating 'linking hypotheses' between model variables for brain regional activities and clinical symptoms data. The success of such challenging projects may further encourage the development of extensive laboratory and clinical data banks for psychiatric disorders, a necessary step towards developing more quantitative models.

Finally, Levine (this volume) describes a model of prefrontal dysfunction. This chapter has been included in the psychiatric disorders' section in light of the central role that abnormalities of the prefrontal cortex are assumed to play in schizophrenia. Levine presents a new theory of executive function in the brain, based on the interaction of three subsystems; reward, working memory and a schemata forming subsystem. The neural networks forming these subsystems are gated by reward and attention cues. Within this framework, the role of various lesions is discussed and compared with the relevant animal experimental data. While not discussing schizophrenia directly, Levine's work addresses some prefrontal tasks similar to those discussed by Cohen & Servan-Schreiber in this volume. It will be of interest to see whether these different models are consistent with each other, and to study their possibly distinct consequences in a comparative manner.

6. Prospects

As the previous sections have illustrated, the last several years have witnessed the development of a wide variety of interesting computational models of neurological, neuropsychological and psychiatric disorders. We now consider the general limitations of these models and what future developments may be anticipated.

6.1 Limitations

The use of neural models to study brain and cognitive disorders currently appears to be very promising. These models have already demonstrated that a small set of fairly simple assumptions can account for phenomena seen in recovery from brain damage and impaired cognitive information processing. However, most previous neural models greatly simplify the true psychological/biological phenomena being studied. For example, many of the models of cognitive disorders that have been discussed characterize patients' symptoms in only general terms, relying on syndrome classification labels such as "agrammatic aphasia", "deep dyslexia", etc. The point has been made repeatedly in the neuropsychological literature that these syndrome labels frequently present an erroneous picture of symptom homogeneity among patients. Modeling based on such syndrome labels will be subject to the same criticisms that are leveled against other uses of syndrome labels as a basis for scientific investigation.

Another limitation of neural models relates to their size. Many of the models discussed here are quite small in scope. Even with this simplification, many are computationally very expensive to run on conventional computer architectures (e.g., they require very large amounts of processing time). Further, past work in this area has only attempted to model a very small fraction of the clinical problems that are potentially amenable to study with neural networks.

With all of these limitations of current neural modeling technology, why has there been such a rapidly growing interest in using neural models to study brain and cognitive disorders? We believe that there are a number of reasons for this, as follows. Traditional medical investigative techniques (clinical trials, animal experiments, etc.) are expensive and face substantial barriers in terms of what can be practically or ethically studied. Computational models, on the other hand, are relatively inexpensive and provide for large numbers of "subjects" without ethical concerns. They allow one, in theory, to vary any aspect of a system to assess its effects, and to record virtually any variable from a system without interfering with the system's behavior. Ultimately, computational models may prove the most effective way to understand the underlying mechanisms of brain and cognitive disorders. They may become important factors in suggesting new treatments or in their preliminary assessment. To a great extent, it is this hope of deeper understanding of pathophysiology and of potential therapeutic guidance that motivates much of current modeling work in this area.

6.2 Future Expectations

It can be anticipated that the technological base supporting the development and use of neural models of cognitive and brain disorders will continue to grow, both in terms of hardware and software. Computer hardware suitable for supporting "massive" explicit parallelism of the sort used in neural models already exists, and should be increasingly available in the future. Computer chips based on analog VLSI technology that mimic nervous system structure and functionality are also a very active research area, and should greatly reduce the cost of access to such technology. Research is under way to understand better the parallel hardware architectures needed for neural models and should produce future systems that are especially suited for neural computations (Nordstrom and Svensson, 1992). In addition to these hardware implementations, investigation of more radical concepts is under way that could have a dramatic impact if successful. Examples of these latter endeavors include the development of "wetware" (biological neurons grown in culture on a chip and interfaced to electrical circuitry (Gross et al., 1985)), optical computing (Psaltis and Farhat, 1985), connectionist control of prostheses (Wan et al., 1990), and "nanotechnology" (technology on a nanometer scale). It can be anticipated that progressively more powerful parallel processing computers will become available, allowing the development of larger, more realistic applications.

Software developments can also be anticipated, not only in terms of new methods for controlling network functionality, but also in terms of more widespread availability of general purpose software environments for implementing and using neural networks. Many general connectionist software environments now exist (Schwartz, 1988; Reid & Zeichick, 1992; Wilson et al., 1989). Software like this can greatly expedite development of neural models.

Another important issue is the acceptance of computational modeling efforts as potentially useful by more traditional investigators. Physicians and neuroscientists have readily embraced mathematical formulations of single cell behavior in the past, but have been relatively reluctant to accept mathematical and computational neural modeling at the network level as "good science." As we have noted, these reservations have been appropriate in the sense that most neural modeling efforts greatly simplify the biological phenomena being studied. On the other hand, this criticism misses the point that even fairly simple neural network models can exhibit interesting behaviors and can generate hypotheses about important neurophysiological phenomena, suggesting that some emergent behaviors are quite robust in the context of simplified simulations. As the many articles in this book illustrate, this also appears to be true with respect to brain and cognitive disorders.

With regard to the modeling of cognitive disorders specifically, connectionist models provide a means for evaluating a number of hypotheses about the functional impairments that underlie neuropsychological deficits that are not easily investigated using other means. As noted earlier, these models have already suggested some non-obvious effects that alteration of a single parameter (e.g., an information decay parameter) can have on the operation of other cognitive functions. Future efforts can be expected to focus on manipulation of dynamic aspects of information processing, and on interactions among relatively independent cognitive components, both of which are elements of cognition that are difficult to address using behavioral testing.

Much progress is needed to make neural models of brain and cognitive disorders more powerful. In addition, there is a need for increased education of neuroscientists, physicians, and others about this technology. However, if these models live up to their apparent potential during the coming decades, they will make a major contribution to the understanding and treatment of many important clinical disorders.

7. Acknowledgements: Preparation of this chapter was supported in part by NIH grants NS29414, NS35460, and DC00699.

8. References

Amit D.J. *Modeling brain function: the world of attractor neural networks.* Cambridge University Press, 1989.

Anderson J. *IEEE Trans. Systems, Man and Cybernetics*, 13, 1983, 799-815.

Andreasen N.C. *Current Opinion in Neurobiology*, 4,245–251, 1994.

Armentrout S., Reggia J. & Weinrich M. *Artificial Intelligence in Medicine*, 6, 1994, 383-400.

Avni A., Ruppin E. and Stern M. 1995. Preprint.

Barth D, Baumgartner C, & Sutherling W. *Electroenceph. and Clin. Neurophys.*, 73, 1989, 389-402.

Beauvois M. and Derouesne J. *Journal of Neurology, Neurosurgery, and Psychology*, 42, 1115-1124, 1979.

Berndt R., Reggia J. & Mitchum C. *Behavior Research Methods, Instruments and Computers.* 19, 1987, 1-9.

Besner D., Twilley L., McCann R. and Seergobin K. *Psychol Rev*, 97, 1990, 432.

Borrett D, Yeap T, & Kwan H. *Canadian J. Neurological Sciences*, 20, 1993, 107-113.

Brain W & Walton J, *Brain's Diseases of Nervous System*, Oxford Univ Press, 1969.

Broadbent D.E. *Decision and Stress.* Academic Press, 1971.

Callaway E. and Naghdi S. *Arch. of Gen. Psych.*, 39,339–347, 1982.

Callaway E., Halliday R., Naylor H.,et al *Neuropsychopharmacology*, 10, 9–19, 1994.

Callaway E. *Arch. of Gen. Psych.*, 22, 193–208, 1970.

Carlsson M. and Carlsson A. *Trends in Neuroscience*, 13, 272–276, 1990.

Carpenter W.T. and Buchanan R.W. Schizophrenia. *New England Journal of Medicine*, 330, 681–690, 1994.

Carrie J.R. *British Journal of Psychiatry*, 163, 217–222, 1993.

Chen Y. & Reggia J. *Neural Computation*, 8, 1996, 731-755.

Cohen J. and Servan-Schreiber D. *Psychiatric Annals*, 22, 1992a, 131-136.

Cohen J. and Servan-Schreiber D. *Psych. Rev.*, 99, 1992b, 45-77.

Cohen J.D. and Servan-Schreiber D. *Psychiatric Annals*, 22, 113–118, 1992c.

Cohen J.D., Servan-Schreiber D., and McClelland J.L. *American Journal of Psychology*, 105, 239–269, 1992d.

Cohen J.D. and Servan-Schreiber D. *Schizophrenia Bulletin*, 19, 85–104, 1993.

Cohen J.D., Romero R.D., Servan-Schreiber D. and Farah M.J. *Journal of Cognitive Neuroscience*, 1995. In press.

Coltheart M. *Attention and Performance XI*, eds. M.I. Posner and O.S.M. Marin, Lawrence Erlbaum, 3-37, 1985.

Coltheart M., Curtis B. and Atkins P. *Psychological Review*, 100, 589-608, 1993.

Coltheart, M., Patterson, K. and Marshall, J., eds. *Deep Dyslexia*, Lawrence Erlbaum Assoc., London, 1980.

Contreras-Vidal J & Stelmach G, *Biol. Cyb.*, 73, 1995, 467.

Cottrell G. *Proc. Ninth Symp. Comp. Applic. Med. Care*, M. Ackerman (ed.), 1985, 237-241.

Dean P. *Psychol. Review*, 87, 1980, 470-473.

Dell G. *Psychol. Review*, 93, 1986, 283-321.

Farah M. and McClelland J. *J. Exper. Psychol*, 120, 1991, 339-357.

Fodor J and Pylyshyn z, *Cognition*, 28, 1988, 3-71.

Forster, K.I. *J. Exp. Psychol., Human Percep. Perform.*, 20, 1292-1310, 1994.

Funnel E. *British Journal of Psychology*, 74, 159-180, 1983.

Gigley H. *Cognition and Brain Theory*, 6, 39-88, 1983.

Globus G.G. and Arpia J.P. *Biological Psychiatry*, 35, 352–364, 1994.

Glosser G. & Friedman R. *Cortex*, 26, 1990, 343-359.

Glushko R. *Journal of Experimental Psychology: Human Perception and Performance*, 6, 674-691, 1979.

Goodall S., Reggia J., Peng Y. and Berndt R. *Proc. 14th Symp. Comp. Applic. Med. Care*, IEEE, 1990, 294-298.

Gordon B. *Neural Models of Language Processes*, M. Arbib, D. Caplan, and J. Marshall, Eds. New York, NY: Academic Press, 1982, 511-530.

Grajski K. and Merzenich M., *Neural Computation*, 2, 1990, 71-84.a

Gross G., Wen W. and Jacob L., *J. Neuroscience Methods*, 15, 243-252, 1985.

Haarman, H.J., Just, M.A. and Carpenter, P.A. *Brain Lang.*, 1996.

Haarman, J.J. and Kolk, H. *Cog. Sci.*, 15, 49-87, 1991.

Harley, T.A. *Language Cognitive Processes*, 10, 47-58, 1995.

Hasselmo M.E. and Barkai E. *Soc. Neurosci. Abstr.*, 18, 521, 1992.

Hasselmo M.E. and Bower J.M. *Journal of Neurophysiology*, 67(5), 1222–1229, 1992.

Hasselmo M.E., Anderson B.P. and Bower J.M. *Journal of Neurophsiology*, 67(5), 1230–1246, 1992.

Hasselmo M.E. *Neural computation*, 5, 32, 1993.

Hasselmo M.E. *Neural Networks*, 7, 13–40, 1994.

Heilman K. & Valenstein E., *Clinical Neuropsychology*, 1979, Oxford Univ. Press, 477.

Hestenes D. In D.S. Levine and S.J. Leven, editors, *Motivation, Emotion and Goal Direction in Neural Networks*. Erlbaum, 1992.

Hinton G. and Shallice T. *Psychol. Review*, 98, 1991, 74-95.

Hoffman R. *Arch. Gen. Psychiatry*, 44, 1987, 178-188.

Hoffman R. and Dobscha S. *Schizophrenia Bulletin*, 15, 477, 1989.

Hoffman R. *Psych. Annals*, 22, 1992, 119-124.

Hoffman R.E. and McGlashan T.H. *Schizophrenia Bulletin*, 19, 119–140, 1993.

Hoffman R.E., Rapaport J., Ameli R., McGlashan T.H., Harcherik D. and Servan-Schreiber D. 1994. Preprint.

Horn D. and Ruppin E. *Medical Hypothesis*, 39, 316–318, 1992.

Horn D. and Ruppin E. *Neural Computation*, 7, 182–205, 1995.

Horn D., Ruppin E., Usher M. and Herrmann M. *Neural Computation*, 5, 736–749, 1993.

Jenkins W. & Merzenich M. *Progress in Brain Research*, 71, Seil F., Herbert E. & Carlson B. (eds.), Elsevier, 1987, 249-266.

Jenkins W., Merzenich M., Allard T. and Guic-Robels E. *J. Neurophys*, 63, 1990, 82-104.

Jobe T.H., Harrow M., Martin E.M., Whitfield H.J., and Sands J.R. *Schizophrenia Bulletin*, 20, 413–416, 1994.

Joseph M.H., Frith C.D. and Waddington J.L. *Psychopharmacology*, 63, 273–280, 1979.

Kaas J. *Ann. Rev. Neuroscience*, 14, 1991, 137-167.

Katzman R. *New England Journal of Medicine*, 314, 964–973, 1986.

Kay J. and Marcel A. *Quarterly Journal of Experimental Psychology*, 33A, 397-413, 1981.

Knudsen E., du Lac S. & Esterly S. *Annual Review of Neuroscience*, 10, 1987, 41-65.

Kohonen T. *Biological Cybernetics*, 43, 1982, 59-69.

Kohonen T. *Self-Organization and Associative Memory*, Springer-Verlag, 1989.

Leven S.J. In D.S. Levine and S.J. Leven, editors, *Motivation, Emotion and Goal Direction in neural networks*. Lawrence Erlbaum Associates, Publishers, 1992.

Levine D.S. and Prueitt P.S. *Neural Networks*, 2, 103–116, 1989.

Luciano J.S., Cohen M.A. and Samson J.A. In *Irish Neural Network Conference*, September 12-13 1994.

Luciano J.S., Cohen M.A., Samson J.A., and Hagan P.G. In *Irish Neural Network Conference*, September 12-13 1994.

Martin N., Saffran E., and Dell G. *Brain Lang*, 52, 83-113, 1996

Martin, N., Dell, G.S., Saffran, E.M. and Schwartz, M.F. *Brain Lang.*, 47, 609-660, 1994.

McClelland J. and Rumelhart D. In J. McClelland, D. Rumelhart, et al, *Parallel Distributed Processing*, Vol. 2, 1986, 503-527.

McClelland J. and Rumelhart D. *Psychol. Rev*, 88, 1981, 375-407.

McClelland J.L., McNaughton B.L., and O'Reilly R.C. *Psychological Review*, 1995, to appear.

McCloskey, M. *Psychol. Sci.*, 2, 397-395, 1991.

Mehta M, Dasgupta C, & Ullal G. *Biol. Cybernet.*, 68, 1993, 335-340.

Merzenich M., Kaas J., et al. *Neuroscience*, 8, 1983a, 33-55.

Merzenich M., Kaas J., et al. *Neuroscience*, 10, 1983b, 639-665.

Mozer M. and Behrmann M. *Cognitive Neuroscience*, 2, 1990, 96-123.

Nordstrom T. and Svensson B. *J. Par. and Distrib. Comp.*, 14, 1992, 260-285.

Obermayer K., Ritter H. & Schulten K. *Proceedings of International Joint Conference on Neural Networks*, Vol. II, 1990, 423-429. San Diego, CA.

Olson A and Caramazza A. *Handbook of Spelling: Theory, Process and Intervention*, G. Brown & N. Ellis (eds.), John Wiley & Sons, 1994.

Pascual-Leone A., Wassermann E, Sadato N & Hallett M. *Ann. Neurol.*, 38, 1995, 910-915.

Patterson, K., Marshall, J. and Coltheart, M. (Eds.), *Surface Dyslexia*, Lawrence Erlbaum Assoc., London, 1985.

Patterson K., Seidenberg M. and McClelland J. P. Morris (Ed.), *Connectionism: The*

Oxford Symposium, Cambridge University Press, 1989.

Pearsón J., Finkel L. and Edelman B. *Journal of Neuroscience*, 7, 1987, 4209-4233.

Pinker S. and Prince A. *Cognition*, 28, 1988, 73-184.

Pinsky P. & Rinzel J. *J. Comp. Neurosci.*, 1, 1994, 39-60.

Plaut, D.C. *Brain Lang.*, 52, 25-82, 1996.

Plaut, D.C., McClelland, J., Seidenberg, M.S. and Patterson, K. *Psychol. Rev.*, 103, 56-115, 1996.

Plaut, D.C. and Shallice, T. *Cognitive Neuropsychol.*, 10, 377-500, 1993.

Pons T., Garraghty P. & Mishkim M. *Proc. Nat. Acad. Sci.*, 85, 1988,5279-5281.

Psaltis D. and Farhat N. Networks, *Optics Letters*, 10, 1985, 98-100.

Reggia J, D'Autrechy C, Sutton G & Weinrich M. *Neural Computation* 4, 1992 287-317.

Reggia J., Marsland P. and Berndt R. *Complex Systems*, 2, 1988, 509-547.

Reggia J. & Montgomery D. *Comp. Biol. Medicine*, 26, 1996, 133-141.

Reid K. and Zeichick A. *AI Expert*, June 1992, 5-56.

Ritter H., Martinetz T. & Schulten K. *Neural Networks*, 2, 1989, 159-168.

Roberts G. *Trends in Neuroscience*, 13, 207–211, 1990.

Ruppin E. *Network*, 6, 1995, 1-22.

Ruppin E. and Reggia J. *Br. Jour. of Psychiatry*, 166, 19–28, 1995a.

Ruppin E. and Reggia J. *Neural Computation*, 7, 1105-1127, 1995b.

Ruppin E., Reggia J. and Horn D. *Schizophrenia Bulletin*, 1996. To appear.

Sanes J., Suner S., Lando J. and Donoghue J. *Proc. National Acad. Sci.*, 85, 1988, 2003-2007.

Schwartz T. *AI Expert*, August 1988, 73-85.

Seidenberg M. and McClelland J. *Psychological Review*, 96, 1989, 523-568.

Seidenberg, M.S., Plaut, D.C., Petersen, A.S., McClelland, J.L. and McRae, K. *J. Exp. Psychol.: Human Percept. Perform.*, 20, 1177-1196, 1994.

Seidenberg M, Waters G, Barnes M, & Tanenhaus M. *J. Verbal Learning and Verbal Behavior*, 23, 1984, 383-404.

Servan-Schreiber D. and Cohen J.C. *Psychiatric Annals*, 22, 125–130, 1992.

Servan-Schreiber D., Printz H. and Cohen J.D. *Science*, 249, 892–895, 1990.

Shallice T. and McCarthy R. *Surface Dyslexia*, K. Patterson, J. Marshall and M. Coltheart (eds.), Lawrence Erlbaum Associates, 1985, 361-397.

Shallice, T., Glasspool, D.W. and Houghton, G. *Language Cognitive Processes*, 10, 195-225, 1995.

Shrager J., Hogg T., Huberman B.A. *Science*, 236, 1092–1094, 1987.

Sklar, E. *Proc Intl Joint Conf Neural Networks*, III, 1990, 727-732.

Small S, Hart J, Nguyen T and Gordon B, *Brain*, 118, 441-453, 1995.

Spitzer M, et al. *Biol. Cybernet*, 72, 1995, 197-206.

Stevens J.R. *Arch. of Gen. Psych.*, 29, 177–189, 1973.

Stevens J.R. *Arch. of Gen. Psychiatry*, 49, 238–243, 1992.

Sutton G., Reggia J., Armentrout S. & D'Autrechy L. *Neural Computation*, 6, 1993, 1-13.

Thaler S.L. *Neural Networks*, 8, 55–65, 1995.

Traub R. *J. Comp. Neurosci.*, 2, 1995, 283-289.

Udin S. & Fawcett J. *Annual Review of Neuroscience*, 11, 1988, 289-327.

Venezky, R.L. *The Structure of English Orthography*, Mouton, The Hague, 1970.

Vinograd S., King R.J. and Huberman B.A. *Psychiatry*, 55, 79–94, 1992.

von der Malsburg C. *Kybernetic*, 14, 1973, 85-100.

Waddington J.L. *Schizophrenia Bulletin*, 19, 55–69, 1993.

Walsh, K., *Neuropsychology*, Churchill Livingston, NY, 1978, p. 284.

Wan E., Kovacs G., Rosen J. and Widrow B. *Proc. Intl. Joint Conf. on Neural Networks*, Washington DC, II, Lawrence Erlbaum, 1990, 3-21.

Webster C., Glass R. and Banks G. *Proc. Twelfth Symp. on Comp. Applic. in Med. Care*, R. Greenes (ed.), IEEE, 1988, 287-291.

Weinrich M., Sutton G., Reggia J. & D'Autrechy C. *J. Artif. Neural Networks*, 1993, 51-60.

Weinberger D.R. *Arch. of Gen. Psych.*, 44, 660–669, 1987.

Wilson M., Bhalla U., Uhley J. and Bower J. Touretzky D (ed): *Adv. in Neural Network Information Processing Sys.*, Morgan Kaufman Publ., 1989, 485-492. ~

Wong R., Traub R. and Miles R., *Advances in Neurology*, 44, 583-592, 1986.

Wood C., Silverstein, Ritz and Jones, *Psychological Review*, 85, 582-591, 1978.

Wood C. *Psychological Review*, 87, 1980, 474-476.

Xing J and Gerstein G. *Journal of Neurophysiology*, 75, 1996, 184–232.

Zepka R. and Sabbatini R. *Mathematical Approaches to Brain Functioning Diagnostics*, Dvorak I & Holden A (eds.), Manchester University Press, 1991, 249.

MEMORY
DISORDERS

DOES THE SPREAD OF ALZHEIMER'S DISEASE NEUROPATHOLOGY INVOLVE THE MECHANISMS OF CONSOLIDATION?

MICHAEL E. HASSELMO and BRADLEY P. WYBLE

Dept. of Psychology and Program in Neuroscience
Harvard University, 33 Kirkland St., Cambridge, MA 02138
E-mail: hasselmo@katla.harvard.edu

ABSTRACT

A model of the hippocampus allows analysis of the role of network dynamics in the initiation and progression of neuropathology in Alzheimers disease. The model is neutral with respect to etiology, focusing on a final common breakdown in function termed runaway synaptic modification. This phenomenon could account for evidence showing that the neurofibrillary tangles associated with Alzheimers disease first appear and attain their highest concentration in subregions of the hippocampal formation, then successively spread into temporal lobe cortex and the cortex of the frontal and parietal lobes. The model demonstrates how the spread of neuropathology from the hippocampus into neocortical structures could result from the mechanisms of consolidation. Initial sensitivity of the hippocampus and entorhinal cortex to the development of neurofibrillary tangles is proposed to result from an imbalance of parameters regulating the influence of synaptic transmission on synaptic modification. Degeneration of cortical cholinergic innervation is proposed to result from exponentially increased demands on the feedback regulation of cholinergic modulation. Increased levels of amyloid are attributed to exponential increases in the modification and maintenance of synaptic connections, while development of paired helical filaments is ascribed to exponentially increased demands on the mechanisms of axonal transport or remodeling. Memory deficits are described as due to increased interference effects in recent memory caused by runaway synaptic modification which ultimately progresses to cause impairments of remote memory and semantic memory.

1. Introduction

In the popular consciousness, Alzheimer's disease is identified as a disorder of memory function. While research on Alzheimer's disease has produced a range of etiological theories, ranging from the improper splicing of the amyloid precursor protein (Selkoe 1993) to epidemiological factors such as aluminum exposure (Crapper McLachlan and Van Berkum 1986) or prions (Goudsmit and Van der Waals 1986), these etiological theories have not explicitly accounted for why this disorder should show its earliest symptoms as a disorder of memory function (Jolles 1986; Morris and Kopelman 1986; Albert et al. 1991), and should so severely affect those structures associated with memory function (Arnold et al. 1991; Arriagada et al. 1992; Hyman et al. 1984; 1990). As it stands, the early effect on memory function is attributed to the unexplained specificity of Alzheimer's disease for hippocampal region CA1, the subiculum, and layers II and IV of entorhinal cortex (Hyman et al. 1984, 1990; Arnold et al. 1991; Braak and Braak 1991). Here it will be proposed that the causality is in fact reversed. The selective cortical neuropathology associated with the progression of this disorder may be rooted in the breakdown of the essential mechanisms of cortical memory function.

This paper presents a computational theory of the initiation and progression of Alzheimer's disease which attempts to account for evidence on the progression of Alzheimer's disease not in terms of a specific etiological factor, but in terms of the processing characteristics of cortical structures, and the stability of the learning mechanisms within these structures. This theory was inspired by the phenomenon of runaway synaptic modification, as demonstrated in models of cortical associative memory function (Hasselmo et al. 1992; Hasselmo 1993a, 1994; Hasselmo and Bower 1993; Barkai et al. 1994; Hasselmo and Barkai, 1995). In these models, interference during learning can lead to the exponential growth of a large number of synaptic connections within the network. Runaway synaptic modification of this sort may underlie the neuropathological characteristics of Alzheimer's disease. The theory provides a framework showing why this neuropathology should appear initially in particular cortical regions associated with memory function (Braak and Braak 1991; Arriagada et al. 1992), and why it should appear to progress into adjacent regions of association cortex along the observed anatomical connections (Pearson et al. 1985; Arnold et al. 1991; Arriagada et al. 1992). Finally, the theory suggests that the apparent degeneration of cortical cholinergic innervation in this disease (Davies and Maloney 1976; Perry et al. 1977; Whitehouse et al. 1982; Coyle et al. 1983; Saper et al. 1985) may result from feedback mechanisms placing too great a demand on the cholinergic modulation of learning processes.

In terms of specific causative factors, this theory is neutral in many respects. The phenomenon of runaway synaptic modification could be initiated by a variety of changes in the parameters of cortical function, due to either a genetic predisposition or environmental influences. The initial appearance of runaway synaptic modification is attributed to an imbalance of cortical parameters, which could result from insufficient normalization of synaptic strength within each neuron, from a lowering of the threshold of synaptic modification, from insufficient feedback inhibition, from an imbalance of the sensitivity of pre-synaptic and post-synaptic cholinergic receptors, or from direct overload of the information capacity of cortical structures.

2. Experimental data.

2.1. Selective distribution and progression of neuropathology

A vast range of research on Alzheimer's disease has provided a body of empirical evidence which must be explained by any theory of the progression of Alzheimer's disease. Alzheimer's disease is diagnosed post-mortem on the basis the density of the neuropathological characteristics including neuritic plaques and neurofibrillary tangles (for review, see Price 1986; Katzman 1986; Hyman et al. 1990; Selkoe 1993). Neuritic plaques tend to be broadly distributed, appearing throughout the cortex, with a greater density in regions of frontal, parietal and temporal association cortex distant from the primary sensory and motor cortices (Pearson et al. 1985; Arnold et al. 1991). In addition, neuritic plaques appear in subcortical regions receiving projections from the cortex (Pearson et al. 1985). The distribution and component features of neuritic plaques have led to the suggestion that they reflect the degeneration of axonal processes from the same set of neurons which develop neurofibrillary tangles (Hyman et al. 1984). Here it is proposed that neuritic plaques result from a breakdown in the normal mechanisms for modification of synaptic strength.

Neurofibrillary tangles show a more localized initial distribution than plaques and spread in a characteristic sequence (Hyman et al. 1990; Arnold et al. 1991; Braak and Braak 1991). Tangles appear initially and attain their highest concentration in layer II of entorhinal cortex, region CA1 of the hippocampus, and the portions of the subiculum adjacent to region CA1 (Ball 1972; Hyman et al. 1984; Hyman et al. 1990; Arriagada et al. 1992; Braak & Braak 1991). As the severity of the disease progresses, tangles appear in regions receiving projections from these areas, initially in portions of the temporal lobe adjacent to the entorhinal cortex, and later in regions of parietal lobe and frontal cortex which are closely linked to entorhinal cortex (Brun & Gustafson 1976; Pearson et al. 1985; Arnold et al. 1991; Arriagada et al. 1992; Braak & Braak 1991). Tangles appear to be distributed in almost columnar fashion, with tangles in layer 2 and 3 appearing in register with tangles in layers 5 and 6 (Pearson et al., 1985). The primary sensory and motor cortices typically show the lowest density of neurofibrillary tangles, suggesting they are the least sensitive to the mechanisms underlying this disorder (Brun & Gustafson 1976; Pearson et al. 1985; Esiri et al. 1986). These patterns of distribution suggest that the disease progresses from the hippocampus along back-projections into cortical regions. In addition, it suggests that susceptibility to degeneration is somehow correlated with the level of involvement in higher order cognitive processes and associations between modalities -- processes which involve ongoing remodeling of cortical representations.

2.2. Loss of neuromodulatory agents

Studies have shown decreases in the levels of various cortical neuromodulatory agents in Alzheimer's disease, with a primary focus on enzymatic markers for acetylcholine. Acetylcholinesterase (AChE) and cholineacetyltransferase (ChAT) show marked decreases in concentration in the cortex of patients diagnosed with Alzheimer's disease (Davies & Maloney 1976; Perry et al. 1977; Coyle et al. 1983). In addition, the regions of the basal forebrain which provide the cholinergic innervation of cortical structures show decreases in the number of neurons, suggesting a degeneration in Alzheimer's disease (Whitehouse et al. 1982; Rapp & Amaral 1992). This evidence, coupled with research showing that cholinergic muscarinic antagonists such as scopolamine impair memory function in normal subjects (for review, see Hasselmo, 1995), led to the suggestion that the memory deficits of Alzheimer's disease might somehow be specifically related to the loss of cortical cholinergic innervation. Administration of acetylcholinesterase blockers cause a small but significant alleviation of the memory impairment associated with Alzheimer's disease.

2.3. Theories of the progession of Alzheimer's disease

Research on potential causes of Alzheimer's disease at the molecular level do not attempt to systematically describe the spread of pathology between different regions.

Many forms of familial Alzheimer's disease have been linked to specific inherited differences in protein structure (Schellenberg et al. 1992), though the fact that monozygotic twins can show different susceptibility for the disease suggests the disease is not entirely genetic (Breitner et al. 1993). This class of theories depends upon the assumption that one of the protein components of the Alzheimer neuropathology, such as amyloid or tau, is a causative agent in the disease (see e.g. Hardy and Higgins 1992). The characteristic distribution of neuropathology places extra demands on this theory, suggesting a particular susceptibility of the hippocampus and association cortex but not the primary motor and sensory cortices. Theories based on environmental factors must also account for this selective sensitivity.

The theory presented here focuses on relating initiation and progression of the disease to functional characteristics of cortical regions. In this framework, the initial imbalance of cortical parameters which results in pathology could be due to defects of the genetic code, the spread of toxic factors, an infection by a prion, or a combination of different factors. But this theory proposes that the final effect of this imbalance is the initiation of runaway synaptic modification within cortical regions with a strong capacity for synaptic modification, such as the hippocampal formation. In this context, the progression of the disease depends upon the functional interaction of cortical regions. Rather than depending on the transmission of some substance from the axon terminal of an affected cell to an as yet unaffected post-synaptic neuron, this theory depends only on the normal mechanisms of synaptic transmission and synaptic modification at these connections. The basis of this theory is that the pattern of activity propagated from affected to unaffected regions may be pathological in itself. That is, runaway synaptic modification may cause a breakdown of function in one region, and the patterns of activity elicited can induce runaway synaptic modification in connected regions.

The focus of this model differs from other models of Alzheimer's disease (Horn et al., 1993; Herrmann et al., 1993), which do not attempt to address the dynamics of spread of cortical neuropathology. These previous models start with the assumption of loss of neurons or synaptic connections within models of cortex, and then analyze how the effects of this loss on memory function may be affected by synaptic compensation mechanisms.

3. Runaway synaptic modification in models of cortex.

This theory of Alzheimers disease focuses on the phenomenon of runaway synaptic modification as the final common pathway by which different etiological influences can result in Alzheimer neuropathology (Hasselmo, 1994). Runaway synaptic modification can occur in any system in which synaptic modification depends upon synaptic transmission. Thus, most neural network models of cortical function have the potential to undergo runaway synaptic modification.

Models of cortical associative memory function (Anderson 1972; Grossberg 1970; Hopfield 1982; Kohonen 1984; McClelland & Rumelhart 1988; Amit et al. 1990) focus on the anatomical evidence for widely distributed excitatory intrinsic and associational connections linking pyramidal cells within cortical structures, including neocortex and hippocampus. While they differ in detail, the function of all these models depends upon the synaptic modification of excitatory connections using some modification of the Hebb rule (Hebb 1949; Wigstrom et al., 1986). The basic feature of the Hebb rule is a change in synaptic strength proportional to pre-synaptic and post-synaptic activity during learning. These modified excitatory synapses can then form the basis for recalling associations between different patterns of activity. A simple example of this associative memory function is shown in Figure 1.

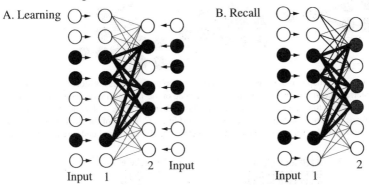

Figure 1. Associative memory function. A. Learning: Separate input patterns are presented to region 1 and region 2. The synapses between active neurons are strengthened using a Hebbian learning rule (dependent on pre and post-synaptic activity). Strengthened synapses are represented by thicker lines between neurons. B. Recall: Input is presented to region 1 only. The spread of activity along previously strengthened connections (thick lines) induces activity in region 2 resembling the pattern previously associated with pattern 1.

Neurophysiological data suggests that Hebbian synaptic modification depends upon combining post-synaptic depolarization with synaptic transmission to activate NMDA receptors at the synapse being modified (Wigstrom et al. 1986). However, if a modifiable synapse can influence post-synaptic activity during learning, strengthening this synapse will increase post-synaptic activity, and thereby increase subsequent strengthening of the synapse. This positive feedback effect can very rapidly lead to exponential growth of undesired synapses within the network, i.e. runaway synaptic modification.

The mechanism for runaway synaptic modification is illustrated in Figure 2. This figure shows that if synaptic transmission at modifiable synapses is allowed during learning, the spread of activity across previously modified connections causes the new synaptic modification to contain elements of proactive interference from previously learned memories (Hasselmo et al. 1992; Hasselmo & Bower 1993; Hasselmo 1993; 1994; Hasselmo et al., 1995). Without the proper balance of parameters of cortical function, this interference during learning can have disastrous effects in models of cortical memory function . Though the effect of interference during learning in any particular stage of learning may be small, this phenomenon can severely affect the function of the network over time, because the effects are compounded by subsequent learning. The progressive buildup of interference from previous retrieval leads to a malignant nostalgia resulting in runaway synaptic modification throughout the whole network. In this case, severe proactive and retroactive interference results in a complete breakdown of normal memory function. This runaway interference during learning has been described previously in detail using mathematical analysis (Hasselmo 1994) and computational models (Hasselmo et al. 1992; Hasselmo 1993; Barkai et al., 1994).

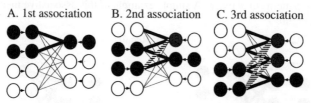

Figure 2. Runaway synaptic modification. As more overlapping memories are stored within the network, greater interference during learning occurs. A: Learning of the 1st association shows no interference. B: Interference due to recall of the 1st association during learning of the 2nd association causes strengthening of one additional undesired connection (dashed line). C: Recall of the 1st and the 2nd association during learning of the 3rd association causes strengthening of 2 additional undesired connections.

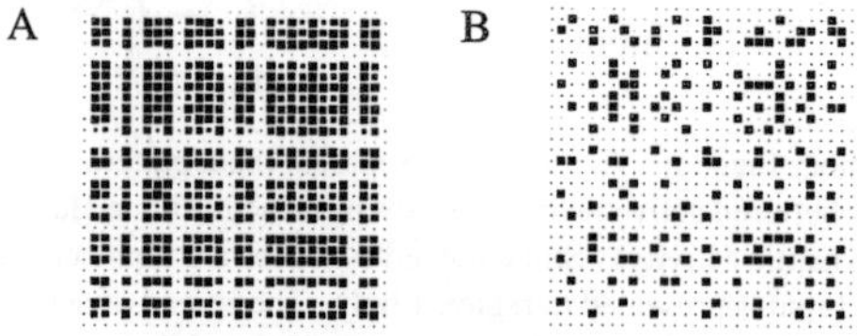

Figure 3. Matrix of synaptic connectivity within an associative memory model. Size of black squares represents strength of synapses. A. After runaway synaptic modification. B. After normal learning.

Because of the problems caused by synaptic transmission during learning, most associative memory models ignore the effects of synaptic transmission at modifiable synapses during learning (Kohonen 1972; Anderson 1972; Hopfield 1982; McClelland & Rumelhart 1988; Amit et al. 1990), allowing synaptic transmission only during recall. In computational models, this suppression of synaptic transmission at intrinsic and association fiber synapses during learning can prevent runaway synaptic modification (Hasselmo et al. 1992; Hasselmo 1993; 1994; Hasselmo & Bower 1993; Barkai et al., 1994; Hasselmo and Barkai, 1995). Though this suppression of synaptic transmission during learning has been used for decades in neural network models, researchers did not provide a neurophysiological mechanism for this effect until recently. Recently, it has been shown that acetylcholine has the capacity to selectively suppress intrinsic and association fiber synaptic transmission, while leaving afferent fiber synaptic transmission unaffected (Hasselmo & Bower 1992; Hasselmo and Schnell, 1994; Hasselmo et al., 1995). In addition, acetylcholine enhances the excitability of cortical neurons to the afferent synaptic input (Cole & Nicoll 1984; Barkai & Hasselmo 1994). In computational models of cortical associative memory function, application of this selective suppression of intrinsic fiber synaptic transmission during learning prevents interference from previously learned memories (Hasselmo et al. 1992; Hasselmo 1993, 1994; Hasselmo and Bower 1993; Hasselmo and Barkai, 1995). While the examples shown here are highly simplified, the prevention of runaway synaptic modification has also been explored in detailed biophysical simulations of cortical associative memory function (Hasselmo and Barkai, 1995; Barkai et al., 1994). Prevention of runaway synaptic modification by cholinergic suppression of synaptic transmission is illustrated in simplified form in Figure 4.

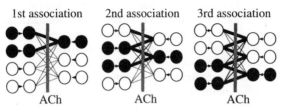

Figure 4. Cholinergic suppression of synaptic transmission during learning can prevent runaway synaptic modification. The thick gray line represents diffuse cholinergic suppression of transmission at modifiable synapses, preventing the spread of excitation across previously modified synapses from bringing post-synaptic neurons above threshold. This allows Hebbian synaptic modification to occur only between neurons receiving direct afferent input (only these neurons have sufficient post-synaptic activity). Strengthening of additional undesired connections does not occur (compare with Figure 2).

In this new framework for learning, synaptic modification must be maximal during the cholinergic suppression of synaptic transmission. But how does this allow activation of post-synaptic NMDA receptors? The activation of NMDA receptors and the mechanisms of synaptic modification are still possible because the cholinergic suppression of synaptic transmission is not complete. In neurophysiological experiments, the cholinergic suppression of synaptic transmission is usually less than 70% (Hasselmo & Bower 1992). Analysis of associative memory models incorporating feedback inhibition, a threshold for synaptic modification and gated decay of synaptic strength shows that this level of suppression is sufficient to prevent interference during learning, while allowing sufficient synaptic transmission for the modification of synapses (Hasselmo 1993; 1994). In models of cortical associative memory function, interference during learning can be prevented by the proper balance of cortical physiological parameters including 1.) pre-synaptic cholinergic modulation of synaptic transmission, 2.) Regulated decay of synaptic connectivity strength, 3.) post-synaptic cholinergic modulation of cellular excitability, 4.) the level of inhibition within the network, 5.) the threshold for synaptic modification, and 6.) the nature of the patterns being stored within the network. In addition, cholinergic agonists have been shown to enhance synaptic modification in cortical structures (Hasselmo and Barkai, 1995; Huerta and Lisman, 1994).

Associative memory models with fixed-point attractor dynamics have been utilized in other modeling work focused on Alzheimer's disease (Horn et al., 1993; Herrmann et al., 1993). In that work, the accuracy of memory recall is analyzed as different numbers of synaptic connections or processing units are deleted within the network. This causes a gradual impairment in memory function which can be offset by postulating various processes for synaptic compensation, in which strengthening of existing synapses offsets the loss of other synapses. Thus, this research focuses on compensatory mechanisms for decreasing the impaired memory function associated with Alzheimer's disease, rather than addressing the spread of pathology directly.

Synaptic transmission at synapses undergoing Hebbian synaptic modification is a regular feature of a different class of models, focused on self-organization of feature detectors in cortical structures (Linsker, 1988; Miller et al., 1990). These models avoid the exponential growth of the full population of synapses by using techniques such as normalization. However, even slight imbalances in the mechanism of normalization of synaptic strength causes a breakdown of function and runaway synaptic modification in these networks. Here it is proposed that neuronal degeneration in Alzheimer's disease may result from runaway synaptic modification due to an imbalance of synaptic normalization, which could include overproduction or flaws in the function of the amyloid precursor protein, or improper phosphorylation of the tau protein.

4. Runaway synaptic modification and the progression of Alzheimer's disease.

The phenomenon of runaway synaptic modification would greatly increase the metabolic and structural demands on the mechanisms of synaptic modification within cortical regions. As shown in Figures 2 and 3, runaway synaptic modification results in the strengthening of many additional connections -- in proportion to the number of associations stored in the network.   Thus, runaway synaptic modification in a network storing 100 different associations would result in synaptic modification at a 100-fold greater number of synapses. While cortical structures do not show the complete connectivity used in these models, the axon collaterals of each pyramidal cell within a cortical region makes from 1000 to 10,000 excitatory synapses on other pyramidal cells. An exponential increase in the demands on synaptic modification might explain neuronal degeneration of the sort seen in Alzheimer's disease. This theory does not stand in opposition to any specific theory of the etiology of the disease, since it suggests that the progression of Alzheimer's disease could start from any one of a number of imbalances in cortical function. In fact, this theory could even allow for multiple different initiating factors -- including the gradual overload of the capacity of cortical networks.

4.1. Time course of onset of neuropathology.

Evidence for specific genetic markers of Alzheimer's disease raises the question: Why does the disease appear late in life? This question might be answered by analysis of how an imbalance of cortical parameters can result in the initiation of runaway synaptic modification. This analysis shows the relative importance of different parameters in preventing runaway synaptic modification, and how the magnitude of the imbalance relates to the speed of progression of runaway synaptic modification. As noted above, the imbalance could result from changes in the strength of any of a number of factors. As a specific example, a simplified analysis of an associative memory model suggests that runaway synaptic modification will appear if cholinergic suppression of synaptic transmission is not sufficient to bring the level of post-synaptic activity for undesired connections below the level of inhibition and the threshold of synaptic modification (Hasselmo 1993; 1994). Another important factor in determining whether runaway synaptic modification appears within the network is the normalization of synaptic weights. If the mechanisms of normalization of synaptic weights are somehow impaired, then runaway synaptic modification can be initiated.

In cortical function, the relative strength of any of these parameters could change due to toxic factors, or these parameters could be improperly balanced due to genetic predisposition. For low cholinergic suppression, low inhibition, and a low threshold of synaptic modification, runaway synaptic modification will occur after a smaller number of patterns are stored. For strong cholinergic suppression, strong inhibition, and a high threshold of synaptic modification, runaway synaptic modification will take longer to appear, or may be prevented entirely. It is the relative balance of these different parameters which determines how well the network resists the initiation of runaway synaptic modification.

The breakdown of function can take one of two forms: 1) The network can start with a given balance of parameters, and when the capacity of the network is exceeded, runaway synaptic modification will cause a breakdown of function, or 2) The network could start with a given balance of parameters, and suffer some change in this balance which causes the breakdown of function. In either case, the larger the imbalance, the earlier the breakdown appears, and the more rapidly it will progress. A simplified analysis of a linear associative memory model shows that the undesired connections strengthened due to interference during learning will grow exponentially. If cholinergic suppression is very low relative to other cortical parameters, interference will appear sooner within the network, and the spread of interference throughout the network will be more rapid. If there is only a slight imbalance, interference will take much longer to appear, and once it appears, it will progress more slowly (Hasselmo, 1994).

This phenomenon could underlie the evidence for differences in the time course of progression of presenile dementia of the Alzheimer type as compared with senile dementia of the Alzheimer type. It has been shown that quantitative measures of anatomical markers of Alzheimer's disease suggest greater severity in presenile dementia as compared with senile dementia of the Alzheimer type (Hansen et al. 1988). In addition, some studies show a correlation between age and cognitive performance on memory tasks, with younger Alzheimer's patients performing more poorly (Kopelman 1985), and clinical evidence suggests that the rate of progression from onset of symptoms to death may be more rapid in presenile dementia (Selzter & Sherwin 1983). However, other evidence suggests that the progression of neuropsychological deterioration is actually slower in presenile dementia (Huff et al. 1987).

This model of the initiation of Alzheimer's disease pathology could also be used to address the epidemiology of this disease. Alzheimer's disease has been characterized as a disease of old age primarily because the frequency of the disease increases rapidly with increasing age. The exponential progression of runaway synaptic modification in these computational models could be used as a model of the epidemiology of Alzheimer's disease. Since the risk factors for onset of runaway synaptic modification include many components of normal cortical function, all humans may have some probability of induction of these pathological effects. Depending upon individual variation in certain parameters, the induction will take place at different time points, but once initiated, it will progress exponentially. This means that the percentage of cases of senile dementia of the Alzheimer type should increase exponentially with increasing age (though an epidemiological prediction of this sort must take into account the reduction of the population at each age level due to death from Alzheimer's disease and death from other factors). There is certainly a rapid increase in the number of cases of Alzheimer's disease in later life (Katzman, 1986), and neuropathological data from normal elderly subjects suggest a rapid increase in the density of tangles with increasing age, even in tissue from subjects who have not been diagnosed with Alzheimer's disease (Arriagada et al., 1992). A more radical prediction of the model is that runaway synaptic modification will appear more rapidly in proportion to the greater overlap between stored patterns. This suggests that the amount of correlation in the environment could influence the propensity for development of Alzheimer's disease.

4.2. Selective distribution of neuropathology.

If the neuropathology associated with Alzheimer's disease results from runaway synaptic modification, this suggests that the apparent early and severe involvement of layers II and IV of the lateral entorhinal cortex, region CA1 of the hippocampus and the adjacent regions of the subiculum (Hyman et al. 1984; 1990; Arnold et al. 1991; Braak & Braak 1991; Arriagada et al. 1992) results from a particular sensitivity of these regions to runaway synaptic modification. For example, it is possible that sensitivity to runaway synaptic modification might be associated with 2 features: 1.) a strong capacity for Hebbian synaptic modification, and 2.) absence of the cholinergic suppression of synaptic transmission during learning. Considerable research has focused on the how subregions of the hippocampus resemble the structures of associative memory models (Marr 1971; McNaughton & Morris 1987). As noted above, this region shows robust Hebbian synaptic modification (Wigstrom et al. 1986) and has been implicated in memory function in extensive research (Scoville & Milner 1957; Squire & Zola-Morgan 1991). The greater propensity for synaptic modification could underlie the early sensitivity of the hippocampal formation. The early sensitivity of lateral entorhinal cortex could be linked to the absence of cholinergic suppression at synapses arising from this region and terminating in the outer molecular layer of the dentate gyrus (Kahle and Cotman, 1990), while the relative sparing of region CA3 could result from the robust cholinergic suppression of synaptic transmission at synapses arising from CA3 pyramidal cells (Hasselmo and Schnell, 1994; Hasselmo et al., 1995).

4.3. Spread of degeneration between cortical regions.

The neuropathology of Alzheimer's disease appears to spread from hippocampus into the neocortex along well-established anatomical connections, the back projections from the subiculum and entorhinal cortex to association cortex (Pearson et al. 1985; Hyman et al. 1990; Arnold et al. 1991). In later stages of the disease, neurofibrillary tangles appear in regions of the temporal, parietal and frontal neocortex (Hirano and Zimmerman 1962; Pearson et al. 1985; Arnold et al. 1991). Neurofibrillary tangles primarily spread into cortical regions, though the plaques associated with terminal degeneration appear in subcortical regions as well (Pearson et al. 1985). This spread of degeneration is here proposed to result from the spread of runaway synaptic modification between cortical regions. This would use the same mechanisms important for transferring information stored in the hippocampus back into the neocortex -- the process of consolidation (Wilson and McNaughton, 1994; McClelland et al., 1995). A network simulation of the hippocampus (Hasselmo, 1995b; Hasselmo et al., 1996) has been used to model the process of consolidation, as shown in Figure 5.

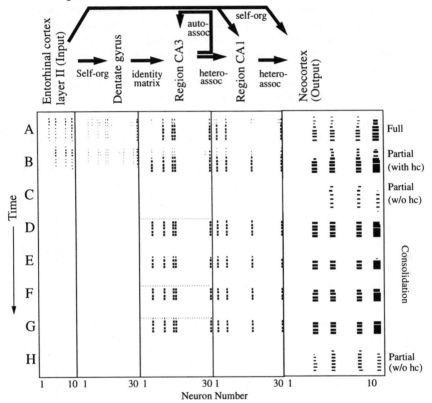

Figure 5. Consolidation of a single pattern in a network model of the hippocampal formation. Size of black squares represents the activity of individual neurons. A. Presentation of input to entorhinal cortex layer II. Synaptic modification in dentate gyrus forms a sparse self-organized representation, and modification in region CA3 forms an attractor state. B. Testing recall with degraded (partial) input with hippocampus present (with hc). Representations are activated in dentate gyrus and region CA3. Attractor dynamics in region CA3 drive recall activity in CA1 and neocortex. C. With a simulated hippocampal lesion (w/o hc), no recall can occur. Input to neocortex alone does not result in recall before consolidation. This corresponds to temporally limited retrograde amnesia. D. -G. Consolidation. Homogeneous depolarization of region CA3 results in activation of the previously stored attractor state. This activates the full pattern in neocortex, allowing gradual strengthening of synapses in neocortex. H. The preceding period of consolidation allows neocortex to respond to the partial input cue with the full learned pattern. Thus, after consolidation, memory recall is not impaired by lesions of the hippocampus.

Runaway synaptic modification could spread from hippocampus back into neocortical structures using the same mechanisms as consolidation. It has been shown in simulations that if runaway synaptic modification occurs during the initial formation of representations of new memories in the hippocampus, then subsequent retrieval of these representations will result in a spread of runaway synaptic modification. For example, as shown in Figure 6, a decrease in the mechanisms of synaptic decay of the input from entorhinal cortex layer II to dentate gyrus results in the initiation of runaway synaptic modification in this pathway. Even if the parameters of other connections have not been altered, the initiation of runaway synaptic modification at these perforant path synapses results in the spread of runaway synaptic modification into back projections from region CA1 to neocortex. In simulations with multiple interacting layers, the initiation of runaway synaptic modification in one layer results in the progressive spread to other layers, even if those layers would not undergo runaway synaptic modification independently.

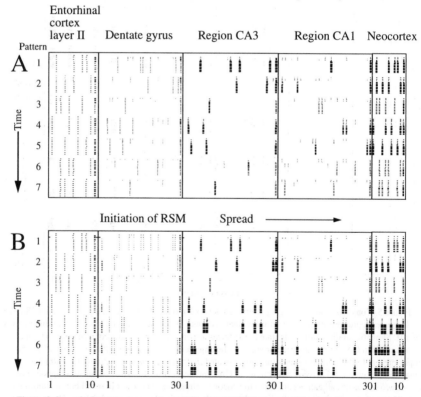

Figure 6. Spread of runaway synaptic modification (RSM) between different regions. A. Normal function of the network. B. Initiation of runaway synaptic modification due to insufficient synaptic decay in the dentate gyrus rapidly results in a spread of runaway synaptic modification through regions CA3 and CA1. Excessive strengthening of backprojections from CA1 to neocortex result in broadly distributed activity in response to presentation of later patterns (e.g. pattern 7).

Modeling suggests that runaway synaptic modification will spread according to functional boundaries. That is, after occurring in neurons encoding a particular category of information, it will more rapidly influence similar or strongly associated information before influencing unrelated information. This might explain the apparent heterogeneous distribution of tangles in Alzheimer's disease and the apparent specificity for specific modalities in some cases. In particular, the distribution of neurofibrillary tangles may be on the order of the size of cortical columns, with tangles in layers 2 and 3 in register with tangles in layers 5 and 6 (Pearson et al. 1985).

The rate of spread of runaway synaptic modification depends upon the ongoing capacity for Hebbian synaptic modification and the amount of excitatory associative connectivity. Primary sensory and motor cortices have more restricted and specific connectivity of excitatory intrinsic and associational connections (Lund 1988), and are further removed from the highly plastic structures of the hippocampal formation. This may explain why the neuropathology in Alzheimer's disease is far less pronounced in the primary sensory cortices (Hirano and Zimmerman 1962; Brun and Gustafson 1976; Pearson et al. 1985; Esiri et al. 1986).

Based on the distribution of neuropathology in cortical regions and impairments in olfactory identification (Koss et al. 1988), it has been suggested that a pathogen for Alzheimer's disease enters via the olfactory epithelium (Pearson et al. 1985; Talamo et al. 1989). The olfactory epithelium does show changes which may be associated with Alzheimer's disease (Talamo et al. 1989), but the relative lack of pathology within the mitral cell layer of the olfactory bulb does not support the hypothesis that the disease spreads through these neurons (Hyman et al 1991). Even if an environmental factor arriving along this pathway is responsible, its effects appear highly specific to regions with modifiable excitatory intrinsic connections. For example, high concentrations of tangles have been found in regions with intrinsic excitatory synapses which may be modifiable such as the anterior olfactory nucleus (Esiri and Wilcock 1984; Hyman et al. 1991) and the piriform cortex (Reyes et al. 1987). In contrast, much lower concentrations of tangles are found in the olfactory bulb, which contains primarily inhibitory feedback connections (Kauer 1991).

4.4. Breakdown of cholinergic modulation.

A range of evidence suggests the degeneration of cortical cholinergic innervation in Alzheimer's disease, including decreased levels of AChE and ChAT in cortical structures (Davies and Maloney 1976; Perry et al. 1977) and decreased cell counts in basal forebrain nuclei (Whitehouse et al. 1982). However, other evidence shows increased sprouting of the cholinergic innervation of the dentate gyrus (Geddes et al. 1985) and increases in ChAT staining levels in the dentate gyrus and stratum moleculare of the subiculum (Hyman et al. 1986). In addition, memory impairment has been correlated with hypertrophy of basal forebrain neurons in aged non-human primates (Rapp and Amaral 1992). The latter effects have been suggested to reflect the reafferentation of hippocampal neurons which have lost their innervation from the entorhinal cortex. However, the effects of acetylcholine on dentate gyrus granule cells is considerably different from the effects of the glutamate released by the terminals of the perforant path. It is unclear why sprouting would occur to replace such innervation. The model presented here provides a different perpsective on this data.

As shown above, cholinergic modulation can help prevent runaway synaptic modification in models of cortical associative memory. While deficiencies of cholinergic modulation could underlie the initiation of runaway synaptic modification, runaway synaptic modification could also be due to changes in other parameters, without any significant change in the level of cholinergic modulation. However, once runaway synaptic modification begins to appear, it is likely that the normal feedback mechanisms which regulate the level of cholinergic modulation would be significantly increased as a mechanism for preventing the breakdown of function. This might place increasingly greater demands on cortical cholinergic modulation, initially resulting in a strong enhancement of cholinergic modulation. This effect could underlie the increased sprouting of cholinergic axons in the dentate gyrus (Geddes et al. 1985) and the increases in AChE staining in the dentate gyrus and subiculum (Hyman et al. 1986). The increases in AChE staining appear in exactly those regions where insufficient cholinergic modulation during learning might underlie the initiation of runaway synaptic modification.

While a large increase in cholinergic modulation might slow the progression of runaway synaptic modification, once the breakdown has been initiated it is very difficult to forestall. Even at very high concentrations of acetylcholine some synaptic transmission remains (Hasselmo and Bower 1992), allowing continued runaway synaptic modification. This would result in continually increasing demands which could lead to an initial hypertrophy and eventual degeneration of cells of the basal forebrain nuclei from which this innervation arises (Whitehouse et al. 1982). Thus, the model suggests two phases: an initial increase of innervation followed by degeneration.

4.5. Molecular components of the neuropathology of Alzheimer's disease.

The phenomenon of runaway synaptic modification in models suggests how the molecular components of the neuropathology of Alzheimer's disease might underlie the initiation of runaway synaptic modification, and how runaway synaptic modification could result in large scale deposits of these particular substances.

4.5.1. Amyloid precursor protein and runaway synaptic modification.

Neuritic plaques have as their main component feature the accumulation of the b-amyloid protein (BAP). BAP apparently arises from a normal component protein of the brain referred to as amyloid precursor protein (APP). The APP has a transmembrane domain, with the bulk of the protein being extracellular (Selkoe 1993; Marotta et al. 1992). Some forms of the protein contain a segment which can act as a protease inhibitor in the extracellular portion (Wagner et al. 1992; Hyman et al. 1992). Unfortunately, the functional role of the amyloid precursor protein has not yet been determined. However, the known properties of the APP are compatible with some role in the growth and maintenance of synaptic connections (Milward et al. 1992; Leblanc et al. 1992; Saitoh et al. 1989). For example, APP may prevent proteolysis of existing or newly strengthened synapses by extracellular proteases.

In this framework, if post-synaptic activity is not correlated with the activity of the pre-synaptic terminal, the APP will be cleaved at its usual site just outside the cell membrane (at amino acid 16 of the BAP), and will allow extracellular proteases to break down the components of the synaptic contact. However, if all synaptic connections are showing increased correlation of pre and post-synaptic activity, as would occur with the feedback mechanisms of interference during learning, then the APP will not be removed, but will continue to accumulate on the pre-synaptic terminals. This will allow runaway growth of the synaptic connection, protected from proteolysis by the protease inhibitors of the membranous APP, and could ultimately lead to high concentrations of APP throughout cortical regions with excessive synaptic modification. The pathways concerned with the breakdown of APP would come under increasing demands, possibly leading to a build-up of BAP in the region of the synapse. Alternately, the cell giving rise to the synapse might be unable to cope with the excessive metabolic demands of thousands of growing synapses. Its death would lead to the degeneration of a synaptic terminal with high concentrations of APP which might be broken down into BAP.

In this framework, the build-up of BAP is seen as a by-product of the runaway synaptic modification due to interference during learning, but this framework could also account for a causal role in Alzheimer's disease not of BAP, but of the overproduction of the precursor of BAP, APP. Over-production of APP due to genetic mutations, or the additional copy of chromosome 21 associated with Downs syndrome, would lead to excessive APP on the pre-synaptic terminal. This would slow the normal breakdown or weakening of synaptic connections not associated with correlation of pre and post-synaptic activity, and could ultimately trigger the initiation of runaway synaptic modification. This would account for the apparent linkage of some forms of familiar Alzheimer's disease with genetic defects within the APP or in other portions of chromosome 21 as well as the apparent development of Alzheimer's type symptoms in people with Downs syndrome. Perhaps the mental retardation found in Downs syndrome might also result from the insufficient breakdown of existing synaptic connections. Any influence of APP on the mechanisms of synaptic modification could result in runaway synaptic modification if that influence is somehow altered by mutations in the APP gene.

4.5.2. Tau protein and runaway synaptic modification

Neurofibrillary tangles appear to contain considerable levels of paired helical filaments, of which a primary component is an abnormally phosphorylated form of the tau protein (Grundkeiqbal et al. 1986) . The tau protein may play a role in the assembly of microtubules. Blockade of the expression of tau protein impairs the development of axons in culture (Kosik and Caceres 1991), suggesting possible involvement in the growth and remodeling of axonal connectivity, or in axonal transport mechanisms. Thus, the tau protein may be involved in formation and regulation of synaptic connections. A breakdown in the normal function of the tau protein, possibly due to improper phosphorylation, might lead to a slowing of the normal mechanisms of normalization of synaptic strength arising from a single neuron. A slowdown in this redistribution of synaptic strength could allow the initiation of runaway synaptic modification in a self-organizing network.

Once runaway synaptic modification begins to occur, it could place increasing demands on this aspect of cellular function, since it would require increased transport of substances produced in the cell body to the thousands of growing synapses. Ultimately, this could overload the capacity of the axonal transport system, leading to excessive production of structural elements of cellular transport, and ultimately an increased accumulation of the byproducts of this system, the paired helical filaments. Ultimately, the increased demands on each individual neuron might cause a complete breakdown of function, and the ulti-mate the death of neurons, leaving behind neurofibrillary tangles.

4.6. Neuropsychology of Alzheimer's disease

In its initial stages, a major characteristic of Alzheimer's disease is the impairment of memory function. The most common early symptoms of this impairment appear to prima-rily involve episodic or declarative recent memory. In later stages, the symptoms progress to impairments of semantic memory and other factors such as emotional disturbances.

In neuropsychological tests, a clear deficit can be shown in a range of memory tasks. The overall characteristics of memory loss in Alzheimer's disease have been reviewed elsewhere (Morris and Kopelman 1986). Impairments appear to be particularly severe on memory for recent events. The computational modeling presented here suggest that run-away synaptic modification could cause increased interference between stored representa-tions, causing impairments in short-term memory tasks requiring free recall (Corkin 1982; Morris 1986) and increasing the number of intrusions reported in other tasks (Fuld et al. 1986; Troster et al. 1989; Jacobs et al. 1990; Delis et al. 1991). Continued interference effects during learning could eventually lead to the spread of runaway synaptic modifica-tion into neocortex via the mechanisms of consolidation. This would lead to impairments of remote memory (Wilson et al. 1981; Corkin et al. 1984) and semantic memory (Huff et al. 1986; Ober et al. 1986). It is important to discriminate the neuropsychological effects at different stages of the disease. In the early stages of the disease, the interference effects predicted by the model should be evident. However, in later stages of the disease, the degeneration of cortical structures could have memory effects which are less directly related to interference during learning.

The model predicts that interference between stored memories should impair memory function in early stages of the syndrome. Thus, storage and retrieval of information will still be possible, but the encoding of information should be impaired, particularly for over-lapping memories. The effect of interference may not only result in erroneous answers due to intrusions from previously learned information. In some situations, interference could lead to the activation of many conflicting associations, so that the subject is unable to recall any particular association. In any case, this model predicts that in the early stages of Alzheimer's disease, interference effects should become more severe.

The notion of interference between memories is compatible with the presenting charac-teristics of Alzheimer's disease. The most common complaints refer to loss of memory for the location of simple household objects, loss of topographical memory, loss of orientation in time, and loss of recognition memory for acquaintances. All of these forms of memory require accurate memory for complex associations with a high degree of similarity. Development of higher order spurious associations between these items would severely interfere with day to day memory. A similar effect might underlie associations for days of the week or the various streets in a neighborhood. As summarized in previous work (Hasselmo, 1994), the model can account for the following neuropsychological data on Alzheimer's disease: 1. Increased intrusion errors. 2. Interference effects in short-term retention, 3. Sparing of implicit memory. 4. Homogeneous impairment of remote memory. 5. Impairments of semantic memory. However, this theory is far from complete. The predictions of the model must be tested experimentally using techniques ranging from brain slice physiology to behavioral memory tasks. In addition, more detailed biophysical simulations of the cortical structures affected by the disorder must be analyzed. However, computational modeling of the breakdown of function in cortical structures provides a unique means for linking evidence on this disorder across a range of different experimental techniques. Use of these types of modeling techniques will be vital to bringing together the disparate disciplines of neuroscience research in the understanding of Alzheimer's disease.

References

Albert, M., Smith, L.A., Scherr, P.A., Taylor, J.O., Evans, D.A. and Funkenstein, H.H. (1991) International Journal of Neuroscience 57: 167-178.

Amit, D.J., Evans, M.R. and Abeles, M. (1990) Network 1: 381-405.

Anderson, J.A. (1972) Mathematical Biosciences 14: 197-220.

Arnold, S.E., Hyman, B.T., Flory, J., Damasio, A.R., and Van Hoesen, G.W. (1991) T Cerebral Cortex 1: 103-116.

Arriagada, P.V., Marzloff, B.A. and Hyman, B.T. (1992) Neurology 42: 1681-1688.

Ball, M.J. (1972) Neuropathology and Applied Neurobiology 2: 395-410.

Barkai, E. and Hasselmo M.E. (1994) Journal of Neurophysiology 72: 644-658.

Barkai, E., Horwitz, G., Bergman, R.E. and Hasselmo, M.E. (1994) Journal of Neurophysiology. 72: 659-677.

Braak, J. and Braak, E. (1991) Acta Neuropathologica. 82: 239-259.

Breitner, J.C.S., Gatz, M., Bergem, A.L.M., Christian, J.C., Mortimer, J.A., McClearn, G.E., Heston, L.L., Welsh, K.A., Anthony, J.C., Folstein, M.F. and Radebaugh, T.S. (1993) Neurology 43: 261-267.

Brun, A., Gustafson, L. (1976) Archiv fur Psychiatrie und Nervenkrankheiten 223: 15-33, 1976.

Cole, A.E. and Nicoll, R.A. (1984) Journal of Physiology 352: 173-188.

Corkin, S. (1982) In: S. Corkin, K.L. Davis, J.H. Growdown, E. Usdin and R.J. Wurtman (eds.), Alzheimer's disease: A report of research in progress. New York: Raven Press.

Corkin, S., Growdown, J.H., Nissen, M.J., Huff, F.J., Freed, D.M. and Sagar, H.J. (1984) In: R.J. Wurtman, S. Corkin and J.H. Growdown (eds.) Alzheimer's disease: Advances in basic research and therapies. Center for Brain Sciences: Cambridge, MA.

Coyle J.T., Price, D.L. and DeLong, M.R. (1983) Science 219: 1184-1190.

Crapper McLachlan, D.R. and Van Berkum, M.F.A. (1986) In: D.F. Swaab, E. Fliers, M. Mirmiran, W.A. Van Gool and F. Van Haaren (eds) Progress in Brain Research 70: 399-409.

Davies, P. and Maloney, A.J.F. (1976) Lancet 2: 1403.

Delis, D.C., Massman, P.J., Butters, N., Salmon, D.P., Cermak, L.S. and Kramer, J.H. (1991) Psychological Assessment 3: 19-26.

Esiri, M.M. and Wilcock, G.K. (1984) Journal of Neurology Neurosurgery and Psychiatry 47: 56-60.

Esiri, M.M., Pearson, R.C.A., Powell, T.P.S. (1986) Brain Research 366: 385-387.

Fuld, P.A., Katzman, R., Davies, P. and Terry, R.D. (1982) Annals of Neurology 11: 155-159.

Geddes, J.W., Monaghan, D.T., Cotman, C.W., Loh, I.T., Kim, R.C., Chui, H.C. (1985) Science 230: 1179-1181.

Goudsmit, J. and Van der Waals, F.W. (1986) In: D.F. Swaab, E. Fliers, M. Mirmiran, W.A. Van Gool and F. Van Haaren (eds) Progress in Brain Research 70: 399-409.

Grossberg, S. (1970) Studies in Applied Mathematics 49: 135-166.

Grundkeiqbal, I., Iqbal, K., Tung, Y.C., Quinlan, M., Wisneiwski, H.M. and Binder, L.I. (1986) Proceedings of the National Academy of Sciences, U.S.A. 83: 4913-4917.

Hansen, L.A., DeTeresa, R., Davies, P. and Terry, R.D. (1988) Neurology 38: 48-54.

Hardy, J.A. and Higgins, G.A. (1992) Science 256: 184-185.

Hasselmo, M.E. (1993) Neural Computation. 5(1): 32-44.

Hasselmo, M.E. (1994) Neural Networks. 7(1): 13-40.

Hasselmo, M.E. (1995a) Behav. Brain Res. 67: 1-27.

Hasselmo, M.E. (1995b) In L. Niklasson, M.B. Boden (eds.) Current Trends in Connectionism. Lawrence Erlbaum Assoc.; Hillsdale, N.J. pp.15-32..

Hasselmo, M.E. and Barkai, E. (1995) J. Neurosci. 15(10); 6592-6604.

Hasselmo M.E., Anderson B.P. and Bower J.M. (1992) Journal of Neurophysiology 67: 1230-1246.

Hasselmo M.E. and Bower J.M. (1992) Journal of Neurophysiology 67: 1222-1229.

Hasselmo M.E. and Bower, J.M. (1993) Trends in Neurosciences 16: 218-222.

Hasselmo, M.E. and Schnell, E. (1994) J. Neurosci. 14(6): 3898-3914.

Hasselmo, M.E., Schnell, E., Barkai, E. (1995) J. Neurosci. 15(7): 5249-5262.

Hasselmo, M.E., Schnell, E., Berke, J. and Barkai, E. (1995) In G. Tesauro, D. Touretzky, T. Leen (eds.) Advances in Neural Information Processing Systems, Vol. 7. MIT Press: Cambridge, MA.

Hebb, D.O. (1949) The organization of behavior. New York.: Wiley.

Herrmann, M., Ruppin, E., Usher, M. (1993) Biol. Cybern. 68: 455-463.

Hirano, A. and Zimmerman, H.M. (1962) Archives of Neurology 7: 73-88.

Hopfield, J. J. (1982) Proceedings of the National Academy of Sciences USA 79: 2554-2559.

Horn, D., Ruppin, E., Usher, M. and Herrmann, M. (1993) Neural Comp. 5: 736-749.

Huerta, P.T., Lisman, J.E. (1994) Nature 364: 723-725.

Huff, F.J., Corkin, S., and Growdon, J.H. (1986) Brain and Language 34: 269-278.

Huff, F.J., Growdown, J.H., Corkin, S. and Rosen, T.J. (1987) Journal of the American Geriatrics Society 35: 27-30.

Hyman, B.T., Damasio, A.R., Van Hoesen, G.W., and Barnes, C.L. (1984) Science 225: 1168-1170.

Hyman, B.T., Van Hoesen, G.W., Kromer, L.J. and Damasio, A.R. (1986) Annals of Neurology 20:472-481.

Hyman, B.T., Kromer, L.J., and Van Hoesen, G.W. (1987) Annals of Neurology. 21: 250-267 1987.

Hyman, B.T., Van Hoesen, G.W., and Damasio, A.R. (1990) Neurology 40: 1721-1730.

Hyman, B.T., Arriagada, P.V. and Van Hoesen, G.W. (1991) Annals of the New York Academy of Sciences. 640: 14-19.

Jacobs, D., Salmon, D.P., Troster, A.I. and Butters, N. (1990) Archives of Clinical Neuropsychology 5: 49-57.

Jolles, J. (1986) In: D.F. Swaab, E. Fliers, M. Mirmiran, W.A. Van Gool and F. Van Haaren (eds) Progress in Brain Research 70: 399-409.

Kahle, J.S. and Cotman, C.W. (1989) Brain Research 482: 159-163.

Katzman, R., (1986) New England Journal of Medicine 314: 964-973.

Kauer, J.S. (1991) Trends in Neuroscience 14: 79-85.

Keane, M.M., Gabrieli, J.D.E., Fennema, A.C., Growdon, J.H. and Corkin, S. (1991) Behavioral Neuroscience 105: 326-342.

Keppel, G. and Underwood, B.J. (1962) Journal of Verbal Learning and Verbal Behavior 1:153-161.

Kopelman, M.D. (1985) Neuropsychologia 23: 623-638 1985.

Kopelman, M.D. (1986) Quarterly Journal of Experimental Psychology 38: 535-573.

Kosik, K.S. and Caceres, A. (1991) Journal of Cell Science S15: 69-74.

Koss, E., Weiffenbach, J.M., Haxby, J.V. and Friedland, R.P. (1988) Neurology 38: 1228-1232.

Leblanc, A.C., Kovacs, D.M., Chen, H.Y., Villare, F., Tykocinski, M., Autiliogambetti, L. and Gambetti, P. (1992) Journal of Neuroscience Research 31: 635-645.

Levy, W.B. and Steward, O. (1979) Brain Research 175: 233-245.

Levy, W.B. and Colbert, C.M. (1992) Soc. Neurosci. Abstr. 18: 628.14.

Liljenstrom H. and Hasselmo M.E. (1995) J. Neurophysiol. 74: 288-297.

Linsker, R. (1988) Computer 21: 105-117.

Lund, J.S. (1988) Annual Review of Neuroscience 11: 253-288.

Marotta, C.A., Majocha, R.E. and Tate, B. (1992) Journal of Molecular Neuroscience 3: 111-125.

Marr, D. (1971) Philosophical Transactions of the Royal Society B 262: 23-81.

McClelland, J.L. and Rumelhart, D.E. (1988) Explorations in Parallel Distributed Processing. Cambridge, MA: MIT Press.

McClelland, J.L., McNaughton, B.L. and O'Reilly, R. (1995) Psych. Rev. 102: 419-457.

McNaughton, B.L. and Morris, R.G.M. (1987) Trends in Neurosciences 10: 408-415.

Miller, K.D., Keller, J.B. and Stryker, M.P. (1989) Science 245: 605-615.

Milward, E.A., Papadopolous, R., Fuller, S.J., Moir, R.D. and Small, D. (1992) Neuron 9: 129-137.

Morris, R.G. (1986) Cognitive Neuropsychology 3: 77-97.

Morris, R.G. and Kopelman, M.D. (1986) Quarterly Journal of Experimental Psychology 38A: 575-602.

Pearson, R.C.A., Esiri, M.M., Hiorns, R.W., Wilcock, G.K. and Powell, T.P.S. (1985) Proceedings of the National Academy of Sciences USA 82: 4531-4534.

Perry, E.K., Gibson, P.H., Blessed, G., Perry R.H. and Tomlinson, B.E. (1977) Journal of Neurological Science 34: 247-265.

Postman, L. and Underwood, B.J. (1973) Memory and Cognition 1:19-40.

Rapp, PR. and Amaral, D.G. (1992) Trends in Neurosciences. 15: 340-345.

Reyes, P.F., Golden, G.T., Fagel, P.L., Fariello, R.G., Katz, L. and Carner, E. (1987) Archives of Neurology 44: 644-645.

Saitoh, T., Sundsmo, M., Roch, J.M., Kimura, N., Cole, G. (1989) Cell 58: 615-622.

Saper, C.B., German, D.C., and White, C.L. (1985) Neurology 35: 1089-1095.

Schellenberg, G.D., Bird, T.D., Wijsman, E.M., Orr, H.T., Anderson, L., Nemens, E., White, J.A., Bonnycastle, L., Weber, J.L., Alonso, M.E., Potter, H., Heston, L.L., Martin, G.M. (1992) Science 258: 668-671.

Scoville, W.B. and Milner, B. (1957) Journal of Neurology, Neurosurgery and Psychiatry 20: 11-21.

Selkoe, D.J. (1993) Trends in Neurosciences 16: 403-409.

Seltzer, B. and Sherwin, I. (1983) Archives of Neurology 40: 143-146.

Squire, L.R. and Zola-Morgan, S. (1991) Science 253: 1380-1386.

Talamo, B.R., Rudel, R., Kosik, K.S., Lee, V.M.Y., Neff, S., Adelman, L. and Kauer, J.S. (1989) Nature 337: 736-739.

Troster, A.I., Jacobs, D., Butters, N., Cullum, C.M., Salmon, D.P. (1989) Clinics in Geriatric Medicine 5: 611-632.

Wagner, S.L., Siegel, R.S., Vedvick, T.S., Raschke, W.C., Vannostrand, W.E. (1992) Biochemical and Biophysical Research Communications 186: 1138-1145.

Whitehouse, P.J., Price, D.L., Struble, R.G., Clark, A.W., Coyle J.T. and DeLong, M.R. (1982) Science 215: 1237-1239.

Wigstrom, H., Gustafsson, B., Huang, Y.-Y. and Abraham, W.C. (1986) Acta Physiologica Scandinavica 126: 317-319.

Wilson, R.S., Kaszniak, A.W. and Fox, J.H. (1981) Cortex 17: 41-48.

Wilson, M.A. and McNaughton, B.L. (1994) Science 265: 676-679.

COMPUTATIONAL STUDIES OF SYNAPTIC ALTERATIONS IN ALZHEIMER'S DISEASE

EYTAN RUPPIN

Departments of Computer Science & Physiology
Tel-Aviv University, Tel Aviv 69978, Israel
ruppin@math.tau.ac.il

and

DAVID HORN and NIR LEVY

School of Physics and Astronomy
Raymond and Beverly Sackler Faculty of Exact Sciences
Tel-Aviv University, Tel Aviv 69978, Israel
horn@vm.tau.ac.il   nirlevy@post.tau.ac.il

and

JAMES A. REGGIA

Departments of Computer Science & Neurology
A.V. Williams Bldg.
University of Maryland
College Park, MD 20742
reggia@cs.umd.edu

ABSTRACT

In the framework of an associative memory model, we study the interplay between synaptic deletion and compensation, and memory deterioration, a clinical hallmark of Alzheimer's disease. We show that deterioration of memory retrieval due to synaptic deletion can be much delayed by multiplying all the remaining synaptic weights by a common factor such that each neuron maintains the profile of its incoming post-synaptic current. This compensatory process can be realized either by global or local mechanisms. Our results show that neural models can account for a large variety of experimental phenomena characterizing memory degradation in Alzheimer patients. They open up the possibility that the primary factor in the pathogenesis of cognitive deficiencies in Alzheimer's disease is the failure of local neuronal regulatory mechanisms.

1. Introduction

Alzheimer's disease (AD) is the major degenerative disease of the brain, responsible for a progressive deterioration of the patient's cognitive and motor function, with a grave prognosis (Adams & Victor 1989). Its clinical course is usually characterized by gradual decay, although both slow and rapidly progressive forms have been reported, exhibiting a large variation in the rate of

AD progression (Drachman et. al. 1990). While remarkable progress has been gained in the investigation of neurochemical processes accompanying AD, their role in neural degeneration, the main pathological feature of AD, is yet unclear (Selkoe 1987, Kosik 1991). The work summarized in this chapter has been motivated by recent investigations studying in detail the neurodegenrative changes accompanying AD, on a neuroanatomical level. Following the paradigm that cognitive processes can be accounted for on the neural level, we examine the effect of these neurodegenerative changes within the context of neural network models. This allows us to obtain a schematic understanding of the clinical course of AD.

Recent investigations have shown that in addition to the traditionally described plaques and tangles found in the AD brain, this disease is characterized by considerable synaptic pathology. There is significant synaptic loss in various cortical regions, termed *synaptic deletion*, accompanied by *synaptic compensation*, an increase of the synaptic size reflecting a functional compensatory increase of synaptic efficacy (Bertoni-Freddari et. al. 1990, DeKosky & Scheff 1990, Scheff et. al. 1993). The combined outcome of these counteracting synaptic degenerative and compensatory processes can be evaluated by measuring the total synaptic area per unit volume (TSA), which is initially preserved but decreases as the disease progresses. The TSA has been shown to strongly correlate with the cognitive function of AD patients (DeKosky & Scheff 1990, Terry et. al. 1991, Masliah et. al. 1994, Masliah & Terry 1994), pointing to the important role that pathological synaptic changes play in the cognitive deterioration of AD patients. In this chapter, we describe and summarize our studies of the functional effects of these synaptic changes (Horn et. al. 1993, Ruppin & Reggia 1995, Horn & Ruppin 1995).

Since memory deterioration is a clinical hallmark of AD, it is natural to investigate the effects of synaptic deletion and compensation on the performance of an associative memory neural model. In particular, we have studied ways of modifying the remaining synapses of an associative memory network undergoing synaptic deletion, such that its performance will be maintained as much as possible. To this end, we used a biologically-motivated variant of a Hopfield-like attractor neural network (Tsodyks & Feigel'man 1988): M memory patterns are stored in an N-neuron network via a Hebbian synaptic matrix, forming fixed points of the network dynamics. The synaptic efficacy J_{ij} between the jth (presynaptic) neuron and the ith (postsynaptic) neuron in this network is

$$J_{ij} = \frac{1}{N} \sum_{\mu=1}^{N} (\eta^{\mu}_{i} - p)(\eta^{\mu}_{j} - p) , \tag{1}$$

where $\eta^\mu{}_i$ are $(0,1)$ binary variables representing the stored memories and p is the activity level of each memory. The updating rule for the state V_i of the ith neuron is given by

$$V_i(t+1) = \Theta\left(h_i\right) , \tag{2}$$

where

$$h_i = \sum_{j \neq i}^{N} J_{ij} V_j(t) - T , \tag{3}$$

Θ is the step function and T, the threshold, is set to its optimal value $T = \frac{1}{2}p(1-p)(1-2p)$. In the intact network, when memory retrieval is modeled by presenting an input cue which is sufficiently similar to one of the memory patterns, the network flows to a stable state identical with that memory. Performance of the network is defined by the average recall of all memories. The latter is measured by the *overlap m^μ*, which denotes the similarity between the final state V the network converges to and the memory pattern η^μ that is cued in each trial (see Horn et. al. 1993). The appeal of attractors, as corresponding to our intuitive notion of the persistence of cognitive concepts along some temporal span, has been fortified by numerous studies testifying to the applicability of attractor neural networks as models of the human memory (for a review see Amit 1989), and also supported by biological findings of delayed, post-stimulus, sustained activity (Fuster & Jervey 1982, Miyashita & Chang 1988).

Synaptic deletion has been carried out by randomly removing a fraction d of all synaptic weights, such that a fraction $w = 1 - d$ of the synapses remains. We have investigated two principle ways of *synaptic compensation*. In the *global compensation* approach (Horn et. al. 1993), synaptic compensation was modeled by multiplying all remaining synaptic weights by a common factor c. Varying c as a function of d specifies a compensation strategy. In the *local compensation* approach (Horn et. al. 1996), a fraction $d_i = 1 - w_i$ of the input synapses to each neuron i are deleted. This is compensated for by a factor c_i which each neuron adjusts individually, based on the sole knowledge of its local field h_i. Correlating synaptic size with synaptic strength, we interpret the TSA as proportional to $c \cdot w$ in in the global-compensation model, and to $1/N \sum_{i=1}^{N} c_i \cdot w_i$ in the local-compensation model.

We turn to describe the study of global compensation strategies in the next Section. In Section 3 we extend this investigation to include memory storage as well as retrieval. In Section 4 we study local compensation algorithms. Our results are summarized in the last Section.

2. Global synaptic compensation

2.1 Compensation strategies

To obtain an intuitive notion of the network's behavior when global synaptic deletion and compensation are incorporated consider Figure 1. The neurons that stand for firing neurons in the stored memory, and the neurons that stand for quiescent neurons in the stored memory, have distinct post-synaptic potential distributions (the full curves in figure 1). When synaptic deletion takes place, by removing a fraction d of the synapses, the mean values of the neurons' post-synaptic potential change, and the threshold is no longer optimal (see dashed curves in figure 1). Multiplying the weights of the remaining synaptic connections by an *optimal performance compensation factor* (OPC) $c = \frac{1}{1-d}$, restores the original mean values of post-synaptic potential, and the optimality of the threshold (dot-dashed curves in figure 1). The accompanying increase in the variance of the post-synaptic potential, which is $\sqrt{\frac{1}{1-d}}$ times larger than the original one, leads however to performance deterioration. This is formally shown in (Horn et. al. 1993).

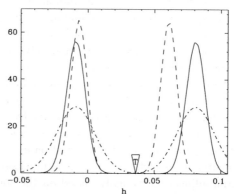

Figure 1: The distribution of the postsynaptic potential ($p = 0.1, \alpha = 0.05$). A. (full line) Initial state: two Gaussian distributions peaked at $-p^2(1-p)$ and $p(1-p)^2$. The *optimal threshold* $T = p(1-p)(\frac{1}{2}-p)$ lies in the middle between the two Gaussian mean values. B. (dashed curve) After deletion ($d = 0.25$), the new peaks of the postsynaptic potential are no longer equidistant from the threshold T. C. (dot-dashed curve) The OPC strategy restores the initial mean values of the postsynaptic potential.

As shown in (Horn et. al. 1993), we can interpolate between the case of deletion without compensation and the OPC within a a class of compensatory strategies, defined by

$$\hat{J}_{ij} = cJ_{ij} \, , \qquad c = 1 + (\frac{1}{1-d} - 1)k = 1 + \frac{dk}{1-d} \, , \qquad (4)$$

with the parameter $0 \le k \le 1$. All the *fixed* k strategies, examined via simulations measuring the performance of the network at various deletion and compensation levels, display a similar sharp transition from the memory-retrieval phase to a non-retrieval phase, as shown in figure 2. Varying the compensation magnitude k merely shifts the location of the transition region. This sharp transition is similar to that reported previously in cases of deletion without compensation in other models (Canning & Gardner 1988, Koscielny-Bunde 1990).

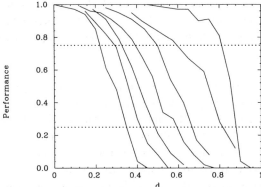

Figure 2: Performance of a network with fixed k compensation. Starting from an initial state that is a corrupted version $(m^1(0) = 0.8)$ of a stored memory pattern, we define performance as the percentage of cases in which the network converged to the correct memory. The simulation parameters are $N = 800$ neurons, $\alpha = 0.05$ and $p = 0.1$. The curves represent (from left to right) the performance of fixed strategies with increasing k values, for $k = 0, 0.25, 0.375, 0.5, 0.625, 0.75, 1$. The horizontal dotted lines represent performance levels of 25% and 75%.

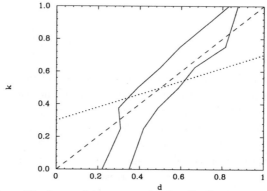

Figure 3: The critical transition range in the (k, d) plane. The full curves represent performance levels of 75% and 25%, derived from figure 2. The straight lines describe the variations employed in two variable compensations presented in figure 4.

Figure 3 describes the transition region as a map in the (k, d) plane. The performance levels read off figure 2 delineate the domain over which deterioration occurs. Staying close to the upper boundary of this domain, defines a compensation strategy which enables the system to maintain its performance, with a much smaller amount of synaptic strengthening than that required by the OPC strategy. In face of restricted compensatory resources, such an *optimal resource compensation* strategy (ORC) could be of vital importance. The essence of such ORC strategy is that k is varied as synaptic deletion progresses, in order to retain maximal performance with minimal resource allocation. In figure 4, we present the performance of two *variable k* compensation strategies, which we propose to view as expressions of (albeit unsuccessful) attempts of maintaining an ORC. These examples, indicated on figure 3, include a 'gradually decreasing' strategy defined by the variation $k = 0.3 + 0.4d$, and the 'plateau' strategy defined by the variation $k = d$.

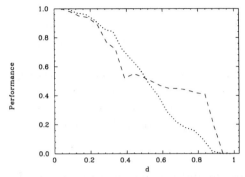

Figure 4: Performance of a network with gradually decreasing (dotted curve) and plateau (dashed curve) compensation strategies.

2.2 Clinical parallels

The analogs of these strategies can be found in clinical observations. As mentioned in the introduction, while synaptic degeneration occurs, the TSA stays constant in some cortical layers at the initial stages of AD. A plausible general scenario seems to involve some initial period of OPC. As AD progresses, synaptic compensation no longer succeeds in maintaining the TSA (Bertoni-Freddari 1990, DeKosky & Scheff 1990). In advanced AD cases, severe compensatory dysfunction has been observed (Buell & Coleman 1979, Flood & Coleman 1986, DeKosky & Scheff 1990).

In accordance with our ideas, young AD patients are likely to have high compensation capacities, and therefore can maintain an OPC strategy ($k = 1$, in figure 2) throughout the course of their disease. This will eventually lead to rapid deterioration when the reserve of synaptic connections is depleted. Indeed, young AD patients have a rapid clinical progression (Heston et. al. 1981, Heyman et. al. 1983), accompanied by severe neuronal and synaptic loss (Hansen 1988). A similar clinical pattern of rapid memory decline, already manifested with less severe neuroanatomical pathology, was found in very old patients (Huff et. al. 1987). We propose that in these old patients, the rapid clinical decline results from the lack of compensatory capacities ($k = 0$, in figure 2), possibly of the kind observed by Buell and Coleman (1979) and Flood and Coleman (1986).

Rapid cognitive decline characterizes a minority of AD patients. Most patients show a continuous gradual pattern of cognitive decline (Katzman 1986, Katzman et. al. 1988, Adams & Victor 1989), taking place along *a broad span* of synaptic deletion (DeKosky & Scheff 1990). As shown in figure 2, this performance decline cannot be accounted for by any network employing fixed k compensation. Variable compensation, such as that defined by the gradually decreasing strategy, is needed to explain the memory decline observed in the majority of AD patients, as shown in figure 4. The clinical state of some AD patients remains stable at mild to moderate levels for several years before finally rapidly decreasing (Cummings & Benson 1983, Katzman 1985, Botwinick et. al. 1986). This can be accounted for by a 'plateau' strategy whose performance, shown in figure 4, stays at an approximately constant level over a large domain of deletion.

3. Memory storage and retrograde amnesia in AD

3.1 Modeling memory storage

The model described in the previous Section has been extended in (Ruppin & Reggia 1995) to address a broader scope of memory alterations in AD, concerning deficient memory storage and the temporal pattern of amnesia typically observed in the disorder. The basic model is similar to the one described in the previous Section. However, the synaptic memory matrix is not prescribed, but memory storage (i.e., learning) is now explicitly modeled via activity-dependent Hebbian mechanisms. Each neurons receive two kinds of connections: 1. *external connections*, via which external input patterns are presented to the network, and 2. *internal connections*, which store the memorized patterns and whose synaptic strengths may change as a function of the neural activity in the network. The input (post-synaptic potential) h_i of neuron i is the sum of internal contributions from other neurons in the network and external contributions F_i^e,

$$h_i(t) = \sum_j J_{ij} V_j(t-1) + F_i^e \tag{5}$$

The network has two behavioral modes:

1. In its *learning* (storage) mode, the memory patterns are stored in the network by sequentially presenting them as inputs to the network one after the other. An input pattern (say η^1) is memorized by orienting the external inputs F^e with it, such that

$$F_i^e = e_l \cdot \eta^1_i \ , \ \ (e_l > 0) \ , \tag{6}$$

where e_l is a scalar denoting the strength of the external inputs during learning. Following the dynamics defined in (5) and (2), the network state evolves until it converges to a stable state. Concomittantly, as the network iterates, the synaptic weights are modified in an activity-dependent, Hebbian-like manner, according to the rule

$$J_{ij}(t) = J_{ij}(t-1) + \frac{\gamma}{N}(\bar{V}_i - p)(\bar{V}_j - p) \ , \tag{7}$$

where $\bar{V}_k$ is 1 (0) only if neuron k has been firing (quiescent) for the last consecutive 5 iterations and γ is a constant determining the magnitude of activity-dependent changes. Subsequent presentation of the same pattern results in stable states with increasing overlap with the learned input pattern. Eventually, the patterns are engraved into the network's synaptic matrix.

2. *Memory retrieval* is modeled in a similar fashion to the way a pattern is engraved into the network, i.e., by making the input pattern be a scaled version of one of the memorized patterns (the *cued* pattern, say η^1), such that

$$F_i^e = e_r \cdot \eta^1{}_i \ , \ (e_r > 0) \ , \tag{8}$$

but e_r is typically smaller than e_l.

3.2 Temporal memory gradient and relearning

In this model, we set to account for experimental psychological data demonstrating a temporal gradient with relative sparing of remotely-stored memories (Beatty et. al. 1988, Sagar et. al. 1989, Kopelman 1989). Twenty-five memory patterns were arbitrarily divided into five sets, each having five memories. Then, five consecutive steps of synaptic degeneration and memory storage were performed; in each such step an additional fraction of incoming synapses were deleted, and a set of five additional memories were stored in the network in an activity-dependent manner. This storage process simulates memory storage over a period of time, in the presence of continued diffuse loss of synaptic connections. After this process was completed, we studied the retrieval of memories from each of the stored sets, and examined the temporal gradient achieved. The results of this experiment are presented in Figure 5. The memory set numbers are displayed on the x-axis, such that set No. 1 denotes the most remotely stored memories and set No. 5 the most recently stored set. As shown, with no synaptic compensation the (low) performance has no temporal gradient. With synaptic compensation, the experimentally observed temporal gradient is obtained for a wide range of synaptic damage. These results are demonstrated both for the case where the external input is the cued pattern applied via a weak external field (A), and for the case where the external input is a subset of the cued pattern (B).

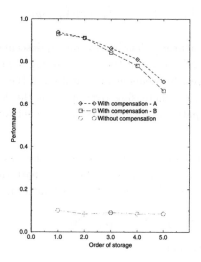

Figure 5: Retrieval performance of memories stored at different levels of synaptic degeneration. $N = 400$, $p = 0.1$, $e_l = 0.075$, $e_r = 0.035$ and $\gamma = 0.02$.

The increasing imprecision of memory storage in damaged networks raises the possibility that even re-learning of memory patterns that have been already stored in the network may cause memory degradation at advanced levels of damage. To examine this, we investigated memory retrieval performance at progressing levels of synaptic deletion and compensation, comparing the performance without re-learning with that achieved with re-learning. Re-learning was performed by presenting the remote memory patterns (i.e., the *same* memory patterns stored in the intact, pre-lesion network) again to the damaged network. The results, shown in Figure 6, demonstrate that while at low levels of damage re-learning improves performance, at high levels of damage it actually worsens it.

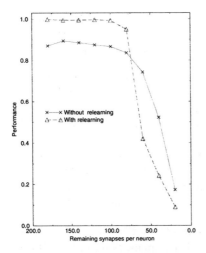

Figure 6: The effect of re-learning on memory performance. Simulation parameters are as in Figure 5.

Simple signal-to-noise considerations show that the relative sparing of remote memories is a general characteristic of our model. This is true if patterns are stored via a repetitive-learning rule like that employed in this work (which makes memory storage more liable to damage than memory retrieval), and only as long as synaptic compensation takes place along with synaptic deletion. Hence, the model provides a solid account of the temporal gradient observed clinically, extending back to the time of onset of the degenerative processes.

The model predicts that Alzheimer's patients with the same level of neurodegenerative changes, but differing in the level of synaptic compensation, will exhibit two distinct manifestations of memory disturbances: Those patients with little compensatory synaptic changes should suffer from a considerable, general decrease in memory retrieval, but should have relatively maintained learning capacities and hence, preserved recent memory (an 'inverse' temporal gradient). Those patients with considerable synaptic compensatory changes should have relatively maintained remote memory, but decreased learning capacities leading to a deteriorated recent memory (and the temporal gradient observed typically).

4. Local, neural-based, synaptic compensation

In the global compensation framework described in Section 2, we have seen that maintaining the premorbid levels of TSA (that is, employing $c = 1/w$) efficiently preserves the performance as synapses are deleted. However, uniform, global compensation strategies suffer from two fundamental drawbacks:

1. They can only work when neurons in the network undergo a similar, uniform, process of synaptic deletion. Otherwise, it is advantageous for the different neurons, which undergo different levels of synaptic deletion, to develop their own suitable compensation factors.

2. While global compensation mechanisms may be carried out in biological networks via the actions of neuromodulators, their biological realization remains problematic, since it requires the *explicit* knowledge of the ongoing level of synaptic deletion in the whole network.

In this Section, based on (Horn et. al. 1996), we present a solution to these problems by showing that synaptic compensation can be performed successfully by *local* mechanisms: a fraction d_i of the input synapses to each neuron i are deleted, and are compensated for by a factor c_i which each neuron adjusts individually. This is equivalent to performing the replacement $J_{ij} \rightarrow c_i w_{ij} J_{ij}$ where w_{ij} is either 0 or 1, and $w_i = 1 - d_i = \sum_j w_{ij}/N$. Our method is based on the neuron's post-synaptic potential h_i, and does not require the explicit knowledge of either global or local levels of synaptic deletion. The local compensatory factor c_i develops dynamically so as to keep the membrane potential and neural activity at their original, premorbid levels. The proposed *neuronal* activity-dependent compensation modifies all the synapses of the neuron concomittantly, in a similar manner, and thus differs fundamentally from conventional Hebbian *synaptic* activity-dependent modification paradigms like long-term potentiation and long-term depression which modify each synapse individually. Our proposal is that while synaptic activity-dependent modification plays a central role in memory storage and learning, neuronal-level synaptic modifications serve to maintain the functional integrity of memory retrieval in the network.

Several biological mechanisms may take part in neural-level synaptic modifications that self-regulate neuronal activity (see van-Ooyen 1994 for an extensive review). These include receptor up-regulation and down-regulation (Turrigiano et. al. 1994), activity-dependent regulation of membranal ion channels (Armstrong & Montminy 1993), and activity-dependent structural changes that reversibly enhance or suppress neuritic outgrowth (Mattson & Kater 1989, Schilling et. al. 1991, Grumbacher-Reinert & Nicholls 1992). Interestingly, while neurotransmitters application may act in isolation on individual dendrites, membrane depolarization simultaneously regulates the size of all growth cones and neurites of a given neuron (Stuart & Sakmann 1994). Taken together, these findings testify that there exist feedback mechanisms that act on the neuronal level, possibly via the expression of immediate early genes (Morgan & Curran 1991) to ensure the homeostasis of neuronal activity. These mechanisms act on a slow time scale and are active also in the normal adult brain.

In the next subsection, we present local compensation algorithms in two classes of associative memory models. First, in the framework of the Tsodyks-Feigelman (TF) model where we have previously studied global strategies, and then in the framework of the Willshaw model (Willshaw et. al. 1969). These models are representatives of two fundamentally different classes of associative networks, differing in the characteristics of the neurons' mean post-synaptic potential and the level of competitiveness in the network. Computer simulations, and their possible clinical implications, are presented further on.

4.1 Locally-driven synaptic compensation

4.1.1 The Tsodyks Feigel'man model

Our local compensation method aims at maintaining the premorbid profile of the postsynaptic potential. In Section 2 it was shown that this profile can be maintained through *TSA conservation*, i.e., by using the compensation $c = 1/w$. Guided by this finding, we now set to implement its local compensation version, $c_i = 1/w_i$. For this purpose we employ the differential equation

$$\frac{dc_i}{dt} = \kappa c_i \left(1 - \hat{w}_i c_i\right) , \tag{9}$$

where κ is a rate parameter and $\hat{w}_i$ is a *field-dependent* estimate of the local connectivity w_i. This equation is then transformed to a difference equation which is used in the simulations

$$c_i(t + \Delta t) = c_i(t) + \tau c_i(t) \left(1 - \hat{w}_i c_i(t)\right) , \tag{10}$$

where $\tau = \kappa \Delta t$.

We are looking for an estimate $\hat{w}_i$ that depends only on information which is available to the single neuron. We propose using moments of the neuronal input field (post-synaptic potential) h_i, after averaging over a set of retrieval trials, and comparing them with their values in the normal, premorbid state. From a biological perspective, such knowledge and computational algorithms may be pre-wired in the neuronal regulatory mechanisms reviewed in the previous Section, which are responsible for homeostasis of neural activity.

There are two possible measurements of the field h_i, either under conditions of random noise input or through a set of trials of memory retrieval from the existing repertoire of memories [1]. In the Tsodyks-Feigelman model, the first moment of the field vanishes, $\langle h_i \rangle = 0$, both for random inputs and memories. So we turn to the second moment, which can be calculated for random noise initial conditions in the premorbid state

$$\left\langle h_i{}^2(w_i) \right\rangle = c_i{}^2 \hat{w}_i \left\langle h_i{}^2(w_i = 1) \right\rangle \equiv c_i{}^2 \hat{w}_i \left\langle R_i{}^2 \right\rangle. \tag{11}$$

When using a set of memories instead of random noise we obtain a different expression which separates into signal and noise terms with different power dependence on deletion

$$\left\langle h_i{}^2(w_i) \right\rangle = c_i{}^2 \hat{w}_i^2 \left\langle S_i{}^2 \right\rangle + c_i{}^2 \hat{w}_i \left\langle R_i{}^2 \right\rangle. \tag{12}$$

Here $\langle S_i{}^2 \rangle$ is the signal term in the premorbid state ($w = 1$) and $\langle R_i{}^2 \rangle$ is the same noise term as in (11). Given these two equations one can solve for $\hat{w}_i$ either by using noise alone, or by using trials of memory retrieval and relying on the separate knowledge of the premorbid magnitude of the signal and noise terms.

To perform local synaptic compensation in our simulations, we proceed in small steps of deletion Δd. At each deletion step the network is presented with all (slightly corrupted) memories and allowed to converge to its fixed points. By averaging the field strengths measured over all memory retrieval trials, we calculate $\hat{w}_i$ via equation (12). Thereafter, synaptic compensation via algorithm (10) is applied. The resulting performance is evaluated by presenting all memory cues again. As demonstrated in Figure 7, dynamic local compensation via algorithm (12) works as well or even better than the local TSA-conserving compensation $c_i = 1/w_i$.

---

[1] One may speculate that the biological realization of such field measurements occurs during dreaming.

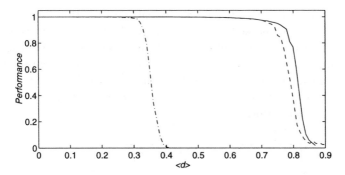

Figure 7: Performance versus deletion for a network that runs the local TF-compensation algorithm via (4) and (6). The result, presented by a solid line, is compared with the performance of local TSA conserving method ($c_i = 1/w_i$, dashed curve) and no compensation ($c_i = 1$, dot-dashed curve). The simulation parameters were $N = 1000, M = 100, p = 0.1, \tau = 0.25, \Delta d = 0.01$.

4.1.2 The Willshaw model

A simpler, and perhaps more biologically plausible mechanism of local synaptic compensation arises in the Willshaw model (Willshaw et. al. 1969), where memory patterns are stored in excitatory synapses through the rule

$$J_{ij} = \frac{1}{Np} \Theta \left(\sum_{\mu=1}^{M} \eta^{\mu}_{i} \eta^{\mu}_{j} \right) . \tag{13}$$

The updating rule is similar to equation (2) and each neuron has a uniform threshold T smaller than 1. In the Willshaw model, unlike the TF model, spurious states with high activity emerge as deletion proceeds. These deviations of the Willshaw network activity level from its premorbid values rule out the possibility to accurately estimate the connectivity $\hat{w}$ in a manner analogous to the way equations (5) and (6) were used in the TF model. However, in the Willshaw model $\langle h_i \rangle \neq 0$ so instead of estimating the connectivity from moments of the field and using it for the compensation algorithm as in equation (9), we can now use the changes in the field itself to correct for the effects of synaptic deletion directly,

$$\frac{dc_i}{dt} = \kappa c_i \left(1 - \frac{\langle h_i(t) \rangle}{\langle h_i(t = 0) \rangle} \right) . \tag{14}$$

When the dynamics remain similar to those of the intact network, this method is close the TSA-conserving strategy ($c_i = 1/w_i$). However, as demonstrated

78

in Figure 8, the new, direct, field-dependent method (the discretized version of equation (14)) is markedly superior to the TSA-conserving strategy ($c_i = 1/w_i$) as changes in the level of activity of the network occur; the high-activity spurious stable states which emerge as deletion proceeds are suppressed by using compensation values that are lesser than those dictated by a TSA-conserving algorithm (which is of course insensitive to the level of activity in the network), resulting in better performance.

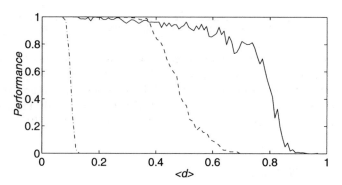

Figure 8: Performance versus deletion for a network that runs the local Willshaw-compensation algorithm (8). The result, presented by a solid line, is compared with the performance of local TSA conservation ($c_i = 1/w_i$, dashed curve) and no compensation ($c_i = 1$, dot-dashed curve) methods. The simulation parameters were $N = 1500, M = 75, p = 0.05, \tau = 0.1, \Delta d = 0.009$.

This simple and efficient algorithm is used in the next subsection to study the effect of synaptic deletion and compensation rates on network performance, and its relevance to AD progression.

4.2 Results and clinical relevance

4.2.1 Compensation rates and AD progression

In this Section we discuss results of simulations of a Willshaw network of $N = 1500$ neurons in which $M = 75$ randomly-generated memory patterns with activity $p = 0.05$ are stored with $T = 0.8$. In every simulation run, a sequence of synaptic deletion and compensation steps is executed, and the performance of the network is traced as deletion progresses. In each simulation step (considered as one time unit) a fraction Δd of the remaining synapses is deleted. Synaptic compensation is performed via the discretized version of algorithm (14) by averaging the local field following the presentation of the stored memories.

We first study the network's performance at various compensation rates τ, as presented in Figure 9a. The performance level is better maintained if the compensation rate is high. As described in Section 2, young and very old AD patients suffer from rapid clinical deterioration characterized by a sharp decline, while the majority of AD patients have a more gradual pattern of decline. These clinical patterns may arise because very old patients have almost no compensation resources (that is, corresponding to low compensation rates illustrated in the leftmost curve in Figure 9a), and young patients still have potent synaptic compensation mechanisms (the rightmost curve). Interestingly, studies of reactive synaptogenesis following experimental hippocampal deafferentation lesions in rodents show indeed that the *rate* of compensatory synaptogenesis decreases as a function of age (Cotman & Anderson 1988, Cotman & Anderson 1989). The dependence of performance on compensation rate τ for a given deletion level d is demonstrated in Figure 9b; while the performance levels obtained in early stages ($d = 0.4$) are almost similar for a broad range of τ values, a more pronounced τ dependence is observed as deletion proceeds ($d = 0.8$).

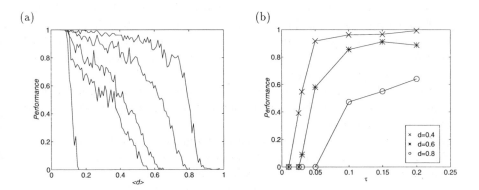

Figure 9: (a) Performance versus deletion for different compensation rates. τ is increased from left to right, with values $0.01, 0.025, 0.03, 0.05, 0.1$. $\Delta d = 0.009$. (b) Performance versus τ for fixed d values.

To examine how the rate of synaptic deletion affects performance, we kept the compensation rate τ constant and varied Δd. The results are basically similar to the results displayed in Figure 9a; the performance decreases as the rate of deletion increases. Hence, when there is a significant 'mismatch' between synaptic deletion and compensation, whether its origin is increased synaptic deletion or decreased compensation rates, the network's performance degrades. In the intermediate range, the network's performance degrades in a fairly gradual manner. Thus, when local compensation is employed, a single compensation mechanism can give rise to a variety of clinically observed patterns of degradation, in contradistinction to the need to assume the existence of several different compensation strategies in the global compensation case.

4.2.2 Two routes to dementia

The pathological synaptic changes in Alzheimer's disease are accompanied by the eventual loss of about $10 - 20\%$ of cortical neurons (Katzman 1986, Masliah 1995). Motivated by developmental studies showing death of hypoactive neurons (see van-Ooyen 1994 for a review), and the assumed degeneration of hypoactive neurons in AD (Bowen et. al. 1994), we incorporated a neuronal degeneration rule that kills neurons as their input field decreases below a *viability-threshold (VT)* value. In addition we set upper bounds on the neuronal compensation factors. Both viability thresholds and compensation bounds may vary within certain limits over the neural population. Figures 10a and 10b illustrate the differential effect of high versus low neuronal viability thresholds: Obviously, different viability thresholds lead to distinct resiliency of the network to damage. But more interesting, they also give rise to different relations between the level of neuronal death and network performance. In general, there are two principal pathological pathways in which performance collapses in the network as deletion proceeds:

1. *Synaptic loss*, i.e. a strong decrease in the synapse/neuron ratio. This requires low viability thresholds, and may lead to large cognitive deficits with little structural damage.

2. *Neuronal loss*, which is expected to occur for higher values of viability thresholds. This will generally cause a faster avalanche of the disease, once it starts to take place, and significant neural death. A qualitatively similar effect may be seen with low versus high compensation rates. Since the primary factor responsible for cortical atrophy in AD is likely to be neural degeneration (synapses occupy a very small fraction of the cortical volume (Bourgeois & Rakic 1993)), the finding that the extent of neural damage depends on the pathological pathway may shed some light on the broad range of cortical atrophy levels observed in AD patients, suffering from similar levels of cognitive deterioration (Wippold et. al. 1991, Murphy et. al. 1993). Severe cognitive deterioration may occur via either route, but the neural route leads to considerably more cortical atrophy

than the synaptic route, while causing similar levels of cognitive deterioration. We hypothesize that the profile of pathological routes taken in a specific AD patient depends on the distribution of his neuronal viability thresholds.

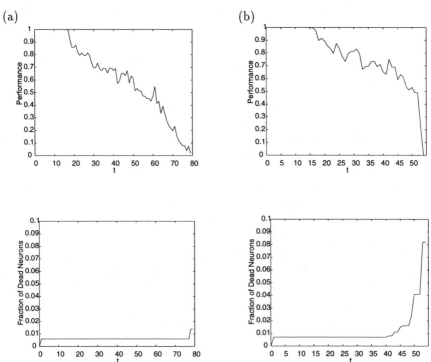

Figure 10: Performance versus time with (a) a low viability threshold ($VT = 0.2$) and (b) a high viability threshold ($VT = 0.5$). $\tau = 0.02$ and the rest of the simulation parameters are as in Figure 7. The bottom figures trace the fraction of dead neurons as a function of time. Neuronal damage is traced until complete performance collapse (the patient's 'death'), i.e., zero overlap.

5. Summary

During the last several years there has been a considerable increase of interest in using neural models to explore potential pathophysiological theories of psychiatric and neuropsychological disorders (see Reggia et. al. 1994 and Ruppin 1995 for recent reviews). In this chapter we have examined how attractor neural network models can qualitatively account for some basic features of memory degradation in AD: the various patterns of memory decline observed in different subgroups of AD patients; the differential sparing of old memories versus recent ones, and the typical temporal gradient of memory decline.

We have begun our studies by investigating the effects of simple, uniform, global compensation strategies. The uniformity of these strategies has enabled us to obtain analytical insight into the effects of synaptic deletion and compensation on the network's performance, and to formulate optimal compensation strategies. We then extended our model to include memory storage as well as retrieval, and thus were able to study the temporal gradient of memory decline. Finally, we reviewed our studies of local compensation mechanisms. These mechanisms introduce the important concept of neurally-based synaptic compensation, as a complementary process of Hebbian synaptic changes which have been in the focus of neural modeling and experimental studies in recent years. We have shown that synaptic compensation can be achieved in a stable manner via local, activity-driven mechanisms, which in many cases are more efficient than their global counterparts. Within the local model, the variation of a single parameter, the compensation rate, can describe the different progression rates of cognitive deterioration observed in AD.

Our work points to the possible important role of synaptic compensation failure in the progression of Alzheimer's disease. This failure probably reflects a breakdown of regulatory mechanisms that play part in maintaining the functional integrity of the aging, *non-demented*, brain (Buell & Coleman 1979, Flood & Coleman 1986, Bertoni-Freddari et. al. 1988, Bertoni-Freddari et. al. 1990). Considerable support to the *functional* significance of structural synaptic compensatory changes has been furnished by electrophysiological studies in the aging rodent hippocampus (see Barnes 1994 for a review), indicating that older rats have fewer, but structurally larger and functionally stronger synapses. Recently, it was also shown that the infusion of nerve growth factor in aged rats causes a significant increase in the TSA per unit volume of cortex, which is correlated with improved cognitive performance (Chen et. al. 1995). This gives further support to the main mechanism which we propose.

We are now continuing our modeling studies of synaptic alterations and cognitive deterioration in AD in two main avenues:

- *Synaptic maintenance:* Investigating the ability of local synaptic compensation mechanisms to preserve the integrity of the synaptic memory matrix in face of ongoing synaptic attrition. In contrast to the local compensation algorithms studied in this chapter, which rely on the explicit representation (and hence, the 'knowledge') of stored memory patterns, the algorithms currently studied function when the network is presented with random patterns of activity. We hypothesize that, whereas Hebbian synaptic modifications occur as a learning process during awakeness and slow-wave sleep, the neural-based regulatory mechanisms take place during REM sleep, where they are driven by bouts of random cortical activity provided by Ponto-Geniculate waves. Our preliminary results indicate that the new compensation mechanisms not only maintain synaptic stability very effectively, but can also suppress the formation of 'pathological' attractors (attractors with very wide basins of attraction) and mixed attractors, which have been known to plague the state-space of attractor neural networks.

- *Combined neural/metabolic models:* As reviewed in detail in (Masliah 1995), there is now a considerable amount of quantitative data that portrays the changes in the levels of numerous pathological markers of AD as the disease progresses. Our goal is to develop an (albeit simplified) model of the pathogenesis of AD that includes these markers (such as plaques and tangles). This model introduces several assumptions about the causal relations between these markers and the synaptic alterations in AD, and our goal is to find a set of relations which will yield a good fit with the experimental data mentioned above. It is hoped that such a model may help in finding the primary pathological processes underlying AD.

Two key ideas arise from the work surveyed in this chapter. First, many aspects of memory decline in AD can be accounted for by studying the synaptic changes occuring in the disease, in the framework of attractor neural network models. Second, synaptic compensation can be performed efficiently by a *neuronal* activity-dependent compensation mechanism, acting to maintain the functional integrity of memory networks in the aging and ailing brain. This mechanism differs fundamentally from Hebbian *synaptic* modifications which are likely to play a central role in memory storage and learning. Our proposal is that both processes are needed for the proper functioning of the brain.

References

L.F. Abbott, G. Turrigiano, G. LeMasson, and E. Marder (1994). Activity-dependent conductances in model and biological neurons. In D. Waltz, editor, *Natural and artificial parallel computing: Proceedings of fifth annula NEC research symposium.*

R.D. Adams and M. Victor (1989). *Principles of Neurology,* McGraw-Hill, New York.

D.J. Amit (1989). *Modeling brain function: the world of attractor neural networks.* Cambridge University Press.

R.C. Armstrong and M.R. Montminy (1993). Trassynaptic control of gene expression. *Ann. Rev. Neurosci.,* 16:17–29.

C.A. Barnes (1994). Normal aging: regionally specific changes in hippocampal synaptic trasnmission. *TINS,* 17(1):13–18.

W. Beatty, D.P. Salmon, N. Butters, W.C. Heindel, and E.L Granholm (1988). Retrograde amnesia in patient's with Alzheimer's disease or Huntington's disease. *Neurobiology of Aging,* 9:181–186.

C. Bertoni-Freddari, W. Meier-Ruge, and J. Ulrich (1988). Quantitative morphology of synaptic plasticity in the aging brain. *Scanning Microsc.,* 2:1027–1034.

C. Bertoni-Freddari, P. Fattoretti, T. Casoli, W. Meier-Ruge, and J. Ulrich (1990). Morphological adaptive response of the synaptic junctional zones in the human dentate gyrus during aging and alzheimer's disease. *Brain Research,* 517:69–75.

J. Botwinick, M. Storandt, and L. Berg (1986). A longitudinal behavioral study of senile dementia of the alzheimer type. *Arch. Neuorol.,* 43:1124–1127.

J.P. Bourgeois and P. Rakic (1993). Changing of synaptic density in the primary visual cortex of the Rhesus monkey from fetal to adult age. *J. Neurosci.,* 13:2801–2820.

D.M. Bowen, P.T. Francis, I.P. Chessell, and M.T. Webster (1994). Neurotransmission-the link integrating Alzheimer research? *TINS,* 17(4).

S. J. Buell and P.D. Coleman (1979). Dendritic growth in the aged human brain and failure of growth in senile dementia. *Science,* 206:854 – 856.

A. Canning and E. Gardner (1988). Partially connected models of neural networks. *J. Phys. A: Math. Gen.,* 214:3275–3284.

K.S. Chen, E. Masliah, M. Mallory, and F.H. Gage (1995). Synaptic loss in cognitively impaired aged rats is ameliorated by chronic human nerve growth factor infusion. *Neuroscience,* 68 (1):19–27.

C.W. Cotman and K.J. Anderson (1988). Synaptic plasticity and functional stabilization in the hippocampal formation: Possible role in alzheimer's disease.

Adv. Neurol., 47:313–336.

C.W. Cotman and K.J. Anderson (1989). Neural plasticity and regeneration. In G.J. Siegel et. al., editor, *Basic Neurochemestry: Molecular, cellular and medical aspects*, pages 507–522. Raven Press.

J.L. Cummings and D.F. Benson (1983). *Demetia: a clinical approach*, Buttersworths.

S. T. DeKosky and S.W. Scheff (1990). Synapse loss in frontal cortex biopsies in alzheimer's disease: Correlation with cognitive severity. *Ann. Neurology*, 27(5):457–464.

D. A. Drachman, B. F. O'Donnell, R. A. Lew, and J.M. Swearer (1990). The prognosis in Alzheimer's disease. *Arch. Neurol.*, 47:851–856.

D.G. Flood and P.D. Coleman (1986). Failed compensatory dendritic growth as a pathophysiological process in alzheimer's disease. *Can. J. Neurol. Sci.*, 13:475–479.

D.G. Flood and P.D. Coleman. Failed compensatory dendritic growth as a pathophysiological process in Alzheimer's disease. *Can. J. Neurol. Sci.*, 13:475–479, 1986.

J.M. Fuster and J.P. Jervey (1982). Neuronal firing in the inferotepmoral cortex of the monkey in a visual memory task. *The Journal of Neuroscience*, 2(3):361–375.

S. Grumbacher-Reinert and J. Nicholls (1992). Influence of substrate on reduction of neurites following electrical activity of leech Retzius cells in culture. *J. Exp. Biol.*, 167:1–14.

L. A. Hansen, R. DeTeresa, P. Davies, and R.D. Terry (1988). Neocortical morphometry, lesion counts, and choline acetyltransferase levels in the age spectrum of alzheimer's disease. *Neurology*, 38:48–54.

L.L. Heston, A.R. Mastri, V.E. Anderson, and J. White. Dimentia of the alzheimer type: clinical genetics, natural history, and associated conditions. *Arch. Gen. Psychiatry*, 38:1085–1090, 1981.

A. Heyman et al (1983). Alzheimer's disease: Genetic aspects and associated clinical disorders. *Ann. Neurol.*, 14 (5):507–515.

F.J. Huff, J.H. Growden, S. Gorkin, and T.J. Rosen (1987) Age of onset and rate of progression of alzheimer's disease. *J. Am. Geriatr. Soc.*, 35:27–30.

D. Horn, E. Ruppin, M. Usher, and M. Herrmann (1993). Neural network modeling of memory deterioration in Alzheimer's disease. *Neural Computation*, 5:736–749.

D. Horn, N. Levy, and E. Ruppin (1996). Neuronal-based synaptic compensation: A computational study in alzheimer's disease. *Neural Computation*, to appear.

R. Katzman. Clinical presentation of the course of alzheimer's disease: the atypical patient. *Interdiscipl. Topics. Gerontol.*, 20:12–18, 1985.

R. Katzman. Alzheimer's disease. *New England Journal of Medicine*, // 314:964–973, 1986.

R. Katzman et al (1988). Comparison of rate of annual change of mental status score in four independent studies of patients with alzheimer's disease. *Ann. Neurology*, 24(3):384–389.

M.D. Kopelman (1989). Remote and autobiographical memory, temporal context memory, and frontal atrophy in Korsakof and Alzheimer patients. *Neuropsychologica*, 27:437–460.

E. Koscielny-Bunde (1990). Effect of damage in neural networks. *Journal of Statistical Physics*, 58:1257 – 1266.

K.S. Kosik (1991). Alzheimer's plaques and tangles: advances in both fronts. *TINS*, 14:218–219.

E. Masliah (1995). Mechanisms of synaptic dysfunction in alzheimer's disease. *Histology and Histopathology*, 10:509–519.

E. Masliah and R. Terry (1994). The role of synaptic pathology in the mechanisms of dementia in alzheimer's disease. *Clinical Neuroscience*, 1:192–198.

E. Masliah, M. Mallory, L. Hansen, R. DeTeresa, M. Alford, and R. Terry (1994). Synaptic and neuritic alterations during the progression of Alzheimer's disease. *Neuroscience Letters*, 174:67–72.

M.P. Mattson and S.B. Kater (1989). Excitatory and inhibitory neurotransmitters in the generation and degeneration of hippocampal neuroarchitecture. *Brain. Res.*, 478:337–348.

Y. Miyashita and H.S. Chang (1988). Neuronal correlate of pictorial short-term memory in the primate temporal cortex. *Nature*, 331:68–71.

J.I. Morgan and T. Curran (1991). Stimulus-transcription coupling in the nervous system: involvement of inducible proto-oncogenes fos and jun. *Annu. Rev. Neurosci.*, 14:421–451.

D.G. Murphy, C.D. DeCarli, E. Daly, J.A. Gillette, A.R. McIntosh, J.V. Haxby, D. Teichberg, M.B. Schapiro, S.I. Rapoport, and B. Horwitz (1993). Volometric magnetic resonance imaging in men with dementia of the Alzheimer type: correlations with disease severity. *Biological Psychiatry*, 34(9):612–621.

J. Reggia, R. Berndt, and L. D'Autrechy (1994). Connectionist models in neuropsychology. In *Handbook of Neuropsychology*, volume (9), pages 297–333. Elsevier Science, Amsterdam.

E. Ruppin (1995). Neural modeling of psychiatric disorders. *Network*, 6:1–22.

E. Ruppin and J. Reggia (1995). A neural model of memory impairment in diffuse cerebral atrophy. *Br. Jour. of Psychiatry*, 166(1):19–28.

H.J. Sagar, N.J. Cohen, E.V. Sullivan, S. Corkin, and J.H. Growdon (1988). Remote memory function in Alzheimer's disease and Parkinson's disease. *Brain*, 111:185–206.

S.W. Scheff, D.L. Sparks, and D.A. Price (1993). Synapse loss in the temporal lobe in Alzheimer's disease. *Annals of Neurology*, 33:190–199.

K. Schilling, M.H. Dickinson, J.A. Connor, and J.I. Morgan (1991). Electrical activity in cerebral cultures determines Purkinje cell dendritic growth patterns. *Neuron*, 7:891–902.

D. J. Selkoe (1987). Deciphering Alzheimer's disease: the pace quickens. *TINS*, 10:181–184.

G.J. Stuart and B. Sakmann (1994). Active propagation of somatic action potentials into neocortical pyramidal cell dendrites. *Nature*, 367:69–72.

R. D. Terry, E. Masliah, D. P. Salmon, N. Butters, R. DeTeresa, R. Hill, L. A. Hansen, and R. Katzman (1991). Physical basis of cognitive alterations in Alzheimer's disease: Synapse loss is the major correlate of cognitive impairment. *Ann. Neurology*, 30:572 – 580.

M.V. Tsodyks and M.V. Feigel'man (1988). The enhanced storage capacity in neural networks with low activity level. *Europhys. Lett.*, 6:101 – 105.

G. Turrigiano, L.F. Abbott, and E. Marder (1994). Activity-dependent changes in intrinsic properties of cultured neurons. *Science*, 264:974–977.

A. van Ooyen (1994). Activity-dependent neural network development. *Network*, 5:401–423.

D. J. Willshaw, O. P. Buneman, and H. C. Longuet-Higgins (1969). Non-holographic associative memory. *Nature*, 222:960 – 962.

F.J. Wippold, M.H. Gado, J.C. Morris, J.M. Duchek, and E.A. Grant (1991). Senile dementia and healthy aging: a longitudinal CT study. *Radiology*, 179(1):215–219.

SEMANTIC KNOWLEDGE IMPAIRMENTS IN ALZHEIMER'S DISEASE INSIGHTS FROM CONNECTIONIST MODELING

MARTHA J. FARAH
Department of Psychology, University of Pennsylvania
3815 Walnut St., Philadelphia PA 19104 USA

and

LYNETTE J. TIPPETT
Department of Psychology, University of Auckland
Private Bag 92019, Auckland NZ

ABSTRACT

How can the effects of Alzheimer's disease on cognition be characterized? Experiments on confrontation naming have produced evidence implicating a wide array of underlying impairments, including visual and lexical impairments as well as impairments of semantic memory knowledge. These and similar experiments have also suggested that semantic memory is subdivided into components representing knowledge of categories and exemplars, and that AD primarily affects knowledge of exemplars. Using the concepts of distributed representation, interactivity and graded processing, we show how this evidence is also consistent with a simpler hypothesis: AD affects a single, undifferentiated semantic memory store. We also indicate the ways in which this simpler hypothesis can account for evidence initially taken to support an attentional impairment in AD, and can explain the apparently paradoxical finding of increased semantic priming in patients with AD.

1. Goals and Methods of Cognitive Neuropsychology

Cognitive neuropsychologists typically study brain-damaged patients for two related reasons: To characterize the effects of brain damage on the mind in terms of current theories of cognition, and to test those theories using the effects of brain damage as a new source of data. In this chapter we will discuss Alzheimer's disease (AD) from the perspective of both of these research goals. We will show how the use of a simple connectionist model can change the way we characterize the underlying cognitive impairment in AD, and also how inferences about normal cognition based on AD must be reconsidered in the light of this model.

The role that connectionist models play in this research is to provide an explicit,

89

mechanistic link between patient performance, on the one hand, and hypotheses concerning both the normal cognitive system and the effects of brain damage on that system, on the other (Farah, 1994). Traditionally, psychologists have assumed that the link between neuropsychological datum and hypothesis is relatively straightforward. For example, error types are assumed to reflect the disrupted processing stage in a direct manner. If the errors in a naming task are visual, in the sense that the name produced belongs to a different but visually similar object, then researchers infer that the locus of processing impairment is visual. Similarly, semantic errors have been taken to suggest breakdowns at semantic stages, and so on. As reasonable as these inferences sound, they are sometimes wrong. We know this because of computer simulation experiments in which connectionist models are lesioned, by the removal of units or weights, and their errors are studied. For example, Hinton and Shallice (1991) and Plaut and Shallice (1993) trained a series of connectionist networks to read, that is to associate printed words with their meanings, and then lesioned the networks at various locations. Semantic lesions were associated with both visual and semantic errors, as were visual lesions. Cognitive neuropsychologists have used the naming errors of AD patients to draw inferences about the normal cognitive system. In this chapter, we will show how one of the inferences thus drawn, concerning the internal structure of semantic memory, is mistaken, and we will provide a simpler explanation of the error data with the help of a connectionist model.

Another traditional approach to inferring the locus of processing impairment is the selective manipulation of the difficulty of individual task components. For example, if the difficulty of a naming task is increased by selecting objects with low frequency names, and this manipulation disproportionately affects patients' naming performance, then researchers infer that the locus of processing impairment is lexical. Alternatively, if a patient is disproportionately affected by reducing the visual quality of a stimulus, this has been taken to suggest an impairment in visual stages of processing. Again, consideration of the mechanisms of information processing in connectionist systems shows that this reasoning is not sound. In the case of AD, this reasoning has led to unnecessarily complex hypotheses concerning the number of different cognitive impairments that must be hypothesized in AD. It is to this issue that we first turn.

2. Naming Impairments in Alzheimer's Disease: Visual, Semantic or Lexical Locus of Damage?

Alzheimer's disease is associated with impairment in a number of different types of cognitive tasks. Although the learning of new information is perhaps the only ability that is universally affected in the earliest stages of the disease (Hodges & Patterson, 1995), AD invariably affects performance in a variety of tasks that do not involve new learning. For example, the naming of visually presented objects, termed by clinicians 'confrontation naming', is frequently impaired early in the progress of AD, and is eventually impaired in all patients. Other tasks involving language and semantic knowledge are also generally impaired, and in some patients striking disorders of vision or executive function have been observed (e.g., Schwartz, 1990). Given the range of manifestations of cognitive impairment in AD, is it possible to delineate a single, core underlying cognitive deficit? Or, does the relatively widespread nature of the disease at an anatomical level cause a cognitively widespread array of impairments?

2.1. The Semantic Memory Hypothesis and Alternative Hypotheses

Our working hypothesis is that patients may well vary in some respects (e.g., see Martin, 1990), but that the one pronounced commonality among patients with AD, aside from the new learning impairment, is an impairment of semantic memory. This hypothesis finds some support in the literature on confrontation naming in AD. According to the semantic memory hypothesis, individuals with AD cannot name objects because their semantic memory knowledge about them is impoverished. One source of evidence for this comes from the qualitative nature of errors made in naming tasks. Typical kinds of errors include calling an object either by the name of its superordinate category (e.g., animal instead of cat) or by the name of a semantically-related object (e.g., lettuce for asparagus) (e.g., Bayles & Tomoeda 1983; Hodges, Salmon & Butters 1991; Martin & Fedio, 1983). These errors suggest that the available semantic representations are degraded or underspecified. In addition to evidence from naming tasks themselves, evidence from other experimental paradigms also implicates semantic memory as a major locus of cognitive impairments in AD (e.g., see Nebes, 1989, 1992 for reviews). As a result of both sources of evidence, impaired semantic memory is currently the predominant explanation for the naming deficit in AD.

Nevertheless, there is evidence that two additional loci of impairment contribute to the confrontation naming impairment. Patients with AD are disproportionately affected by reduction of the visual quality of the stimulus to be named (e.g., line drawings versus objects), (e.g., Kirshner, Webb & Kelly, 1984; Shuttleworth & Huber, 1988), suggesting a deficit of visual perception. In addition, patients with AD are differentially impaired at naming objects whose names are low frequency words, relative to objects whose names occur with high frequency (e.g., Barker & Lawson, 1968; Skelton-Robinson & Jones, 1984; Shuttleworth & Huber, 1988), which suggests a deficit of lexical access. Furthermore, phonemic cuing has been reported to improve AD subjects' naming (e.g., Martin & Fedio, 1983; Neils, Brennan, Cole, Boller & Gerdeman, 1988), again implicating lexical/phonological retrieval as the locus of impairment. Contrary to our working hypothesis of a core semantic memory impairment, these findings appear to implicate three different loci of impairment underlying the naming deficit in AD, namely semantic, visual, and lexical.

2.2 A Connectionist Reinterpretation of the Evidence for Visual and Lexical Impairment

However, from the perspective of connectionism these findings may be perfectly consistent with a single underlying impairment in semantic memory. Two aspects of connectionism are especially relevant here: distributed representation and interactivity. In a highly distributed and interactive system of representation, different components of the system are in a constant give-and-take relation, continually updating each other with the partial, intermediate results of their processing. Each part of an item's representation (e.g., visual, semantic and lexical) depends on other parts for input to become activated, so that damage confined to one part of the system will render all parts less able to attain their proper activation states. In such a system, manipulations of difficulty that are targeted to nondamaged parts of the system would have an increased effect, because the functioning of the nondamaged parts is nevertheless compromised. Thus, if AD patients have a deficit of semantic memory, reducing the quality of the visual input may affect naming performance more than in persons with intact semantic memory because their visual systems are deprived of some of the normal support from semantics. Similarly, producing words that occur with low frequency may be more vulnerable to damage to semantic memory than producing words that occur with high frequency. Providing additional activation to the lexical or phonological components in the form of phonological cuing may facilitate activation of the correct name, regardless of whether there is damage in the lexical component.

In order to test this interpretation of the effects of visual and lexical difficulty manipulations on confrontation naming in AD, we carried out a series of connectionist simulations. Specifically we trained an interactive neural network to produce "name" patterns when presented with "visual" patterns by way of an intermediate set of "semantic" patterns, thus simulating confrontation naming. We then investigated the claim that damage to the "semantic" component will result in enhanced vulnerability to manipulations affecting non-damaged components, specifically the quality of "visual" inputs, frequency of training of patterns, and effects of phonological cuing (Tippett & Farah, 1994).

2.3 Simulations of Confrontation Naming Experiments

Figure 1 shows the architecture of the model. There are five pools of units. The 16 "visual units" subserve visual representations of objects. The 32 "semantic units" subserve representations of the semantic knowledge that can be activated either by "visual inputs", or by "name inputs". The 16 "name units" subserve the representation of names associated with objects. The model is trained to associate the patterns of activity between these three layers. The learning of these associations is assisted by the presence of hidden units located between the visual and semantic layers (the "visual hidden units") and the name and semantic layers (the "name hidden units"). All units within each layer are connected to each other, and all connections, both between and within layers, are bi directional. Thus, there is a high degree of interconnectivity in the model, which allows for extensive interaction among the different components in the course of naming. In addition to weights between units, there were bias weights for each unit, encoding the relative likelihood of each unit's being activated over all trained patterns.

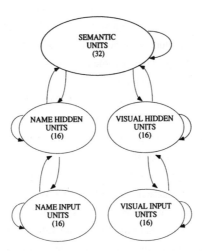

Figure 1. Schematic diagram of connectionist model of confrontation naming.

Twenty patterns consisting of patterns in the visual layer, semantic layer and name layer, were generated. Visual representations and names of objects are represented by randomly generated patterns of activity (-1's and +1's) over the 16 units in each pool. Similarly, the semantic knowledge activated by these inputs is represented by a random pattern of activity over the pool of 32 units in the semantic layer. The representations are distributed, in the sense that an object is represented by a pattern of activation over visual, semantic and name units, and in the sense that within each of these pools of units all of the units participate in representing all of the known patterns. Each unit encodes information that represents some 'microfeature', but there is no attempt to assign units to specific easily-labelled microfeatures (e.g., "red" or "round" for a visual representation). Of course, there is nothing intrinsically visual, semantic, or verbal about these pools of units, aside from the fact that their patterns of mutual connectivity conform to the general notion that semantic representations must be accessed in order to mediate between visual and name representations.

Units in this model can take on continuous activation values between -1 and +1. The weights on the connections between units can take on any real values. Activation levels are updated according to a nonlinear activation function (a hyperbolic tangent). The network was trained to correctly associate the patterns of activity between the three layers, such that when an input pattern was presented to one of the layers (e.g., the visual layer), it was able to produce the correct patterns of activity at the other two layers (the semantic layer and the name layer). During training as well as test, inputs were soft-clamped, that is their activation values were not fixed but were the result of input activation along with activation from other units to which they were connected. Noise was added to each layer to facilitate robustness of learning. To assess the generality of the results, multiple networks were trained with the same patterns but different random starting weights. The learning procedure used during training was the contrastive Hebbian learning algorithm (Movellan, 1990). Note that we are using this algorithm as a means of setting the weights in the network to enable it to perform naming; we are not concerned with the psychological reality of the training procedure as a model of learning.

Confrontation naming was simulated by presenting just the visual pattern to the visual input layer, allowing the network to settle, then looking at the pattern of activation on the name units to see which of the 20 name patterns it matched most closely. The degree of pattern match was simply the number of units whose values (+1 and -1) matched. It was therefore, a forced choice between the 20 patterns representing names.

Damage to semantic memory was simulated by removing randomly chosen subsets of the semantic units. Four levels of damage were used, to explore the effects of increasingly severe damage: 2 units, 4 units, 6 units and 8 units, or 6.25%, 12.5%, 18.75% and 25% of the semantic layer. Although the neuropathological changes in AD are more complex than a simple loss of cells, we chose this means of lesioning the network because it was the simplest and most straightforward. Furthermore, Patterson, Seidenberg, and McClelland (1989) compared the effects on network performance of deleting units, deleting weights, and adding noise, and found them similar.

The first question of interest was whether damage to semantics could render the system more sensitive to manipulations of the visual quality of the stimulus. This was investigated by testing trained undamaged and damaged networks on the production of the correct name patterns with normal visual inputs and impoverished visual inputs. Five undamaged trained networks were used. Twenty different random lesionings at each level of damage were then carried out for each network.

Visual impoverishment of the input patterns was simulated by reducing the inputs of a randomly chosen 50% of the units in the input pattern. For example, if part of the pattern was +1 +1 -1 -1, then the impoverished input might be +.5 +1 -1 -.5. Two levels of visual impoverishment were used for both damaged and undamaged networks. The first level was chosen so that the naming task was as difficult as possible for the intact network without resulting in any errors. The second level of visual impoverishment was selected so that the intact network made at least one error. These levels were motivated by the observation that normal subjects make few or no errors in naming impoverished stimuli.

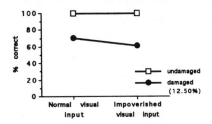

Figure 2. Naming performance by networks with 12.5% damage to semantic layer, with and without visual impoverishment designed to result in no errors with intact network.

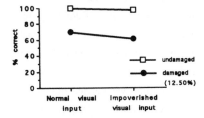

Figure 3. Naming performance by networks with 12.5% damage to semantic layer, with and without visual impoverishment designed to result in some errors with intact network.

While it was expected that damage to the semantic layer would impair network performance on the naming task overall, the question of interest was whether the damaged networks would show enhanced vulnerability to impoverished visual inputs relative to the intact networks. The results showed that although the amount of interaction between visual impoverishment and damage becomes smaller at increasing levels of damage, there is a highly consistent and significant interaction at all levels for the first level of impoverishment (see Figure 2) and for 16 out of 20 of the damaged networks at the second level of impoverishment (see Figure 3) (see Tippett & Farah, 1994 for data from all levels of network damage). In other words, the effect of visual degradation was greater on networks with semantic damage than on intact networks.

In our simulations, normal performance is at or near ceiling. This raises the possibility that the appearance of increased sensitivity to visual impoverishment in the damaged networks is due to a ceiling effect in the intact networks. Of course, the same point can be made about the empirical data from AD subjects and normal controls: Normal subjects invariably perform at or near 100% in confrontation naming, even with the presentation of impoverished visual stimuli (e.g., Kirshner et al., 1984). Furthermore, after semantic memory damage both patients and networks should be at ceiling for the visual stages of processing. Therefore, AD patients should be just as immune to visual manipulations as normal subjects by virtue of the same ceiling effect. Of course, in interactive systems this logic would not apply. As we demonstrated in this simulation, manipulations of difficulty (visual impoverishment) at one level can interact with impairment to a component at another level (semantic damage), while these same manipulations of difficulty have little or no effect on networks with intact semantics.

The second question of interest is the prediction that a naming system with highly interactive components will have more difficulty producing the names of items that have occurred with lower frequency during learning than those that occurred with higher frequency, after damage to the semantic component. This is based on the claim that in an interactive system, names trained with lower frequency will be less robustly represented, and therefore more vulnerable to damage in any component of the system. The investigation was carried out by training a series of 12 networks with stimulus items presented at different frequencies, i.e. ten of the stimulus items were presented at a lower frequency than the other ten items. Six networks were trained with an item-frequency ratio of four to one and six networks with an item frequency ratio of three to one. Networks were then damaged by removing randomly selected units in the semantic layer and were tested on the full set of items used in training. Each network was subjected to 10 different random lesions at each of four levels of damage.

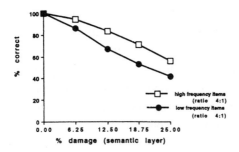

Figure 4. Naming accuracy for high and low frequency items after damage to semantic layer.

As predicted, more errors were made in the production of names for items trained at low frequency, compared with items trained at high frequency for networks trained on each of the two ratios and at each level of semantic damage from 6.25% to 25% (see Figure 4 for results of networks trained at 4:1 ratio). With no damage, all the networks produce all names for the low and high frequency items without error. With damage in the semantic layer, networks make differentially more errors producing names for the low frequency items. These findings were significant on 22 out of 24 tests comparing the performance of networks with semantic damage on the naming of items trained at high frequency and the items trained at low frequency, for networks trained at the ratio of 4:1. For the six networks trained at the ratio of 3:1, 16 out of 24 tests were significant.

These data support the hypothesis that lower frequency items will suffer disproportionately after damage to semantics in an interactive naming system. However, in this simulation the frequency manipulation involved different amounts of training for the visual and semantic, as well as the lexical, levels of representation. In effect, our lexical frequency manipulation was confounded with other types of frequency. However, the same is undoubtedly true, on average, for the concrete nouns used in confrontation naming tasks, even though the degree of correlation among lexical, semantic and visual frequency would be less perfect in reality than it was in our simulation. In fact, without controlling for some nonlexical measure of familiarity, the lexical frequency manipulation cannot be used to implicate a specifically lexical locus of impairment, even in a discrete stage architecture. For this reason, the results of phonemic cuing with AD patients seem a more decisive form of evidence favoring a lexical locus of impairment.

If a phonemic cue helps a patient produce the name of an object, it is generally inferred that the locus of naming impairment is lexical, as opposed to semantic. The final simulation tested the validity of this inference. Will the naming performance of an interactive system, with damage confined to the semantic layer, be facilitated by presentation of a partial "phonemic" pattern, just as the naming of objects by AD patients is facilitated by the provision of a phonemic cue? A random sample of 10 damaged networks from the first experiment was tested, using only those items on which the networks made errors. For each such item, the network was given a "phonemic cue." This was accomplished by soft-clamping 25% of the name units with the correct name pattern while the visual pattern was presented to the visual units, thus simulating, for example, saying "br" to facilitate the naming of a picture of a broom.

Table 1. Effectiveness of simulated phonemic cuing for items not named correctly after semantic layer damage.

Level of damage (percent)	Correct names following a phonemic cue
6.25	68%
12.5	82%
18.75	74%
25	71%

For networks at all levels of damage, phonemic cuing frequently enabled correct naming performance on those items that had previously been failed. Table 1 provides a summary of the mean percentage of correct name responses produced following cuing. The efficacy of cuing ranged from a mean of 67.6% for networks with 6.25% damage to the semantic units, to 81.5% for networks with 12.5% damage. At the highest level of damage to the semantic units (25%) the mean improvement was 71.24%. These findings demonstrate that an unambiguously lexical/phonological manipulation is effective in a semantically-damaged system.

2.4 Summary

These simulations were undertaken to reconcile apparently conflicting data concerning confrontation naming in AD. A number of studies have shown that manipulations of visual or lexical processing difficulty have a disproportionate effect on the naming performance of patients with AD. We used an interactive connectionist model to show that these findings can be accommodated by the hypothesis that semantic memory is impaired in AD. In an interactive system, in which each component depends upon interactions with many others to function properly, damage to one component will impair the functioning of others, and will render them more sensitive to manipulations of difficulty targeted specifically to them. This is true whether the manipulation makes processing harder for a component, as visual degradation does for the visual component of the model, or whether it facilitates it, as phonemic cuing does for the lexical component.

Our findings provide support for the view that, in addition to a new learning impairment, semantic memory impairment is at the core of the cognitive changes in AD, and that additional impairments in vision and lexical access do not need to be hypothesized.

3. Preservation of categorical knowledge in Alzheimer's disease

The semantic memory impairment of AD has the potential to teach us about the nature of semantic memory in normal humans. This is an example of the second type of goal for cognitive neuropsychology, in which the effects of brain damage put constraints on hypotheses about the normal system. One implication that has been drawn from the errors of patients with AD concerns the internal organization of semantic memory. Specifically, the tendency of AD patients to misname objects with the name of a different object in the same category, or the name of the category itself, has led to the proposal that semantic memory is subdivided into knowledge of categories and knowledge of exemplars, and that AD primarily affects the latter. We will show that there is a more parsimonious alternative explanation for this data.

3.1 Dissociations Between Exemplar and Category Knowledge

The dissociation between exemplar and category knowledge can be seen in various measures of semantic memory. In confrontation naming, patients may call a desk "a chair," or simply say "furniture." It thus appears that they have retained knowledge of the desk attributes that are shared with chairs and other furniture in general, that is, category knowledge, but have lost knowledge that distinguishes different exemplars of the category, that is exemplar knowledge. The same pattern shows up in tasks that do not require naming, such as name-picture matching, name-picture verification tasks, and fluency tasks (e.g., Bayles & Tomoeda, 1983; Chertkow, Bub, & Seidenberg, 1989: Hodges et al., 1991; Huff, Corkin, & Growdon, 1986; Martin, 1987; Martin & Fedio, 1983; Ober, Dronkers, Koss, Delis, & Friedland, 1986; Troster, Salmon, McCullough, & Butters, 1989).

The most transparent interpretation of these observations is that the brain honors the distinction between different levels of a hierarchical knowledge system, and that AD primarily affects the neural systems subserving exemplar knowledge while sparing the systems subserving category knowledge.

3.2 A Connectionist Reinterpretation of Spared Category Knowledge

The principles of connectionism give rise to a second interpretation of the dissociation found in AD, however, which does not involve separate systems for representing these two kinds of knowledge. In connectionist systems knowledge representation is distributed and graded. Semantic memory may be thought of as a distributed system in which the same physical substrate represents both categorical and exemplar information. Furthermore, knowledge is graded in that some representations, or some parts of a distributed representations may be better learned than others. In particular, parts of representations that are encountered more frequently will be more overlearned than parts that are encountered less frequently. Each time an object is presented to the network for learning, all of the category attributes (those shared by all members of the category) and all of the exemplar attributes (those unique to the exemplar) are learned. Because the category attributes will be learned every time any member of the category is presented, but the exemplar unique attributes will be learned only when the specific exemplar is presented, the category attributes will be more thoroughly learned or overlearned. This would be expected to render them more resistant to damage, as we saw in the frequency manipulation of the previous confrontation naming simulation. Hence category knowledge will be preserved after damage to a distributed semantic memory system that does not differentiate, architecturally, category from exemplar knowledge.

3.3 Simulations of Experiments Testing Category and Exemplar Knowledge

We tested and confirmed the computational adequacy of this hypothesis in two computer simulations (Tippett, McAuliffe & Farah, 1995). We trained the same interactive network described above (see Figure 1) to associate patterns in "visual" units with patterns in "semantic" and "lexical" units. As before, there is nothing intrinsically visual, semantic, or verbal about these units, aside from the fact that their patterns of mutual connectivity conform to the general notion that semantic representations must be accessed in order to mediate between visual and name representations.

Semantic units:	1-8	9-16	17-24	25-32
CATEGORY 1:	+-+-+-+-	+-+-+-+-	++++++++	++++++++
	+-+-+-+-	+-+-+-+-	--------	++++++++
	+-+-+-+-	+-+-+-+-	++++----	++++----
	+-+-+-+-	+-+-+-+-	----++++	----++++
	+-+-+-+-	+-+-+-+-	+-+-+-+-	-+-+-+-+
CATEGORY 2:	++++++++	-++--++-	-++--++-	++++++++
	--------	-++--++-	-++--++-	++++++++
	++++----	-++--++-	-++--++-	++++----
	----++++	-++--++-	-++--++-	++++----
	+-+-+-+-	-++--++-	-++--++-	-+-+-+-+

Figure 5. Semantic patterns of five exemplars of Category 1 and five exemplars of Category 2. Note that units 1-16 carry the category information for Category 1, and units 9-24 carry the category information for Category 2.

In these simulations the 20 patterns in the semantic layer were constructed so that four categories were represented, each with 5 individual exemplars. Half of each semantic pattern, that is 16 of the 32 units of the semantic representation, represented the properties shared across exemplars within a category. This portion of the pattern was therefore identical across the 5 exemplars. The other 16 units represented the individual exemplar knowledge for each item and overlapped with other exemplars within the category by only 8 of the 16 units. An example is provided in Figure 5, which shows the semantic patterns of the five members of Categories 1 and 2. The other categories were constructed in a similar manner except that they shared different sets of 16 units. Specifically, the category portion of the semantic patterns for Category 1 involved semantic units 1 though 16, Category 2 involved semantic units 9 through 24, Category 3 involved semantic units 17 through 32, and Category 4 involved semantic units 1 through 8 and 24 through 31. Thus, all semantic units functioned equally often to represent category and exemplar knowledge. There is no division of labor, within the semantic layer, for category versus exemplar knowledge.

Ten networks were trained to associate 20 patterns of activity on the visual, naming and semantic layers. Each network was trained with semantic patterns described above, but the visual and naming patterns were different for each of the 10 networks. As before, damage to semantic memory was simulated by removing randomly chosen subsets of the semantic units. Four levels of damage were used to explore the effects of increasingly severe damage: 2 units, 4 units, 6 units and 8 units, or 6.25%, 12.5%, 18.75% and 25% of the semantic layer. At each of these levels of damage, each network was lesioned in 20 different ways, that is, with 20 different random patterns of semantic units eliminated.

The results of this simulation are summarized in Table 2. After damage, the system showed a stronger tendency to within-category errors than between-category errors, as do individuals with AD, even though the damaged representations do not separately implement category and exemplar knowledge. While appearing to confirm our hypothesis as to the greater robustness of category level knowledge, in fact, the reason for these results is ambiguous. It would not be surprising for similar patterns to be confused with one another after network damage, and it is possible that this finding simply reflects the greater similarity among exemplars within a category than among exemplars of different categories, rather than being a result of the greater robustness of the category-level knowledge.

Table 2. Expected and observed number of within-category naming errors following different levels of damage to semantic layer.

Level of damage (percent)	Expected within-category errors	Observed within-category errors	Significance (binomial test)
6.25	.53	.79	<.001
12.5	1.17	1.76	<.001
18.75	1.68	2.39	<.001
25	2.24	2.91	<.001

In order to test this possibility we carried out a second simulation to assess more directly the state of category and exemplar knowledge after semantic layer damage. Instead of looking at the names produced by the damaged network, we looked at the semantic layer itself and compared the relative accuracy of the category versus exemplar portions of the patterns. Table 3 show the average error in category and exemplar portions of the patterns in 10 different networks after 20 different random lesionings at each level of damage. There is a consistent tendency for the categorical information to be more robust to damage than the exemplar-unique information, even though errors in category and exemplar units should be equally likely by chance. In other words, in this simulation the preservation of categorical and exemplar-unique semantic knowledge is assessed directly, without the confounding influence of the greater number of similar and hence confusable patterns within a category than between categories on our error measure. The results support the claim that categorical information is robust to damage because of the greater degree of training enjoyed by categorical information.

Table 3. Average number of erroneous unit activation values per pattern in category and exemplar portions of semantic patterns after different amounts of damage to semantic layer.

Level of damage (percent)	Category portion errors	Exemplar portion errors	Significance (binomial test)
6.25	.20	.29	<.001
12.5	.48	.59	<.001
18.75	.80	.88	<.001
25	1.04	1.12	<.001

In very general terms, our explanation is an instance of the type of explanation noted by Teuber (1955) and Shallice (1988), in which a relatively impaired ability is simply "harder" or less "robust" than the relatively spared ability. "Hard" and "robust" are not mechanistic terms, however, but rather placeholders in an incomplete explanation. Here we have replaced these placeholders with an explicit mechanistic hypothesis.

3.4 Summary

The second set of simulations shows that it is not necessary to hypothesize a two-part structure for semantic memory, with category and exemplar knowledge stored separately, in order to account for the disproportionate effect of AD on knowledge of exemplars. Instead, the concepts of connectionism, particularly distributed representation and graded processing, can explain the phenomenon with a single undifferentiated semantic memory system. A single set of units functions as a distributed semantic memory representation, with the same units representing attributes that are general to some categories and specific to exemplars of other categories. The graded nature of learning allows differences in the degree of learning among representations that are all well-learned from the point of view of the intact system. After damage these differences become manifest, with more overlearned knowledge being more robust. Category general knowledge will be more overlearned than exemplar-specific knowledge because it is learned every time any exemplar of the category is encountered, whereas by definition the exemplar-unique knowledge is learned only when the specific exemplar is encountered.

4. Broader Implications

4.1 For Alzheimer's Disease

Using the framework of connectionism, the semantic memory hypothesis can be extended to account for other aspects of cognition in AD. For example, Nebes (1989) has pointed out that AD patients' semantic memory appears intact in certain tasks, and that a major determinant of AD patients' success in semantic memory tasks is how constrained the task is. Nebes outlines a number of ways in which increasing the constraints on task performance improves outcome: For example, if patients are required to generate as many items as possible from a semantic category, they perform quite poorly, yet if they are asked to sort items by category or to make a decision about whether a particular item belongs to a given category, they perform fairly normally. Similarly, performance is poor when AD patients are asked to list physical attributes and functions of objects, but if they are asked to indicate whether a specific attribute is related to a given object, they are quite accurate. Nebes, Boller, and Holland (1986) directly manipulated the degree of constraint in a sentence completion task with other aspects of the task held constant, and found AD patients to be more keenly sensitive to this task dimension than normal subjects. While all subjects were faster in completing high constraint sentences, such as "Father carved the turkey with a _____," than in low constraint sentences, such as "They went to see the famous _____.", the AD patients were much more affected by the degree of constraint than normal subjects. This body of evidence led Nebes to propose that AD patients are impaired at attention-demanding semantic processing, but not semantic memory per se.

The general principles of connectionism seem well-suited to explaining sensitivity to task constraint as a result of impaired semantic memory, without invoking the concept of attention. Indeed, connectionism is sometimes called "computation by constraint satisfaction." This is because the pattern into which a network settles following presentation of an input is the pattern of activation that best satisfies the simultaneous constraints of the input activation pattern and the pattern of weights within the network. Damage to one component of the network (such as the semantic layer) can be viewed as a loss of the constraints that are needed to push the network towards a correct stable pattern of activation. If constraints from one source are reduced, another source can help compensate. This suggests that the sensitivity of AD patients' semantic memory performance to the degree of constraint imposed by the task on possible answers does not necessarily cast doubt on the reality of their semantic memory deficit. Rather, it is consistent with some degree of semantic memory deficit in which answers are retrieved by a process of constraint satisfaction.

This perspective also resolves a paradox within AD research concerning the effects of semantic priming on speed of lexical decision or naming in AD. On the face of things, one might expect to find smaller effects of semantic priming in AD if semantic memory is a locus of impairment. However, larger than normal semantic priming effects have been observed (e.g., Chertkow et al., 1989). Increased sensitivity to priming after semantic damage makes sense within the framework being developed here: As the constraints needed from semantic memory to perform lexical decision or produce a name are reduced, other sources of constraint will have a larger effect. Priming, in the form of residual activation from a pattern that is at least partly consistent with the target pattern (by virtue of sharing some of its semantic features) would therefore be expected to have an even larger effect than normal, relative to no residual pattern or an inconsistent pattern.

Albert Einstein is credited with having given this advice: Everything should be made as simple as possible, but no simpler. In this chapter we have tried to account for as much of the evidence on cognition in Alzheimer's disease as possible with the hypothesis that there is a single functional lesion to a single undifferentiated semantic memory system. This account is simple, but is it too simple?

We would not want to rule out other loci of cognitive impairment, either in some patients with AD or in all. It is already clear that some patients have pronounced impairments in cognitive capacities other than semantic memory (e.g., Martin, 1990). It is also reasonably clear that as the disease progresses, language, vision, praxis and executive functions are compromised. However, we think that it may be possible to account for many of the phenomena of AD, particularly mild and moderate AD, with the semantic memory hypothesis. In this chapter we have shown that evidence for visual and lexical problems can be explained with the semantic memory hypothesis, and that it is not necessary to subdivide semantic memory into category and exemplar knowledge. We have also sketched out a way in which the semantic memory hypothesis can explain evidence taken to support an attentional impairment over a semantic memory impairment, and can explain the seemingly paradoxical finding of increased semantic priming. In this way we are trying to find out how simple we can make our account of the cognitive impairments in AD, without making it "too simple."

4.2 For Cognitive Neuropsychology

Compared to the methods of cognitive psychology, neuropsychology seems much more direct. Cognitive psychologists study the mind by varying stimuli and instructions on the input end and analyzing responses and response latencies at output. In contrast, neurological disease and injury directly affect the processes that intervene between input and output. However, our data in neuropsychology are the same as in cognitive psychology, namely the behavioral responses of our subjects. Linking those responses to the internal processes that generate them requires an inference. Neuropsychology's manipulations may be in some sense more direct than cognitive psychology's, in that they affect internal cognitive processes themselves rather than affecting the input to those processes, but neither field can escape the need for interpreting its data.

It is nevertheless easy to succumb to the impression that neuropsychological data are generated in such a direct way from the damaged cognitive system that their interpretation is self-evident. For example, there are countless examples in the neuropsychology literature of error types being used to diagnose the locus of impairment (e.g., visual errors indicating damage to the visual system). But error types do not wear their interpretations on their sleeves. We have just seen one example of this, in the tendency of our network to make within-category errors without any architectural distinction between category and exemplar representation. Manipulations of the difficulty of one type of processing, for example degrading visual stimuli or cuing phonological wordforms, cannot resolve the ambiguity concerning the locus of impairment, as we saw in the first section. We have found the concepts of connectionism to be helpful in reasoning about the relations between complex brain-like systems and their behavior, and connectionist models to be an invaluable tool for honing and testing our reasoning.

5. Acknowledgments

The research described here was supported by Alzheimer's Association Pilot Research Grant PRG-93-153, ONR grant N00014-93-I0621, NIH grant R01 NS34030, an NSF STC grant to the Institute for Research in Cognitive Science at the University of Pennsylvania, and the University of Auckland Research Committee.

6. References

M. Barker, & J. Lawson, *Brit. J of Psychiatry* .114 (1968) 1351-1356.

K. A. Bayles, & C. K. Tomoeda, *Brain & Lang.* 19 (1983) 98-114.

A. Caramazza, R. S. Berndt, & H. H. Brownell, *Brain & Lang.* 15 (1982) 161-189.

H. Chertkow, D. Bub, & M. Seidenberg, M. *Brain & Lang.* 36 (1989) 420-446.

M. J. Farah, *Behav & Brain Sci* . 17 (1994) 43-104.

G. E. Hinton, J. L. McClelland, & D.E. Rumelhart, in D. Rumelhart, J. L. McClelland, *Parallel Distributed Processing: Explorations in the Microstructure of Cognition* (MIT Press Cambridge, 1986)

G. E. Hinton, & T. Shallice, *Psych Rev.* 98 (1991) 74-95.

J.R. Hodges & K. Patterson, Neuropsychologia 33 (1995) 441-459.

J. R. Hodges, D. P. Salmon, & N. Butters, *Brain.* 114 (1991) 1547-1558.

J F. Huff, S. Corkin, & J. H. Growdon, *Brain & Lang.* 28 (1986) 235-249.

Kirshner, H. S., Webb, W. G., & Kelly, M. P. *Neuropsychologia*, 22 (1984) 23-30.

A. Martin, *J of Clin. & Exp. Neuropsych.* 9 (1987) 191-224.

A. Martin, in in *Modular Deficits in Alzheimer--Type Dementia*, ed. M. F. Schwartz (MIT Press, Cambridge, 1990) pp. 143-175.

A. Martin, & P. Fedio, *Brain & Lang.* 19 (1983) 124-141.

J. Movellan, in *Proceedings of the 1989 Connectionist Models Summer School* , Eds. D. S. Touretzky, G. E. Hinton, & T. J. Sejnowski (Morgan Kaufman, San Mateo,1990), pp. 10-17.

R. D. Nebes, *Psych Bul.* 106 (1989) 377-394.

R. D. Nebes, in *The Handbook of Aging and Cognition*, eds. F. I. M. Craik & T. A. Salthouse (Lawrence Erlbaum, London, 1992) pp. 373-446.

R. D. Nebes, F. Boller, & A. Holland, *Psych. & Aging.* 1 (1986) 261-269.

J. Neils, M. M. Brennan, M. Cole, F. Boller, & B. Gerdeman, *Neuropsych.* 26 (1988) 351-354.

B. A. Ober, N. F. Dronkers, E. Koss, D. C. Delis & R. P. Friedland, *J of Clin & Exp Neuropsych.* 8 (1986) 75-92.

K. E. Patterson, M. S. Seidenberg & J. L. McClelland, in *Parallel Distributed Processing: Implications for Psychology and Neurobiology* ed. R. G. M. Morris (Oxford University Press, Oxford, 1989).

D. C. Plaut & T. Shallice, *J of Cog Neurosci.* 5 (1993) 89-117.

D. E. Rumelhart, G. E. Hinton & R. J. Williams, in *Parallel Distributed Processing: Explorations in the Microstructure of Cognition*, eds, D. Rumelhart, J. L. McClelland (MIT Press, Cambridge, 1986) pp. 318-362.

D. Rumelhart & J. L. McClelland, *Parallel Distributed Processing: Explorations in the Microstructure of cognition* (MIT Press, Cambridge, 1986).

M. F. Schwartz, & J. A. Stark, in *Modular Deficits in Alzheimer--Type Dementia*, ed. M. F. Schwartz (MIT Press, Cambridge, 1990) pp. 61-82.

T. Shallice, *Neuropsychology to Mental Structure.* (Cambridge University press, Cambridge, 1988).

E.C. Shuttleworth & S.J. Huber, *Brain & Lang.* 34 (1988) 222-234.

M. Skelton-Robinson & S. Jones, *Brit J of Psychiatry.* 145 (1984) 168-171.

L. J. Tippett & M. J. Farah, *Neuropsych.* 8 (1994) 3-13.

L. J. Tippett, S. McAuliffe, & M. J. Farah, *Mem.* 3 (1995) 519-533.

A. I. Troster, D. P. Salmon, D. McCullough, & N. Butters, *Brain & Lang.* 37 (1989) 500-513.

Distributed Representations of Semantic Knowledge in the Brain: Computational Experiments using Feature Based Codes

STEVEN L. SMALL
Department of Neurology, Cognitive Modelling Laboratory, University of Pittsburgh,
325 Scaife Hall, Pittsburgh, PA 15261-2003
Email: small+@pitt.edu

JOHN HART, JR.
Department of Neurology, School of Medicine, The Zanvyl Krieger Mind/Brain Institute,
The Johns Hopkins University, Meyer 222, 600 North Wolfe Street, Baltimore, MD 21287

TRAN NGUYEN
Department of Pediatrics, University of California at Davis, Sacramento, CA

BARRY GORDON
Department of Neurology, School of Medicine, The Zanvyl Krieger Mind/Brain Institute,
The Johns Hopkins University, Meyer 222, 600 North Wolfe Street, Baltimore, MD 21287

ABSTRACT

Category specific language impairments have been postulated to require the existence of an explicit category organization within semantic memory. However, it may be possible to demonstrate analytically that this is not necessary. We hypothesize that category specific organization can emerge from perceptual, functional, and associative feature information about objects that is maintained in order to process language. In this paper, we conduct several experiments to test the computational validity of this hypothesis.

Physical objects were encoded in terms of semantic features, based on basic perceptual and motor modalities and higher level knowledge of function, for use in artificial neural networks. Mathematical methods were used to analyze the encodings and the neural networks. The results demonstrate the emergence of semantic categories in the networks, although such information was not pre-programmed. We conclude that category specific language organization can emerge from the inherent nature of semantic features themselves, and does not require special internal categorical organization of semantic memory.

1. Introduction

Semantic memory supports human language function by encoding word meanings. The neurobiological instantiation of this cognitive structure may comprise aspects of both temporal lobes, especially the left temporal lobe [Damasio et al, 1990; Hart and Gordon, 1992]. Although not all language tasks require access to this semantic memory of word meanings (henceforth referred to simply as "semantic memory"), such conceptual knowledge underlying these lexical descriptors is integral to many linguistic and other cognitive tasks. Focal and diffuse neurological diseases can damage semantic memory and lead to breakdowns in task performance. Neuropsychological and neuroanatomical features of these impairments inform about the structure of semantic memory.

One uncommon type of semantic memory impairment, which typically arises through bilateral temporal lobe damage [Hart and Gordon, 1992], typically of herpes simplex encephalitis or unilateral left temporal lobe damage [Damasio et al, 1990], involves dysnomia restricted to specific categories of knowledge. Category specific semantic deficits have occurred in several different language tasks, implicating functional damage to semantic memory itself.

A categorical organization of semantic memory could be accomplished in several ways. One hypothesis is that word meanings are anatomically arranged so that different categories are located in different brain areas [Goodglass et al, 1966]. Another view suggests that categories of knowledge arise from different channels of physical or functional attributes that converge to form a computational representation of objects and subsequently categories [Warrington and Shallice, 1984; Warrington and McCarthy, 1987]. Further support for this view comes from Shallice [1988] who proposes isolatable semantic systems, including one encompassing the verbal domain. This verbal semantic system would purportedly contain categorical subdomains based upon the distinction between functional and perceptual properties.

Another approach, adapted from a more general model of cognitive processing, has been that objects are identified by their physical properties, the modality in which they are learned (e.g., touch, olfaction), and their frequency of occurrence [Damasio et al, 1990]. In this scheme, category knowledge in the lexical semantic system does not occur by explicit encoding in semantic category labels (e.g., animals, fruit and vegetables), but rather is a byproduct of the regularities of the physical features shared by similar objects.

In keeping with these proposals, it is possible that categories arise in semantic memory from the structure inherent within the more basic

Encoded objects
(57 total objects in 6 categories)
Animals (11)
Fruits and Vegetables (10)
Foods (6)
Transportation (10)
Household Items (10)
Tools (10)

Table 1: A list of the categories of physical objects used in the computational experiments, with an indication of how many objects are in each group. Note that while the objects are summarized by an intuitive class into which they fall, no category information was given to the networks.

information being encoded (e.g., in the semantic features). One plausible categorical organization may emerge from the distributed processing used to link items with their features. As an unexpected effect of this distributed processing, various kinds of neuronal injury (macroscopically diffuse or focal) could selectively affect different "categories" of knowledge. Consequently, the existence of category-specific deficits may not necessitate an explicit categorical partitioning nor a hierarchical, categorical organization of semantic memory. In this paper, we conduct several representational and mathematical experiments to test the computational validity of this hypothesis.

2. Methods

Fifty-seven pictures, each a line drawing of a single physical object, were encoded in terms of 77 semantic features. The pictures are predominantly a subset of those used by Hart and Gordon [1992] in their study of a patient with a category specific deficit, as listed in Table 1. (Appendix A lists all the objects represented).

These features were chosen based upon those used by Hinton and Shallice [1991] to describe precisely all 57 objects in the stimulus set. These features

Semantic Features
(77 Total Features of 11 Types)
Limbs (8)
Color (12)
Size (3)
Cross-Section (2)
Form (8)
Composition (8)
Texture (7)
Noise (3)
Function (10)
Location (11)
Movement (5)

Table 2: A list of the semantic feature types used in the computational experiments. In parentheses are the number of such feature values present in the encoding.

were also derived from several studies of patients with category specific anomias, where explicit knowledge of the features of items were assessed [Hart et al, 1985; Hart and Gordon, 1992]. The feature set was also chosen to depict adequately the specific items in the study based upon their perceptual qualities, physical attributes, motor associations, and functional/associative attributes deemed pertinent to describe the objects verbally. Idiosyncratic associates, features, or qualities were excluded. Table 2 lists the axes along which the specific features were selected. (The features themselves are shown in Appendix B).

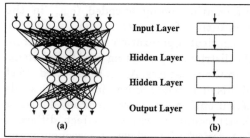

(a)   (b)

Figure 1: The structure of a connectionist (neural) network. Figure 1a shows a fully connected network with an input layer (on top), two hidden layers, and an output layer (on the bottom). All the units comprising each layer are shown explicitly. Figure 1b shows the same network drawn in a standard abbreviated manner.

We employ a connectionist (neural network) modelling approach for the computational studies (see [Small, 1994] for a review). A connectionist model consists of simple neuron-like *units of activation*, which communicate by sharing their activation with other such units to which they are connected. Each such *connection* has an associated strength, called a *weight*. Units thus compute a new level of activation by combining their previous level of activation with the information shared with them through these weighted connections. Input and output of a network are provided by *input units*, that are directly provided with activation levels, and *output units*, which contain the results of the network computation. All other units of activation are referred to as *hidden units* of activation.

A *layer* of units is a collection of activation units with the same pattern of

LIMBS-0	LIMBS-6	LIMBS-0
COLOR-brown	COLOR-green	COLOR-blue
COLOR-silver	SIZE-<1-foot	SIZE->1-foot-and-<2-yards
SIZE-<1-foot	CROSS-SECTION-circular	CROSS-SECTION-circular
CROSS-SECTION-rectangular	FORM-cylindrical	FORM-cylindrical
FORM-cylindrical	MADE-OF-from-animal	MADE-OF-from-animal
MADE-OF-wood	TEXTURE-smooth	TEXTURE-smooth
MADE-OF-metal	NOISE-makes-on-its-own	NOISE-makes-on-its-own
MADE-OF-other-manmade	FUNCTION-makes-waste	FUNCTION-makes-waste
TEXTURE-sharp	FUNCTION-reproduces	FUNCTION-esthetic
NOISE-with-input	LOCATION-yard	FUNCTION-reproduces
FUNCTION-repairs	LOCATION-woods	LOCATION-sea
LOCATION-basement	LOCATION-farm	MOVEMENT-self-moving
MOVEMENT-can-be-propelled	MOVEMENT-self-moving	MOVEMENT-grows
	MOVEMENT-grows	
	MOVEMENT-can-be-propelled	
(a) "Chisel"	(b) "Grasshopper"	(c) "Dolphin"

Figure 2: Semantic feature representations for two of the example pictures from the corpus used in the computational experiments, (a) a chisel; (b) a grasshopper; and (c) a dolphin. All the positive features are shown for both example objects. Note that none of the negative features are shown, although they play an important role in the naming process of the model. The semantic feature vector actually records either the presence and absence of each feature in the set.

receptive fields. Each network thus has a layer of input units, some layers of hidden units, and a layer of output units. Figure 1 shows the organization of such a network, showing connections between adjacent layers of input, hidden, and output units. The overall behavior of a model is determined by the pattern of connections, the weights on these connections, and the ways in which units compute their activation levels.

In our study, the units of the input layer and those of the output layer represent physical objects through specific codes. The simplest code consists of one unit for each object (e.g., motorcycle, dolphin), with a single unit permitted to be active at any time. We call this an *object identification code*, since it is used as the output layer of an identification network. The one active unit in such a code indicates the identification of a particular object. Another code consists of one unit for each semantic feature known to the system (e.g., blue, smooth texture). In this *semantic feature code*, multiple units are allowed to be active simultaneously. The active units in this code indicate the presence of specific semantic features in a particular object. A semantic feature code can be used as the input layer of an identification network. Figure 2 (a-b) shows the active feature units for the objects (a) "chisel" and (b) "grasshopper". (The units coding for other features have no activation).

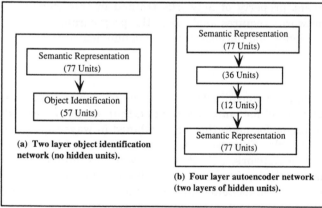

(a) Two layer object identification network (no hidden units).

(b) Four layer autoencoder network (two layers of hidden units).

The two different connectionist networks used in these experiments are shown in Figure 3 (a-b). Figure 3a shows a network that maps semantic feature codes onto object identification codes. The object identification task can be performed with a network having only input and output layers (no

Figure 3: Two connectionist networks that form the basis of the computational experiments and network analysis conducted. Figure 3a shows a two layer network, with a semantic feature vector as input and an object identification vector as output. Figure 3b shows a four layer autoencoder network, which has a semantic feature vector as both input and output. The hidden layers are much smaller in magnitude than the input layer, thus forcing the information encoded in the input layer to become compressed into a distributed code.

hidden units), whereas other complex mappings require hidden units [Rumelhart and McClelland, 1986]. Figure 3b shows an autoassociative network, where the semantic feature codes of the objects are transformed into a distributed code of hidden units prior to being reconstituted back to themselves. Since the intermediate units are far fewer in number than the input units, the input data becomes compressed into a compact distributed form. While it would be imprudent to suggest that the brain uses exactly these structures to perform naming, it is certainly possible that the brain uses some distributed encoding of such knowledge, and for this reason, we believe that investigation of such encodings is valuable.

The networks of Figures 3a-b were trained using a version of the back propagation algorithm [Rumelhart et al, 1985; Fahlman, 1988], which taught the networks to perform the correct mappings by adjusting their connection weights to produce the desired transformations.

How do the networks achieve this result? In the identification network of Figure 3a, the internal functioning of the network is a product of the direct connections from input units to output units. However, the autoassociative network of Figure 3b contains intermediate layers of hidden units between the input and output. When the input unit activations permeate the network, they produce a pattern of values on the hidden units in addition to the desired pattern on the output layer. As this hidden layer of values is not pre-coded, it constitutes an emergent property of networks trained in this way. Thus understanding the networks requires analysis of the preprogrammed input codes, the connection weights, and the emergent hidden unit activations.

3. Analysis

A number of techniques are available for analysis of these codes. Such analysis is particularly useful for units of activation that are not pre-coded, such as the hidden units, or for units that are combined in ways that make them otherwise inaccessible. Five methods were used for analyzing the representations of these networks: (1) direct network examination; (2) hierarchical clustering analysis; (3) unsupervised learning; (4) dependency analysis; and (5) principal components analysis. Each provides separate insights into the hypothesized character of word meanings in the brain.

3.1 Analysis of Feature Codes

The first step involved analysis of the feature representation itself, apart from its specific use in the network models. Three methods of examining these features were employed, including direct examination of these vectors as points in a geometrical space, hierarchical clustering analysis, and competitive learning. Each method of analysis demonstrated commonalities among semantically related items. While one would expect the code for "apple" to be similar to the code for "pear", these analyses revealed numerical measures of just how close each object was to every other. Evaluation of these data demonstrate the extent to which categorical knowledge constitutes an implicit property of the feature based object representations.

3.2 Analysis of Network Behavior

The second step in the analysis involved examination of the connectionist networks that manipulated these codes. The network of Figure 3a that performed the mapping of features to objects was analyzed using a network analysis technique we call "dependency analysis" [Small and Nguyen, 1994].

For each physical object in the corpus, certain features appeared to play a particularly important role in determining its identification. Dependency analysis of the object identification network (Figure 3a) revealed, for example, that whereas the semantic representation of a typical object consists of a dozen or more semantic features (e.g., "dolphin" has fourteen features as shown in Figure 2c), very few of them play a major role in identification. Each object differs in the particular features most important for its identification.

Dependency analysis thus provides a way to understand how a network evolves during the training period, with particular processing units dependent more on the activations of some units than others, despite static connectivity patterns that are similar. It is particularly useful in studying the most complex neural networks, because as an empirical rather than analytical technique, it depends on the functioning rather than the structural details of the network. In multilayer neural networks, it allows the user to study how each unit in a given layer affects each unit in any successive layer, thus revealing information not straightforwardly available from the weights themselves (which would give the same information in systems without hidden layers). In recurrent networks, any unit can be analyzed with respect any number of other units to assess the strength of their dependencies.

The dependency index of output j to an input i, DI_{ji} is the measurement of the extent to which output j is related to changes in input i. In other words, it represents the *dependency* of the final state of output j upon changes in the value of input i.

To obtain DI_{ji} we first train a network using the training input and output patterns, the *standard* sets of values. After the network has converged, we then present it with new test patterns to obtain new output patterns, the *new* sets of values. The new test patterns are generated by taking each input pattern and varying input i over the range of $\{y_{io}, y_{in}\}$ while keeping the remainder of the input units constant. For input pattern p, DI_{ji}^p is calculated as

116

the mean of the ratio of the percentage change in output j to the percentage change in input i, or

$$DI_{ji}^p = \frac{\sum_{x=0}^{x=n} \frac{(y_{jx} - y_{js})/y_{js}}{(y_{ix} - y_{is})/y_{is}}}{n} \quad (1)$$

where y_{ix} is the new value of input i, y_{jx} is the new value of output j obtained using the modified input pattern p that contained y_{ix}, and y_{js} and y_{is} are the standard values of output j and input i for input pattern p, respectively. Finally, the mean of DI_{ji}^p over all input patterns is calculated to give us the final value of DI_{ji},

$$DI_{ji} = \overline{DI_{ji}^p} \quad (2)$$

Thus, once a network is completely trained, each input value (i.e., semantic feature) is varied, while all other values are held constant, and the output (i.e. physical object) recorded. The graphs of these conditions illustrate the importance of each semantic feature in correctly naming each physical object. Note that this characterization does not depend on the number of objects or the number of features in the network.

3.3 Analysis of Hidden Unit Codes

The autoassociative network of Figure 3b compresses and distributes information across two layers of hidden units. Two hidden layers permits greater compression and distribution of information than would a single such layer, and also leads to greater complexity in the nature of the transformation. [Cottrell et al, 1987]. These hidden units were examined both directly [Hinton, 1986] and through an eigenvector analysis [Fukunaga, 1972; Press et al, 1989] with examination of principal components [Elman, 1990]. This *principal components analysis* characterizes the distributed information used by the network to produce desired

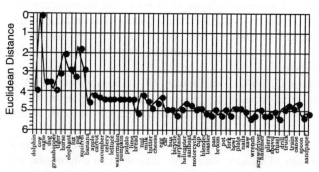

Figure 4: Direct examination of the semantic feature representation as plots on a typical (Euclidean) coordinate system. This plot illustrates the distance from the semantic representation of "cow" to the representation of each other physical object in the experimental corpus.

outputs for particular inputs. In these networks of word meanings, this analysis revealed whether the network used particular commonalities of the feature codes in performing its task.

4. Results

4.1 Direct Network Examination

The input layer of units, i.e., the semantic feature code, was analyzed in simple linear algebraic terms to determine relative distances between objects when plotted in a large dimensional geometric space. Figure 4 compares the location of "cow" to other objects in the experimental corpus. Note that the distances between "cow" and other animals are generally shorter than between "cow" and members of other categories (e.g., fruits and vegetables, tools). For each semantic code of an object, there is greater similarity between objects from a single category than objects from different categories. While this similarity relationship holds in general, Figure 4 also illustrates its imprecision, giving category membership an inexact character.

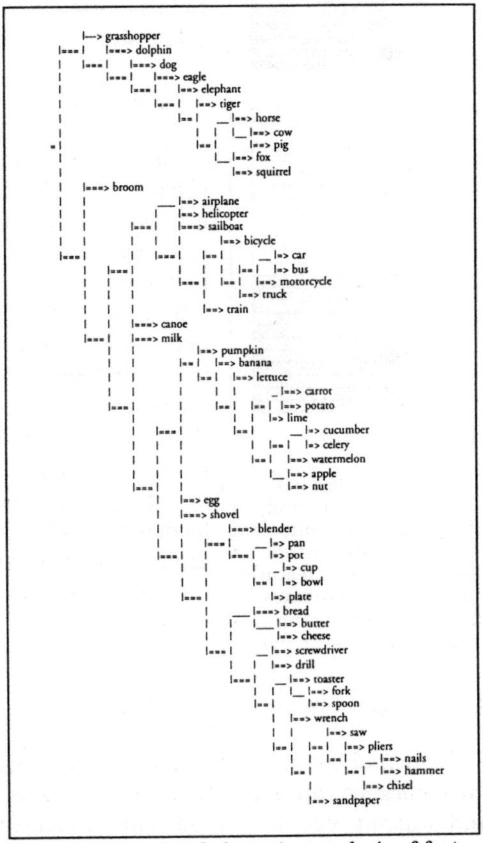

4.2 Hierarchical Clustering Analysis

Figure 5 shows the results of a hierarchical clustering analysis [Tou and Gonzalez, 1974] of the semantic feature code. This method creates a tree

```
                    |--> grasshopper
     |===|   |===> dolphin
     |      |===|    |===> dog
     |      |===|    |===|    |===> eagle
     |      |   |===|    |== |===> elephant
     |      |        |===|  |===> tiger
     |      |             |==|   __|==> horse
     |      |             |   |  |_|==> cow
    -|      |             |==|   |==> pig
     |      |             |_|==> fox
     |      |                  |==> squirrel
     |      |===> broom
     |   |                 __ |==> airplane
     |   |           |    |==> helicopter
     |   |         |===|   |===> sailboat
     |   |         |   |  |  |==> bicycle
     |===|   |     |===| |== |   __|==> car
     |   |===|     | | | |==| |==> bus
     |   |   |     |==| |==|  |===> motorcycle
     |   |   |          |   |==> truck
     |   |   |          |==> train
     |   |   |===> canoe
     |===|   |===> milk
     |   |                 |==> pumpkin
     |   |            |==| |==> banana
     |   |            |  |==| |==> lettuce
     |   |            |   | | |   _|===> carrot
     |===|      |     |==| |==| |==> potato
     |   |===|  |     |   |   | | |==> lime
     |   |   |==|     |==|   __|==> cucumber
     |   |   |           |==| |==> celery
     |   |   |           |==| |==> watermelon
     |===|   |                |__|==> apple
     |   |                   |__|==> nut
     |   |==> egg
     |   |===> shovel
     |   |              |===> blender
     |   |       |===|    __|==> pan
     |===|       |===| |==> pot
     |   |           |   |_|==> cup
     |   |           |==| |=> bowl
     |===|              |==> plate
                 __ |===> bread
             |__|   |===> butter
             |      |===> cheese
     |===|   |===> screwdriver
         | | |==> drill
     |===|   __|==> toaster
         | | |_|==> fork
     |==|    |===> spoon
        |    |==> wrench
        |        |==> saw
     |==|   |==| |==> pliers
         | |  | |==| |==> nails
     |==|  |==| |__|  |===> hammer
        |              |==> chisel
                 |==> sandpaper
```

Figure 5: Hierarchical clustering analysis of feature based representation of physical objects. The analysis results in a tree structure, with more similar objects shown on adjacent branches and less similar objects drawn on more distant branches.

118

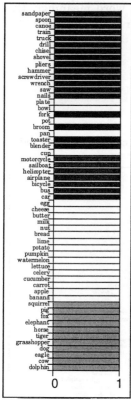

0   1

Figure 6: Result of competitive learning of groupings for physical objects represented in terms of semantic features. Each color indicates a separate grouping of objects (total four groups).

structure, where the items on adjacent branches of the tree have more in common than elements on branches farther apart. With some obvious exceptions (e.g., canoe and milk), this technique also groups the objects in a way that corresponds to our intuitive concept of semantic relatedness, with words having common meanings closer together than those with quite different meanings. In particular, note that animals, vehicles, and fruits and vegetables are clustered into distinct subtrees of the hierarchy. Small household tools and kitchen items are merged into a slightly more heterogeneous cluster.

4.3 Competitive Learning

In competitive learning, a network learns to classify the input vectors into a number of distinct groups based on their relatedness, with each output unit representing one of the groups. We constructed networks that used the algorithm of Rumelhart and Zipser [1985] to sort the feature vectors into four, six, and ten such groups, with similar results in each case (i.e., only four groupings were made regardless of the number of output units). Figure 6 shows the results of this classification, with approximate groupings of hand tools, vehicles, animals, and a fourth grouping including fruits and vegetables, cooking utensils, and food items. With one overly broad category, these groupings otherwise correspond generally to our intuition about the natural categories of the input objects.

4.4 Principal Components Analysis

Principal components analysis [Fukunaga, 1972] was used to investigate the emergent representations of the autoassociative network. While the input and output vectors of an autoassociative network are the same, the intermediate layers can be interesting since they encode the same information in a highly compressed and distributed form. The second hidden layer of our network of Figure 3b encodes all the information of the 77 unit input layer in only 12 units.

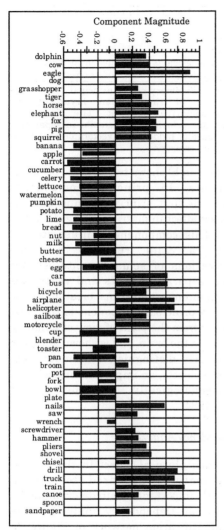

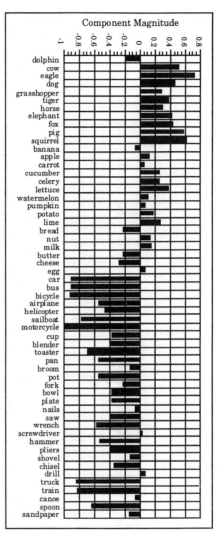

Figure 7: Principal components analysis of the hidden layer of the autoassociative network. Figure 7a shows the magnitude of each object in the experimental corpus along axis defined by the first principal component. Figure 7b shows the magnitude of each object along the axis defined by the fourth principal component. These components demonstrate that even in a distributed compressed encoding of semantic knowledge, certain category distinctions are preserved, and that these categories correspond to those found in empirical studies of human subjects.

Table 3 shows the discriminations performed by the five highest ranked principal components for this highly compressed (hidden) layer of the autoencoder network. These principal components make interesting discriminations, of which four encode for standard categories, including animals and hand tools. The other principal component (#2) distinguishes six seemingly unrelated objects from the rest.

Principal Component Discriminations		
1	animals	plants
2	(6 objects)	other objects
3	animals	plants
4	animate objects	inanimate objects
5	hand tools	other objects

Table 3: Summary of the principal components analysis of the hidden layer of the autoassociative network: The five most important principal components in separating this space of hidden unit vectors demonstrates emergent categories.

Figure 7 (a-b) shows two of these principal components. In principal components analysis, the first principal component has the largest effect in discriminating the input objects. This component is illustrated in Figure 7a, and results in some categorizations of semantic interest, for example, separating fruits and vegetables from both animals and transportation items. The fourth principal component is the most interesting from the point of view of semantic knowledge in the brain, and is shown in Figure 7b. It clearly distinguishes animate from inanimate objects, an important dissociation neuropsychologically [Warrington and Shallice, 1984].

4.5 Dependency Analysis

For each physical object in the corpus, certain features appeared to play a particularly important role in determining its identification. Dependency analysis of the object identification network of Figure 3a revealed, for example, that whereas the semantic representation of such an item as "dolphin" consists of a dozen or more semantic features (see Figure 2c), very few of them play a major role in identification. Each

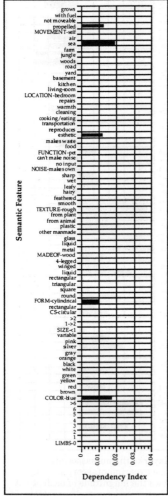

Figure 8: Dependency analysis of the object identification network, showing the indices for "dolphin".

object differs in the particular features most important for its identification.

Figure 8 plots the dependency indices of output unit "dolphin" to the 77 input units (i.e., semantic features) from the object identification network. The network made its decision based primarily on the following features:

COLOR = "blue"
FORM = "cylindrical"
FUNCTION = "esthetic"
LOCATION = "sea"
MOVEMENT = "propelled"

The results clearly indicated that out of the 77 input features, the network recognized five semantic features to be the most indicative of object "dolphin". Nine additional features composing the full semantic representation of "dolphin" do not arise at this level of analysis. While the feature MOVEMENT = "propelled" was not one of the positive features encoded in the input pattern for output "dolphin", the network takes into consideration both negative and positive features of the object for identification purposes. Thus, analysis of the object identification network with Dependency Analysis provides a way to determine the most characteristic and discriminating features of particular entities, given the specific task requested. The characteristic features identified by DA and those found through empirical study [Rosch, 1975] may have some theoretical relationship.

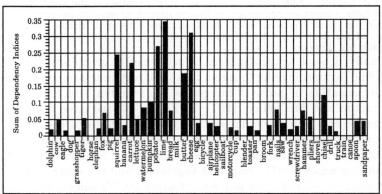

Figure 9: Dependency analysis demonstrates the significance of certain semantic features in performing object identification. In this case, the sum of dependency indices for all COLOR features with respect to the all physical objects represented in the output shows the relative importance of COLOR in the identification of fruits and vegetables over other types of objects.

Dependency analysis can be turned around to examine the individual features used to identify the objects. By grouping the features into classes (e.g., COLOR), associated with verbal system instantiations of particular perceptual, motor, or cognitive modalities, this method can ascertain the most important feature types (and by inference, modalities) in identifying the individual objects. Figure 9 shows the dependency analysis for all COLOR features with respect to each object in the output set. Of particular interest is that identification of fruits and vegetables depends more on aspects of COLOR than does identification of objects in other categories.

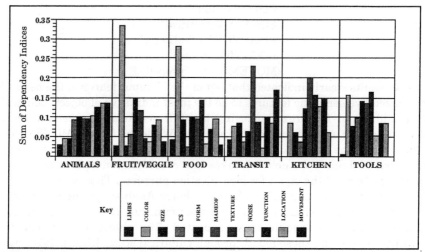

Figure 10: Dependency analysis demonstrates the role of particular semantic feature sets in defining (imprecisely) semantic category groupings of the input objects. Of particular interest are the categories that (a) depend strongly on one or two feature types (e.g., foods depend on color); (b) depend very little on particular feature types (e.g., kitchen items do not depend on movement); and (c) depend on most feature types equally (e.g., animals).

Finally, dependency analysis can be performed on groupings of objects and individual features in order to assess the role of particular semantic features in the organization of natural categories [Warrington and Shallice, 1984; Warrington and McCarthy, 1987]. In Figure 10, we have organized the physical objects into categories and the features into feature sets, and then analyzed the dependencies of each semantic category on each feature set. The dependencies in each category have been normalized to a constant sum. Note that in this analysis, the fruits and vegetables and the other foods depend much more on color than on any other feature set. Vehicles depend more on their composition and characteristics of movement than on other features. Tools and kitchen items depend almost not at all on their number of limbs or movement. Identification of animals depends on a variety of features, without a single predominant contribution.

5. Discussion

The present computational study demonstrates that category specific cognitive behavior can be the byproduct of a representation of physical objects in terms of their semantic features. In the brain, such features constitute a verbal encoding of information that can be concurrently represented in basic perceptual and motor modalities. Although the study shows that object identification for particular categories depends more on certain groups of features than others, it also points out (a) how such apparent categories might arise without any explicit knowledge of the categories themselves; and (b) that the boundaries between categories of features (typically related to particular modalities) and between categories of physical objects can be imprecise.

Each of these characteristics provides valuable flexibility to the human semantic memory of words and their meanings. Different people may classify objects differently, and the same person may change his/her classification over time. If objects are classified by their features, these may change as new features are learned. This imprecision in category boundaries leads to flexibility in use of concepts. Is a knife a weapon or a kitchen utensil? Is a round kitchen container a bowl or a cup? Suppose it has a handle? Suppose it gets wider and wider? [Labov, 1973; Caramazza et al, 1982] We argue that categorical knowledge can be an implicit property of knowledge of features, and that imprecision in the precise composition of specific categories follows as a direct consequence.

Of the five experiments conducted, three investigated the encodings of physical objects through their semantic features, without regard to a specific use in artificial neural networks. Despite the use of three different techniques of analysis, the results were similar, demonstrating that such a semantic feature representation can implicitly encode relationships among the physical objects that may not be completely apparent by direct examination. In fact, the objects are shown to self organize into categories, whether analyzed by hierarchical clustering or competitive learning or even direct plotting on a coordinate grid.

The assumptions underlying any proposed organization of word meanings for object naming have implications for the overall architecture of semantic memory. In order to investigate the consequences of encoding objects in terms of their semantic features, two experiments were conducted with artificial neural networks. The first was a principal components analysis, used to determine the presence of highly compressed information within a hidden layer of an autoassociative network. Despite their integrated compressed nature, these hidden unit activations implicitly encode category specificity in a way that parallels the data on human language processing [Damasio, 1990]. The highest ranked principal components for these particular features appear to encode for animate objects, fruits and vegetables, and small household tools, exactly those categories that have been found in studies of patients with (typically bilateral temporal lobe) brain damage. In the second experiment, a dependency analysis of an object identification network demonstrated that particular features of objects were more important for their identification than others.

The features used in identification, and objects for which they are most relevant, are not discrete sets that are identical for everyone. Labov [1973] suggests that human categories have such an inexact character, and Rosch [1975] shows how human categories might be manifested in different individuals. In our computational formulation, categories depend on the particular set of semantic features and objects known to the system. Certainly within an individual or a single computer system, category boundaries and membership criteria are both idiosyncratic and imprecise.

5.1 Category Specific Impairments

The categories produced in the mathematical analyses have natural analogues in the world. The groupings of "animals", "fruits and vegetables", "tools", and "vehicles" seem to appear in the results of each form of analysis. Other food items and kitchen items sort out slightly differently depending on the technique of analysis. These categories that exist implicitly in the feature vectors are precisely the categories that appear to exist in human behavior, particularly the category specific impairments occurring after brain injury.

Observed loss of one or more language skills related to particular categories of semantic knowledge has motivated discussion of categorical organization. Category-specific deficits have been reported in reading [Warrington, 1981], object naming [Hart et al, 1985; Sartori and Job, 1988], and comprehension [Warrington and Shallice, 1984; Warrington and McCarthy, 1987]. Selective deficits have been demonstrated in particular patients to such categories as concrete objects [Warrington, 1981], inanimate objects [Warrington and McCarthy, 1983] animate objects [Warrington and Shallice, 1984], animals, fruits, and vegetables [Sartori and Job, 1988], fruits and vegetables [Hart et al, 1985], and animals [Hart and Gordon, 1992]. These patients typically have neurological damage involving the left temporal lobe or both temporal lobes.

5.2 Neurological Localization of Categories

Existing evidence from case studies of human language impairment suggests that the anatomical location of semantic feature representations may incorporate both temporal lobes [Pietrini et al, 1988; Sartori and Job, 1988; Hart and Gordon, 1992]. Most reported cases of category specific impairments were caused by bilateral temporal lobe injury, although other examples have arisen in the context of left hemisphere infarction [Warrington and McCarthy, 1983; Hart et al, 1985] or anterior left temporal lobe lesions [Damasio et al, 1990]. Most such patients have had herpes encephalitis [Pietrini et al, 1988; Sartori and Job, 1988], a viral infection that causes diffuse cortical and limbic system damage, particularly involving hemorrhagic infarctions in the temporal lobes [Damasio and van Hoesen, 1985; Price, 1986]. In a recent case, semantic memory loss of animal knowledge was caused by an antibody-mediated paraneoplastic syndrome including both temporal lobes [Hart and Gordon, 1992].

Recent attempts at functional neuroanatomical localizations for aspects of naming have met with great difficulty. Anatomical variability both within and among individuals has been a feature of studies of direct cortical stimulation during naming [Whitaker and Ojemann, 1977; Ojemann et al, 1989; Gordon et al, 1990]. Functional neuroimaging has successfully localized certain visual and auditory components involved in lexical processing [Petersen et al, 1988; Petersen et al, 1990; Howard et al, 1992], but it has been difficult to localize word meanings and other higher-order associative aspects of language processing [Steinmetz and Seitz, 1991; Wise et al, 1991; Small et al, 1994], precisely the type of knowledge that may have a distributed basis.

The rarity of category specific impairments, its frequent co-occurrence with bilateral temporal lobe damage, and the intractability of neuroanatomical localization of aspects of lexical semantic memory using functional techniques, suggests that semantic features may be encoded redundantly and in a distributed fashion throughout the temporal lobes. While primary perceptual and motor functions localize to specific areas of the brain, such as vision in the striate cortex, and oculomotion to several well demarcated areas in the brainstem, parietal lobes, and frontal lobes, the above evidence from cognitive neuroscience suggests that aspects of semantic memory for words may not localize as precisely [Wise et al, 1991]. The distributed representations suggested by the computational experiments described in this paper provide a first step in understanding how this might be neurally encoded.

5.3 Alternative Conceptions

Selective language impairments within semantic categories suggests that in some way human semantic memory respects category information in its internal organization. However, various elaborations on this concept that range from hierarchical to fully distributed are possible. One such conception provides for semantic knowledge to be encoded in a network of semantic nodes [Collins and Quillian, 1969]. Each node encodes a unit of semantic knowledge (e.g., animal, bird, wing) which is organized hierarchically within the network from a feature (e.g., wing) to basic object (e.g., bird) to superordinate category (e.g., animal) levels. Evidence for such a hierarchical network extends from reaction time studies showing that time of semantic processing is related to the number of nodes traversed in the network [Collins and Quillian, 1969]. The presence of neurons with highly tuned receptive fields, in some cases apparently consisting of single units of knowledge [Barlow, 1972; Perrett et al, 1982; Desimone et al, 1985] suggests such an explicit nodal representation of features, objects and categories can be possible in the brain.

Alternatively, Shallice has proposed multiple semantic systems with a distinct verbal semantic subsystem that provides for an internal categorical organization [Shallice, 1988]. The underlying structure for word meanings within this verbal semantic system has been modelled computationally with semantic features mapped through a distributed network into an attractor space [Hinton and Shallice, 1991]. In this conception, the activity pattern of the semantic feature units encodes a word's meaning.

Other studies within the framework advanced by Shallice have specified aspects of the underlying structure of a broadly defined semantic system. For example, Warrington and McCarthy [1987] have proposed multiple such systems encompassing each sensory modality, including language, with categorical organization. These investigators suggest that object comprehension depends on information from all semantic systems, including physical and functional attributes as well as sensory and motor information.

Within the encoding of features for a given object in a semantic subsystem, each unit of feature information is differentially weighted depending upon its saliency for identifying each particular object. By implication from this account, the subsystem that is the focus of our study, i.e., the semantic memory for words, must represent functional and physical attributes in this manner. The findings of our simulations are generally consistent with this view, especially the weighting of all semantic features that are emergent in a network simulation. In addition, the dependency analysis for each feature set (e.g., color) for all categories clearly demonstrates the network's differential representation of a category by a feature (e.g., color for fruits and vegetables) as Warrington and McCarthy postulated.

Damasio and colleagues have further refined this approach by suggesting that man-made objects can be distinguished from living things on a recognition level by the encoding of (1) physical structure; (2) sensorimotor route of learning and object use; and (3) frequency [Damasio et al, 1990]. Natural groupings or subcategorizations emerge based on these three factors within a given modality (e.g., language, vision). Each modality's subcategories may then overlap to yield the conceptual semantic categories that are seen in patients with category-specific deficits. While this model encompasses multiple aspects of cognitive processing and is general in description and specification, it is supported by the outcome of our demonstrations. In essence, our semantic processing demonstration encodes for the language modality aspect of their model, producing the type of emergent subcategorizations that are proposed.

The current evidence from our study of computation does not prove or disprove these alternative hypotheses about semantic memory organization. It simply suggests that a significant degree of semantic memory organization could devolve naturally from the demands of a system that encodes features of objects.

5.4 Weaknesses of the Approach

There are certainly weaknesses of our current theory and demonstration models. First, they are not aimed to explain in detail the neural circuitry involved in semantic memory representations. An account of this complex circuitry awaits further studies of the neuroanatomy, such as those using cortical electrode stimulation [Hart et al, 1992] or functional neuroimaging [Howard et al, 1992; Schneider et al, 1993; Small et al, 1994]. As such data emerges, attempts to build neural network models with more accurate portrayal of neuroanatomy may improve upon the present discussion.

A second weakness of the computational demonstration, and one that we are actively trying to improve, is in the semantic feature representations themselves. While the analyses of these features present robust information, they do depend on how exhaustive and comprehensive the input feature data is. A similar set of analysis techniques can be applied to a richer set of lexical-semantic features and a fuller set of objects, more like those of the human cognitive system. For example, determination of the most characteristic features of a particular object (see previous discussion of dependency analysis) within a larger object set would thus be dependent on the number of features processed and the number of objects that must be discriminated between.

It is not clear at present how these semantic representations relate to the basic perceptual or motor processes that must intervene from other sensory or motor modalities [Damasio, 1990]. Improving theoretical notions on the relationship between perception and semantics, based on empirical studies that interrelate the two, will serve to clarify the issues surrounding categories of knowledge, categories of features, and perceptual modalities. Questions on this topic have been the focus of hotly contested debates [Riddoch et al, 1988; Sartori and Job, 1988; Shallice, 1988].

6. Conclusion

The computational study and results presented here provide one explanation for the cognitive neurological manifestations of diseases such as herpes simplex encephalitis that affect primarily the temporal neocortex and limbic system. The computational evidence demonstrates that if physical objects are encoded in terms of their features, categorical information emerges, without any explicit semantic memory for categories. Furthermore, a distributed and redundant encoding of this knowledge suggests an explanation for the rarity of category specific impairments.

7. Acknowledgments

This work was supported by the National Institute of Deafness and other Communication Disorders (NIDCD) of the National Institutes of Health (NIH) under a Clinical Investigator Development Award (K08-DC-00054) to the first author and (K08-DC-00099) to the second author. The following people provided tremendous assistance in reading and critiquing earlier drafts of the manuscript and this is greatly appreciated: Rita Sloan Berndt, Anthony Harris, Gloria E. Hoffman, Audrey L. Holland, Laurie Knepper, and Oscar M. Reinmuth. Elissa Kinch provided invaluable technical support in encoding the feature sets.

8. References

Barlow HB. Single Units and Sensation: A Neuron Doctrine for Perceptual Psychology. Perception 1972;1:371-394.

Caramazza A, Berndt RS, Brownell HH. The Semantic Deficit Hypothesis: Perceptual Parsing and Object Classification by Aphasic Patients. Brain Lang 1982;15:161-189.

Collins AM, Quillian MR. Retrieval Time from Semantic Memory. J Verb Learn Verb Behav 1969;8:240-247.

Cottrell GW, Munro P, Zipser D. Learning Internal Representations from Grey Scale Images: An Example of Extensional Programming. Proceedings of the Ninth Annual Conference of the Cognitive Science Society. Seattle, Washington: Lawrence Erlbaum Associates, 1987:462-473.

Damasio AR. Category-Related Recognition Defects as a Clue to the Neural Substrates of Knowledge. Trend Neurosci 1990;13:95-98.

Damasio AR, Damasio H, Tranel D, Brandt JP. Neural Regionalization of Knowledge Access: Preliminary Evidence. Cold Spring Harbor Symposia on Quantitative Biology: Cold Spring Harbor Laboratory Press, 1990:1039-1047.

Damasio AR, van Hoesen GW. The Limbic System and the Localization of Herpes Simplex Encephalitis. J Neurol Neurosurg Psychiatry 1985;48:297-301.

Desimone R, Schein SJ, Moran J, Ungerleider LG. Contour, Color, and Shape Analysis Beyond the Striate Cortex. Vision Res 1985;25(3):441-452.

Elman JL. Finding Structure in Time. Cog Sci 1990;14:179-211.

Fahlman SE. Faster-learning Variations on Back-propagation: An Empirical Study. Proceedings of 1988 Connectionist Models Summer School. San Mateo, California: Morgan Kaufmann Publishers, 1988:38-51.

Fukunaga K. Introduction to Statistical Pattern Recognition. New York: Academic Press, 1972.

Goodglass H, Klein B, Carey P, Jones K. Specific Semantic Word Categories in Aphasia. Cortex 1966;2:74-89.

Gordon B, Hart J, Lesser R, et al. Individual Variations in Perisylvian Language Representation. Neurology 1990;40 (Supplement 1)(4):172.

Hart J, Jr., Berndt RS, Caramazza A. Category-Specific Naming Deficit following Cerebral Infarction. Nature 1985;316:439-440.

Hart J, Jr., Gordon B. Neural Subsystems for Object Knowledge. Nature 1992;359:60-64.

Hart J, Jr., Lesser RP, Gordon B. Selective Interference with the Representation of Size in the Human by Direct Cortical Electrical Stimulation. J Cog Neurosci 1992;4(4):337-344.

Hinton GE. Learning Distributed Representations of Concepts. Proceedings of the Eighth Annual Meeting of the Cognitive Science Society: Lawrence Erlbaum Associates, 1986:1-12.

Hinton GE, Shallice T. Lesioning an Attractor Network: Investigations of Acquired Dyslexia. Psych Rev 1991;98(1):74-95.

Howard D, Patterson K, Wise R, et al. The Cortical Localization of the Lexicons: Positron Emission Tomography Evidence. Brain 1992;115:1769-1782.

Labov W. The Boundaries of Words and their Meanings. In: Bailey C-JN, Shuy RW, eds. New Ways of Analyzing Variation in English. Washington, D. C.: Georgetown University Press, 1973:340-373.

Ojemann G, Ojemann J, Lettich E, Berger M. Cortical Language Localization in Left, Dominant Hemisphere: An Electrical Stimulation Mapping Investigation in 117 Patients. J Neurosurg 1989;71:316-326.

Perrett DI, Rolls ET, Caan W. Visual Neurones Responsive to Faces in the Monkey Temporal Cortex. Experimental Brain Research 1982;47:329-342.

Petersen SE, Fox PT, Posner MI, Mintun MA, Raichle ME. Positron Emission Tomographic Studies of the Cortical Anatomy of Single-Word Processing. Nature 1988;331:585-589.

Petersen SE, Fox PT, Snyder AZ, Raichle ME. Activation of Extrastriate and Frontal Cortical Areas by Visual Words and Word-Like Stimuli. Science 1990;249:1041-1043.

Pietrini V, Nertempi P, Vaglia A, Revello MG, Pinna V, Ferro-Milone F. Recovery from Herpes Simplex Encephalitis: Selective Impairment of Specific Semantic Categories with Neuroradiological Correlation. J Neurol Neurosurg Psychiatry 1988;51:1284-1293.

Press WH, Flannery BP, Teukolsky SA, Vetterling WT. Numerical Recipes in Pascal: The Art of Scientific Computing. Cambridge: Cambridge University Press, 1989.

Price RW. Neurobiology of Human Herpesvirus Infections. CRC Cr Rev Clin Neuro 1986;2(1):61-123.

Riddoch MJ, Humphreys GW, Coltheart M, Funnell E. Semantic Systems or System? Neuropsychological Evidence Re-examined. Cog Neuropsych 1988;5(1):3-25.

Rosch E. Cognitive Representations of Semantic Categories. J Exp Psy Gen 1975;104(3):192-233.

Rumelhart DE, Hinton GE, Williams RJ. Learning Internal Representations by Error Propagation. Report # ICS-8506, Institute for Cognitive Science: University of California San Diego, 1985.

Rumelhart DE, McClelland JL. Parallel Distributed Processing: Explorations in the Microstructure of Cognition: Volume 1: Foundations. Cambridge, Massachusetts: The MIT Press, 1986.

Rumelhart DE, Zipser D. Feature Discovery by Competitive Learning. Cog Sci 1985;9:95-112.

Sartori G, Job R. The Oyster with Four Legs: A Neuropsychological Study on the Interaction of Visual and Semantic Information. Cog Neuropsych 1988;5(1):105-132.

Schneider W, Noll D, Cohen J. Functional Topographic Mapping of the Cortical Ribbon in Human Vision with Conventional MRI Scanners. Nature 1993;365(September 9, 1993):150-154.

Shallice T. Specialisation Within the Semantic System. Cog Neuropsych 1988;5(1):133-142.

Small SL. Connectionist Networks and Language Disorders. J Comm Dis 1994;27:305-323.

Small SL, Nguyen T. Dependency Analysis: Assessing the Functional Relationships among Processing Units in Artificial Neural Networks. World Congress on Neural Networks. San Diego, California: IEEE Press, 1994:506-511.

Small SL, Noll DC, Perfetti CA, Xu B, Schneider W. Activation of Left Frontal Operculum and Motor Cortex with Functional MRI of Language Processing (abstract). Society for Neuroscience Abstracts 1994;20:6.

Steinmetz H, Seitz RJ. Functional Anatomy of Language Processing: Neuroimaging and the Problem of Individual Variability. Neuropsychologia 1991;29(12):1149-1161.

Tou JT, Gonzalez RC. Pattern Recognition Principles. New York: Addison Wesley Publishing Company, 1974.

Warrington EK. Concrete Word Dyslexia. Br J Psych 1981;72:175-196.

Warrington EK, McCarthy R. Category Specific Access Dysphasia. Brain 1983;106:859-878.

Warrington EK, McCarthy R. Categories of Knowledge: Further Fractionation and an Attempted Integration. Brain 1987;110:1273-1296.

Warrington EK, Shallice T. Category Specific Semantic Impairments. Brain 1984;102:43-63.

Whitaker HA, Ojemann GA. Graded Localization of Naming from Electrical Stimulation Mapping of Left Cerebral Cortex. Nature 1977;270(5632):50-51.

Wise R, Chollet F, Hadar U, Friston K, Hoffner E, Frackowiak R. Distribution of Cortical Neural Networks Involved in Word Comprehension and Word Retrieval. Brain 1991;114:1803-1817.

Appendix A: Complete list of physical objects used in the computational study (in alphabetical order)

airplane	milk
apple	motorcycle
banana	nails
bicycle	nut
blender	pan
bowl	pig
bread	plate
broom	pliers
bus	pot
butter	potato
canoe	pumpkin
car	sailboat
carrot	sandpaper
celery	saw
cheese	screwdriver
chisel	shovel
cow	spoon
cucumber	squirrel
cup	tiger
dog	toaster
dolphin	train
drill	truck
eagle	watermelon
egg	wrench
elephant	
fork	
fox	
grasshopper	
hammer	
helicopter	
horse	
lettuce	
lime	

Appendix B: Complete list of semantic features used to encode objects for the computational study (in order of position in semantic vectors)

LIMBS-0	MADE-OF-from-animal
LIMBS-1	MADE-OF-from-plant
LIMBS-2	TEXTURE-rough
LIMBS-3	TEXTURE-smooth
LIMBS-4	TEXTURE-feathered
LIMBS-5	TEXTURE-hairy
LIMBS-6	TEXTURE-leafy
LIMBS->6	TEXTURE-wet
COLOR-blue	TEXTURE-sharp
COLOR-brown	NOISE-makes-on-its-own
COLOR-red	NOISE-can-make-noise-with-input
COLOR-yellow	NOISE-can't-make-noise
COLOR-green	FUNCTION-pet
COLOR-white	FUNCTION-food
COLOR-black	FUNCTION-makes-waste
COLOR-orange	FUNCTION-esthetic
COLOR-gray	FUNCTION-reproduces
COLOR-silver	FUNCTION-transportation
COLOR-pink	FUNCTION-cooking-and-or-eating
COLOR-variable	FUNCTION-cleaning
SIZE-<1-foot	FUNCTION-warmth
SIZE->1-foot-and-<2-yards	FUNCTION-repairs
SIZE->2-yards	LOCATION-bedroom
CROSS-SECTION-circular	LOCATION-living-room
CROSS-SECTION-rectangular	LOCATION-kitchen
FORM-cylindrical	LOCATION-basement
FORM-round	LOCATION-yard
FORM-square	LOCATION-road
FORM-triangular	LOCATION-woods
FORM-rectangular	LOCATION-jungle
FORM-liquid	LOCATION-farm
FORM-winged	LOCATION-sea
FORM-four-legged	LOCATION-air
MADE-OF-wood	MOVEMENT-self-moving
MADE-OF-metal	MOVEMENT-can-be-propelled
MADE-OF-liquid	MOVEMENT-not-moveable
MADE-OF-glass	MOVEMENT-can-move-with-fuel
MADE-OF-other-manmade	MOVEMENT-grows
MADE-OF-plastic	

LANGUAGE
DISORDERS

A CONNECTIONIST MODEL OF NAMING ERRORS IN APHASIA

GARY S. DELL*

MYRNA F. SCHWARTZ†

NADINE MARTIN‡

ELEANOR M. SAFFRAN† and

DEBORAH A. GAGNON‡

ABSTRACT

An interactive activation theory of word retrieval in speaking is applied to the picture naming errors of aphasic patients. First, a model was parameterized to fit the probabilities of the major kinds of errors that normal speakers make in a picture naming task. Then, the model was fit to the error patterns of 21 fluent aphasic patients by altering its connection weight and/or decay rate parameters, each patient being fit individually. The fits were then used to derive predictions about other aspects of the patients' behavior, in particular the influence of syntactic categories on the patients' formal errors, the effect of phonology on semantic errors, error patterns after recovery, and patient performance on a single-word repetition task. Tests of these predictions were successful. Aphasic error patterns appear to be the result of quantitative alterations to normal processing parameters.

The most pervasive symptom of language breakdown in aphasia is a difficulty in finding and articulating words. When aphasic patients are unsuccessful at retrieving a target word, they often produce errors or *paraphasias*. These errors exhibit a tremendous variety, not only across patients, but often within a single patient. Sometimes, paraphasias are words that resemble the target word along some dimension. For example, when searching for the target "swan", patients may retrieve semantic or formal relatives such as "duck", or "sun". It is also possible for paraphasias to be both semantically and formally related to the target; "swim" for "swan" would be an example. Or the incorrect word could bear no apparent resemblance to the target, as occurred when one of our patients came up with the word "brain" when searching for "pig". On closer inspection, though, some of these unrelated word errors reveal distant relations to the target. A patient who said "house" for "unicorn" perhaps initially retrieved "horse". Paraphasias can be nonwords as well as words. These may deviate from the target by a single speech sound, for example, /swam/ for "swan", or they may alter the word to such an extent that there are almost no sounds of the target present at all (e.g., "vitchers" for "pyramid"). Clearly, the lexical retrieval errors of aphasic patients provide a rich and challenging data source for theories of language processing.

*Department of Psychology, University of Illinois, 603 E. Daniel St., Champaign, IL 61801, E-mail: gdell@s.psych.uiuc.edu

†Moss Rehabilitation Research Institute, 1200 W. Tabor Road, Philadelphia, PA 19141

‡Temple University School of Medicine, 3401 N. Broad Street, Philadelphia, PA 19140

The first step in understanding pathological language has been the realization that paraphasias are similar to normal speech errors or "slips of the tongue". This similarity has often been remarked upon by students of aphasia, including Freud,[9] who claimed that "the paraphasia in aphasic patients does not differ from the incorrect use and the distortion of words which the healthy person can observe in himself in states of fatigue or divided attention...".[2,15] We have called this claim the *continuity thesis*.[7] More specifically, the thesis is that aphasic error patterns reflect the same forces that create normal speech errors. In this chapter, we make the continuity thesis concrete by showing that patient error patterns can be explained by altering the parameters of a theory of normal lexical retrieval.

The simplest way to study lexical retrieval disorders in aphasia is a picture naming task. A picture of an object is presented and the patient must name it. Object picture naming, hereafter just called naming, provides both a natural and well controlled assessment of a person's ability to retrieve concrete nouns. Here we present a theory of performance on a naming task. We start with a general model of retrieval in production–a model based on interactive activation principles–and develop it so that it can account for the quantitative pattern of naming errors in normal speakers. Then we show that simple changes in the model's processing parameters can account for aphasic performance. In particular, we attempt to fit the naming error pattern of 23 fluent aphasic patients who differ considerably among themselves in overall percentage correct and in the particular pattern of errors. Finally, we predict other characteristics of the patients from the fits, including the syntactic and semantic properties of their formal errors, changes in their error patterns as they recover, and their performance in a different task, single-word repetition.

1. An Interactive Two-Step Theory of Lexical Access in Production

The model that forms the basis of our work was initially developed to account for normal speech error patterns and experimental studies of the time-course of lexicalization.[4,5,6] So, it has considerable motivation as an account of normal performance. Like several other accounts of normal language production, our model is based on interactive activation principles.[1,8,13,17,26] Lexical knowledge is contained in a network of units or nodes, each unit representing an identifiable component of knowledge (see Figure 1). There are distinct levels of representation with excitatory links between units on adjacent levels that permit both feedforward and feedback during the retrieval of a word. The representational levels consist of semantic units (the input), word units, and phonological units (the output). Consequently, the model is concerned only with lexical access–the mapping from a semantic representation of the pictured object to the phonological form of the object's name–rather than the visual processes that come up with the semantic representation, and articulatory processes that convert the phonological representation into speech.

Semantics

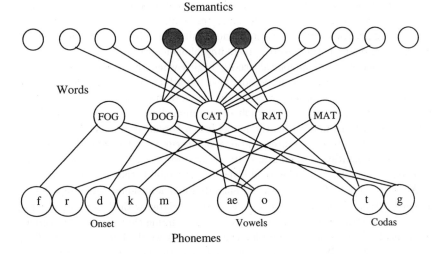

Figure 1: A three-layer model of lexical knowledge

A crucial aspect of the model is that lexical retrieval has two steps, *lemma access* and *phonological access*. Two-step theories of word retrieval have considerable support from studies of normal and aphasic speech errors and a number of experiments.[3,10,12,14,25,19,23] Here we explain the two steps by showing how the lexical item CAT is retrieved.

Lemma access begins by activating the semantic nodes corresponding to the concept to be named. The 10 semantic nodes of CAT are given a "jolt" of 100 arbitrary units of activation, 10 units per node. This activation spreads for n time steps according to a linear activation rule:

$$A(j,t) = A(j,t-1)(1-q) + \sum w(i,j)A(i,t-1) + NOISE \qquad (1)$$

where $A(j,t)$ is the activation of unit j at time step t, q is a decay parameter, and $w(i,j)$ is the connection weight from unit i to unit j. For the implemented model, we assumed that each of the connections has exactly the same weight, designated by p. The noise is normally distributed and is the sum of two components: intrinsic noise, which has a mean of zero and standard deviation $SD1$, and activation noise, whose mean is also zero, and whose standard deviation is $SD2 * A(j,t)$.

After activation has spread for n time steps, the most highly activated word node of the proper syntactic category is *selected*. In a naming task, that category would be nouns. If a sentence were being produced, selection would entail linkage to a slot in a syntactic frame, a data structure that defines that word's ordinal and hierarchical relations to other planned words. With a naming task, however, there is only one word to be produced and so the syntactic frame consists of a single noun slot. The selection of the most activated noun completes lemma access. It is important to note that, during lemma access, activation is not limited to only semantic and word units, it spreads throughout the network, including phonological units.

The second step, phonological access, begins when the selected word node (for CAT) is given a large jolt of activation, also 100 arbitrary units worth. If a sentence is being produced, the jolt occurs when the syntactic frame says that it should occur. In a single-word naming task, the jolt occurs immediately upon selection. The jolt to the selected word node turns the model into a nonlinear system. To map between semantic and phonological representations, one needs a hidden layer that computes a nonlinear combination of semantic units because words with similar meaning do not have similar sounds.[20,24] The word layer in this model is that hidden layer.

After the jolt to CAT, activation spreads for n additional time steps and then the most activated phonemes are selected and associated with slots in a phonological frame, a data structure analogous to the syntactic frame that dictates the order and hierarchical relations among the phonemes within a word. For a word like CAT, a frame for a single CVC syllable is retrieved, and the most highly activated initial consonant (k), the most highly activated vowel (ae), and the most highly activated final consonant (t) are selected and linked to slots in the frame. This completes phonological access.

The model gives a good account of the kinds of errors that can happen in word retrieval. A *semantic error*, such as DOG for CAT, occurs because the concepts for *dog* and *cat* share semantic units. The word node for DOG therefore gets some activation directly from the semantics and has a chance of being selected. More interesting is the case of a word related in form to the target, such as MAT. MAT becomes activated through feedback from the shared phonemes of the target. If MAT is in the same syntactic category as the target–in this case they are both nouns–it could be selected creating what we call a *formal error*. Notice that this happens only if the word is in the same syntactic category as the target. A verb such as SAT could not be produced by this mechanism if the target is a noun. If a word shares both meaning and form, such as RAT, it is especially likely according to the model because the top-down semantic effect and the bottom-up effect from shared phonemes combine to make these errors particularly likely.[6,13,18] We call these *mixed errors*. The three categories of semantic, formal, and mixed errors, together with a fourth category for *unrelated word errors*, are hypothesized to occur during lemma access.

In addition to errors of lemma access, one can also have errors of phonological access. These happen when the wrong phonemes are selected. *Nonword errors* such as LAT occur during this stage. It is also possible for phonological access to create formal errors such as MAT. Unlike the formal errors that occur during lemma access, though, these do not have to be in the same syntactic category as the target. A verb, SAT, could replace a noun target in an error of phonological access. Because the selection of phonemes is governed by the constraints inhabiting the phonological frames, rather than by syntactic constraints, the selection is indifferent to the syntactic properties of the resulting strings In this respect, the model follows speech error models based on the classic linguistic distinction between syntax and phonology.[12] Phonological generalizations tend not to refer to syntactic categories.

2. Implementing the Model

Our goal is to instantiate the model so that it fits normal error data, and then lesion it to fit patient data. The first step is to specify the network, because the opportunities for error afforded by the particular semantic and phonological neighborhoods put into the network greatly influence error probabilities. Our approach is to use very small networks that nonetheless match the relative *error opportunities* afforded by English. We are concerned with the opportunities associated with five categories of error: semantic, formal, mixed, nonwords, and unrelated words. The question is this: If the output of the lexical access process is "random", that is, it is governed entirely by noise as opposed to the target picture, how likely would the various error categories be? Answering this question requires a definition of random outputs, and an assessment of what the English lexicon affords. For us, a random output is a phonotactically acceptable (i.e. pronounceable) string of the length of the typical response in a naming task. Given this definition, we have estimated, from a variety of sources, the error opportunities for the five error categories.[7] If a system randomly produces phonotactically acceptable strings of English at about the average length of naming-response outputs, about 80% of these will be nonwords. The next most common category–10% of the time–will be words that bear no direct relation to the target, the unrelated category. A word that is formally related to the target will occur 9% of the time. We use a rather loose definition of a formally related word; two phonemes in any position or one phoneme in the same structural position must be shared with the target. That is why the opportunities for formal errors are so high. The opportunities for a semantic error (1%) or a mixed error (substantially less than 1%) are quite small.

Next, we configured the model so that it matched these proportions. We used two six-word networks, as shown in Table 1, and we sample from the first of these 90% of the time and the second 10% of the time. The main difference between the two neighborhoods is that the second one provides an opportunity for a mixed error. With these networks and the sampling assumption, the model's error opportunities are similar to those of English (see Figure 2). When the model produces random outputs and errs, 78% of the strings are nonwords, 9% are unrelated words, 8% are formally related words, 4% are semantically related words, and 0.4% are mixed. The similarity between the model and real opportunities will turn out to be important. As patients' naming becomes more and more disrupted, their error probabilities gradually

Neighborhood 1
1 target (e.g., CAT)
1 semantic (e.g., DOG)
2 formals (e.g., HAT, MAT)
2 unrelated (e.g., LOG, FOG)
Neighborhood 2
1 target (e.g., CAT)
1 semantic (e.g., DOG)
1 formal (e.g., MAT)
1 mixed (e.g., RAT)
2 unrelated (e.g., LOG, FOG)
Phonology
Each neighborhood defines 24 legal strings
(6 onsets × 2 vowels × 2 codas).
Of these 6 are words and 18 are legal nonwords (e.g., CAG, FOT)
Semantics
Each word connects to 10 features. Semantically
related words share 3 features with the target.

Table 1: Network Structures Used in the Model

approach the random error opportunity pattern. So, the implemented model's random pattern has to be similar.

The next step is to parameterize the model so that its performance matches those of normal speakers. We gave 60 control speakers the 175 pictures of the Philadelphia Naming Test (PNT) to name and categorized responses into 7 groups—Correct, Semantic, Formal, Nonwords, Mixed, Unrelated, and a Miscellaneous category for responses outside the domain of the model. (See Roach et al,[22] for a description of the PNT, and Dell et al.[7] for the coding rules employed in this study.) Table 2 shows the data and the result of the model's fit. In both the normal speakers and the model, just about all the errors are semantic or mixed. The model's parameters include connection weight, p (.1), decay rate, q (.5), n, the number of time steps for each phase of lexicalization (8), and the two parameters that are associated with noise in the system. Technically speaking, all errors in the model are due to the noise because the selection procedure is deterministic–it always picks the most activated unit of the appropriate category during both lemma and phonological access–and the retrieval process is effective–the correct word and the correct phonemes are always more active than competing words and phonemes when there is no noise in the system.

Although our main goal in parameterizing the model was to fit the naming error data, a secondary goal was to create a model that is consistent with recent experi-

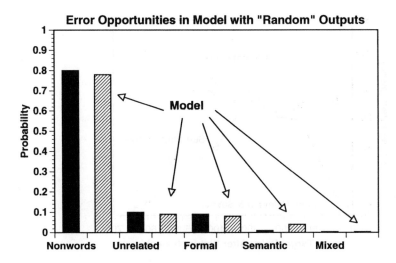

Figure 2: Estimated error opportunities for the English lexicon and the model's error opportunities

mental data dealing with the time course of naming.[16,21,25]   These studies track the extent to which semantic and formal neighbors of a target are activated during picture naming, by presenting probe words at various times while subjects are attempting to name. The probes are semantically or formally related to the picture's name, or they are unrelated, and the subject must either pronounce the probe, make a lexical decision to it,or ignore it.[16,25,21]   Figure 3 shows the data of Peterson and Savoy,[21] in which activation is assessed by the time to name related probes relative to unrelated ones. The figure suggests that early in the retrieval process, semantic competitors of

		Response Category				
	correct	semantic	formal	nonword	mixed	unrelated
Control data	.969	.011	.001	.000	.009	.003
Model	.966	.021	.000	.001	.012	.000

Chosen parameters: $p=.1$; $q=.5$; $SD1=.01$; $SD2=.16$; $n=8$
Simulated probabilities are based on 100,000 trials from each neighborhood.

Table 2: Error Probabilities from 60 Control Patients

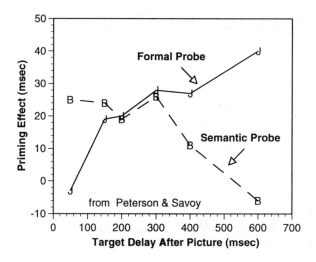

Figure 3: The difference in response time to related probes (either semantic or formal) and unrelated probes as a function of the delay between picture and probe onset (from Peterson & Savoy[21]). The effects show the evolution of the naming process from meaning to sound.

a target are active, but no formal ones are. Later on, both semantic and formal competitors are active, and late in the process, only formal competitors are active. With its present parameters, the model mimics this time course reasonably well. Figure 4 presents the relative amount of activation in non-target lemmas at various points in time for the model. Initially, the activation pattern contains only semantic competitors, but it gradually evolves to one that is dominated by formal competitors.

3. Fitting the Model to Aphasic Patients

Next, we attempt to account for aphasic naming deficits. We tested 23 aphasic patients with naming problems on the Philadelphia Naming Test. The group included patients from the "fluent" categories, specifically, Wernicke, conduction, anomic, and transcortical-sensory. We excluded nonfluent patients because we felt that it would be difficult to separate their phonological errors, which we hypothesize occur during phonological access, from their phonetic/articulatory errors, which are outside the scope of the model. Fluent patients tend to make fewer phonetic/articulatory errors.

Naming performance ranged from 8% correct to a near normal 95% correct, and the error pattern showed considerable variability, as well. For some patients, non-

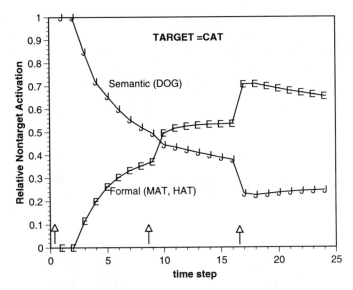

Figure 4: The evolution from meaning to sound in the model. The relative amount of activation of non-target lemmas in presented as a function of time steps. The first arrow indicates the time of the jolt to semantic units; the second arrow, the jolt to the selected word node or lemma; and the third, the jolt to the selected onset, vowel, and coda phonemes.

word errors predominated, while for others semantic or formal errors were the most common.

We modeled the error pattern of each individual patient by altering model parameters. Specifically our theory of naming deficits is this: Brain damage reduces the ability to transmit activation from one level to another; and it also reduces the integrity of the representations at each level. The first of these, the transmission of activation, is tied to connection weight, p. The second of these, the integrity of the representation, can be associated with either variation in intrinsic noise, or the decay rate. It doesn't really matter—lesioning either of these parameters has much the same effect. For the sake of simplicity, we lesioned the decay rate. Hence, our attempt to simulate patients was carried out by reducing connection weight, and/or increasing decay rate.

A critical feature of our theory of naming deficits is that the lesions in connection weight and/or decay rate are global. Each patient is assigned a p that applies to all connections at all levels, and a q that characterizes all the nodes. We adopt this globality assumption because it is both easier and more parsimonious to work with a small parameter space. If decay and connection weight can be lesioned independently on each layer of the model, the space becomes very hard to search and, perhaps more importantly, the model becomes difficult to falsify. Ultimately, though, we expect that level-specific lesions will be needed to relate the model to some patients. If the proportion of such patients is small, it may be worth the loss in explanatory completeness to secure the parsimony associated with the globality assumption.

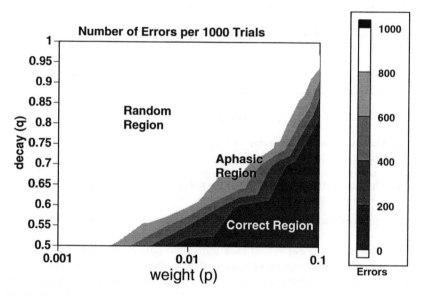

Figure 5: Error rate in the model as a function of connection weight (p) and decay rate (q).

Given the globality assumption, we are now in a position to identify the error patterns that the model allows. Connection weight and decay lesions both increase errors because they cause activation to get small relative to noise. Figure 5 presents a contour map of overall correctness in the model's parameter space. The point associated with normal parameters is in the lower right corner. As either p decreases, or q increases, errors begin to occur. There is a band that we call the *aphasic region* in which performance is disrupted, but not completely random, and finally there is a large area in which performance is completely dominated by noise. Our goal is to place patients in the aphasic region.

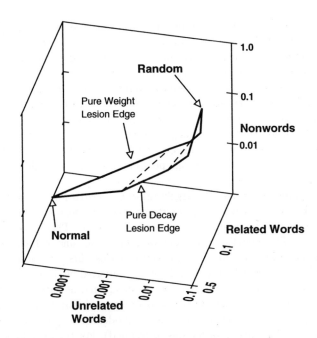

Figure 6: The model's error pattern space. Each point on the surface represents a combination of error proportions allowed by the model. The dotted lines connect points of the two edges that have the same level of correctness.

Figure 6 shows another picture of the model's characteristics, by presenting a map of error-pattern space rather than parameter space. This space collapses the five error response categories into three error probability dimensions: nonwords, related word errors (semantic, mixed & formal), and unrelated word errors. The surface that resembles a twisted piece of metal represents the error patterns that can occur in the model. At one end of the region is the normal point. It has some related word errors, but almost no nonwords or unrelated word errors. At the other end is the random point. Here the error pattern is completely determined by the opportunities. Most of the errors are nonwords, but there are many unrelated word errors and a few related word errors. Between these points, the region expands a bit. One edge of the region corresponds to a lesion that only involves p, and the other edge corresponds to a lesion that only involves q. The surface between the edges represents lesions of both p and q.

The error space figure illustrates two important features of the model. First, the error patterns allowed by the model are quite restricted. Not every logically possible combination of errors is allowed. Second, one can describe the variation in allowed error patterns along two largely orthogonal dimensions, overall severity of the lesion and the type of lesion. Of these, severity accounts for most of the variation. As we move from the normal to the random point, severity increases, and the error pattern evolves by increasing, primarily, the probability of nonword and unrelated errors. The second dimension concerns the degree to which p or q is involved. Lesions that affect activation transmission do something a bit different than lesions that affect the integrity of the representations. We shall postpone a discussion of this difference until particular patients are presented.

The fitting process involved a (largely informal) search for values of p and q for each patient that make the model's proportions of correct, semantic, formal, nonword, mixed, and unrelated, as close to that patient as possible. There are, therefore, two free parameters. The model's proportions were based on runs of 1000 trials for each of its two neighborhoods. To arbitrate between close fits, we picked the fit that minimized χ^2, or in cases where χ^2 could not be computed because of a zero expected value, we chose the fit that minimized root mean squared deviation (RMSD).

We elected not to fit 2 of the 23 patients because more than 15% of their responses were not attempts to name the pictures, and the model has no provision for these non-attempts (picture descriptions or failures to respond). For the remaining 21 patients we were, on balance, successful at fitting the error pattern. The median RMSD was .026, and the worst case was .102. Figure 7 shows the distribution of RMSD's. Table 3 illustrates the fit by presenting four patients.

First consider patient GL, whose performance was at 28% correct, and patient IG, who did much better, 69% correct. Both patients had fits near the median RMSD, .030 and .027, respectively. GL's lesion was primarily in decay, and secondarily in connection weight, and IG's was a pure decay lesion. The main difference between these two is along the severity dimension, and the differences in their error patterns illustrate how severity interacts with the error categories in the patients and the model. Notice that the the proportions of semantic and mixed errors are *not* related to severity, whereas the proportion of formal, nonword, and unrelated errors increase dramatically with severity. IG and GL have about the same number of semantic and mixed errors, but GL's nonword, formal and unrelated errors are much more prevalent. The model exhibits this behavior, too. The reasons for the model's severity interactions lie with the nature of the normal point–which allows mostly semantic and mixed errors—and the random point, at which the opportunities for nonwords, unrelated, and formals far outstrip those for semantic and mixed errors. As severity increases, the overwhelming number of opportunities for nonwords, unrelated words, and to a lesser extent, formally related words, cause these errors to increase dramatically.

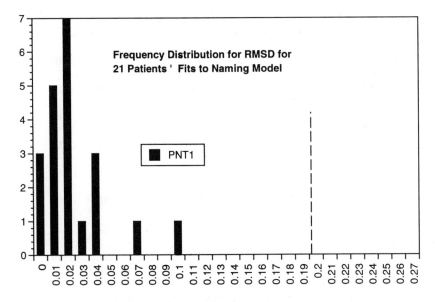

Figure 7: The distribution of root mean squared deviations between each patient's error pattern and the fit of the model. The dotted line shows the mean RMSD for the model's fit to "pseudopatients," error patterns generated at random.

The next example patient, LH, is chosen because he has the same degree of correctness as IG, but a different error pattern. Whereas IG's most common error is semantic, LH's is nonwords. It is exactly this variation that is associated with whether the model's fit involves primarily a decay lesion or a weight lesion. LH is very nicely fit by a pure weight lesion. Notice the differences between LH's weight lesion and IG's decay lesion: The weight lesion promotes nonwords, at the expense of lexically related errors, whereas the decay lesion promotes semantic and mixed errors. In the model, reducing connection weights reduces the extent to which different levels of representations are *consistent* with one another. This promotes what we might call "stupid" errors. For example, the production of a nonword reflects a circumstance in which the phonological level is not consistent with the lexical level. The production of an unrelated word error happens when the semantic and lexical levels are not communicating.

In contrast, when the lesion involves the decay rate, instead of destroying the consistency among representations, the lesion diminishes the representations themselves.

	Response Category					
	correct	semantic	formal	nonword	mixed	unrelated
Patient GL	.28	.04	.21	.30	.03	.09
Model(RMSD=.030)						
p=.08; q=.85	.29	.11	.20	.29	.03	.08
Patient IG	.69	.09	.05	.02	.03	.01
Model(RMSD=.027)						
p=.1; q=.86	.73	.13	.04	.05	.04	.01
Patient LH	.69	.03	.07	.15	.01	.02
Model(RMSD=.019)						
p=.0053; q=.5	.67	.07	.07	.15	.01	.03
Patient WR	.08	.06	.15	.28	.05	.33
Model(RMSD=.102)						
p=.1; q=.94	.18	.09	.20	.37	.03	.13

Simulated probabilities are based on 1000 trials per neighborhood.
Patient data are from 175 pictures in the Philadelphia Naming Test.

Table 3: Naming Data and Model Fits for Four Patients

As a result, there are many errors, but they show evidence of activation transmission among the levels. In particular, there are a great many mixed, semantic, and formal errors, errors which are "smart", in that the phonological level is consistent with the word level, and the chosen word bears some resemblance to the intended word.

To round out our patient sample in Table 3, we have included, in the spirit of airing our dirtiest laundry, the patient who has the worst fit, WR. The model is off somewhat for the unrelated and nonword categories but, otherwise, it fits well.

4. Tests of Predictions from the Fits

The most exciting aspect of the modelling is the possibility of using the fits to predict other aspects of the patients' performance. We have done this with respect to four effects—the influence of syntactic category on errors, the extent to which semantic errors show phonological influences, the pattern of recovery in naming, and the patients' abilities to repeat.

One of the main features of the fit for each patient is whether or not the parameter values allow for a large amount of interaction among the processing levels in the model. Recall that the model's assumption of excitatory feedback provides a mechanism for formal errors to occur at lemma access, and for the increased probability of mixed

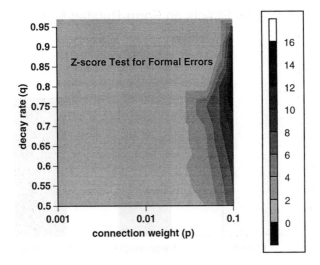

Figure 8: A measure of the amount of interactive feedback in the model as a function of model parameters (see Dell et al.[7] for details). Interaction is confined to cases with near normal ($>.05$) values of p.

errors. We studied the model's performance under many possible parameters with regard to the extent to which feedback affects the activation of competitor words. Figure 8 shows the results of these tests. The darker the shading, the greater the extent to which there are true feedback effects at work at generating errors for those parameter settings. This study allows us to divide the patients into two categories on the basis of their fitted parameters. If the value of connection weight is greater than .05 then the patient should have the potential to generate error effects that are related to interactive feedback. If the weight is less than .05, there should be little tendency for these effects. This partitioning is the basis for some of our predictions.

The first prediction concerns syntactic-class effects on formal errors, such as MAT for CAT. According to our theory, many of these errors are caused when feedback from activated phoneme nodes contacts formally-related word nodes during lemma access. If these words are in the syntactic category of noun, they may be selected. Hence, form-related errors that result from feedback should, according to the theory, be nouns. There is another way that one can get form-related errors in the theory, though. They could be phonological errors that just happen to make words. These should not tend to be nouns more than chance. Therefore, patients with large-weight

150

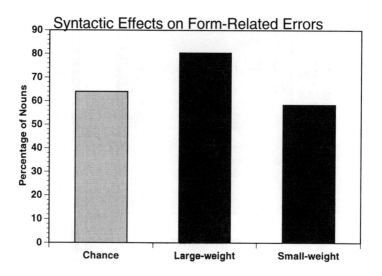

Figure 9: The percentage of form-related errors that were nouns for patients with large-weight fits (>.05), small weight fits (<.05) and the percentage expected by chance.

fits should have form-related errors that are nouns in excess of chance. Patients with small-weight fits should produce form-related nouns at chance. The data, shown in Figure 9, are exactly as predicted. The form-related errors with large-weight patients (N=13) were nouns 80.4% of the time, and the ones from small-weight patients (N=10) were nouns 58.5% of the time. The difference is significant $t(21)=3.32$, $p<.004$, and the small-weight patients are right about at chance which we estimated at 64% (Most words are, in fact, nouns; see Gagnon, Schwartz, Martin, Dell, & Saffran,[11] for chance estimation procedures).

Our second prediction concerns the interaction between phonological and semantic similarity in causing errors at lemma access. Large-weight patients should have a genuine tendency for semantic errors to also show phonological similarity, because the phonological effects derive from feedback. Small-weight patients should not. We took all of the lexical errors that bore a semantic relation to the target (except for morphological errors) and determined whether the first, second, or third phonemes of the target and the error were the same. We did this separately for the large- and small-weight patients. The number of matches was compared to the number expected by chance, using the procedures of Dell and Reich[6] to determine chance. For the large weight patients, one expects 34 of 594 comparisons to match by chance. The actual

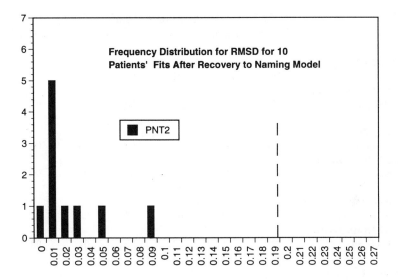

Figure 10: The distribution of root mean squared deviations between patients and the model for the ten patients retested on the Philadelphia Naming Test.

number was 70, which is significantly greater (95% confidence limits are 34 ± 12). For the small-weight patients, one expects 13 of 222 comparisons to match by chance; the result was 18 and was not different from chance (13 ± 7). This is good support for the prediction, and in general, supports the idea that semantic and phonological aspects of words work together in determining errors–an idea which is consistent with interactive two-step models but which requires additional assumptions to explain in non-interactive models.[16]

Thus far, it looks as if the division of patients into small-weight and large-weight groups predicts syntactic and other aspects of the errors. Our third prediction concerns recovery. Of the patients who did the naming test, we were able to retest 10 of them an average of three months after the original test to assess their recovery. The 10 recovered error patterns were then fit to the model. The prediction is that the recovered fits should not alter the model's original characterization of the patient. If a patient was a large-weight patient initially–that is, the lesion is primarily in the decay rate–then that patient should be a large-weight patient after recovery. The recovery should improve the decay rate, rather than move the patient to the small-weight region of parameter space.

The fits for the recovered patients were, as before, good. Figure 10 gives the distribution of RMSD's. Table 4 presents a sample patient, JB. First are JB's results

	Response Category					
	correct	semantic	formal	nonword	mixed	unrelated
Patient JB						
before recovery	.76	.06	.01	.05	.02	.01
Model (RMSD=.021)						
p=.0065; q=.5	.78	.06	.04	.08	.01	.03
Patient JB						
after recovery	87	.01	.01	.03	.03	.00
Model (RMSD=.018)						
p=.0085; q=.5	.89	.04	.01	.04	.01	.00
Patient AF						
before recovery	.75	.02	.03	.07	.06	.04
Model (RMSD=.043)						
p=.1; q=.86	.77	.11	.03	.05	.04	.00
Patient AF						
after recovery	.94	.01	.01	.02	.02	.01
Model (RMSD=.012)						
p=.01; q=.5	.94	.03	.01	.02	.00	.00

Naming data are from 175 pictures of the Philadelphia Naming Test.
Simulated data are from 1000 trials per neighborhood.

Table 4: Naming Data and Model Fits for Two Patients Before and After Recovery

on the earlier test; the fit indicates a small-weight category, in particular a pure connection-weight lesion. After recovery, performance is better, but the character of the fit is the same; it is still a pure connection-weight lesion. Across the 10 patients that we tested again, eight had fits that were of the same character as before, and one had a fit that changed character. The tenth patient recovered to normal performance and hence there is no lesion. So, eight out of nine retained character. This shows that the model's categorization is somewhat stable across recovery. The table also presents the data from patient AF, the single patient who did not conform to the prediction. AF was originally fit to a decay lesion, and had 75% correct. After recovery she went up to 94% correct, and a pure weight lesion fit slightly better than a decay lesion. However, the recovery was to such a high level that the fits for weight and decay lesions are nearly identical. Recall that the model's error pattern surface (Figure 6) collapses around the normal point. Moreover, with a high degrees of correctness there are few errors to work with anyway, and so the ability of the model to identify reliably whether a mildly aphasic patient is high or low-weight is poor.

Our final prediction concerns a different task than naming, single word repetition. The patient hears a word and must repeat it. Because the language production system is involved in both repetition and naming, one ought to be able to use the naming model to make some predictions about repetition. Our theory of repetition is unorthodox, but it worked quite well for most of the patients. We assume that the word is correctly perceived, with the result that the correct word node in the production network is given a full jolt of activation. Then the network attempts to pronounce this word by using the phonological access step of the naming model. Thus, for each patient, we can make strong and precise predictions. If the parameter values for that patient are used, and the model is run just through the phonological access step, one obtains the predicted degree of correctness and the error pattern for the patient's repetition. Because there are no free parameters here, the predictions are absolute.

	Response Category					
	correct	semantic	formal	nonword	mixed	unrelated
Patient JL	.89	.00	.02	.03	.00	.00
Model (RMSD=.015)						
p=.025; q=.6	.92	.00	.03	.05	.00	.00
Patient JF	.94	.00	.02	.03	.01	.00
Model (RMSD=.023)						
p=.1; q=.86	.89	.00	.03	.05	.02	.00
Patient WR	.90	.00	.03	.06	.01	.00
Model (RMSD=.273)						
p=.1; q=.94	.36	.00	.19	.42	.03	.00

Table 5: Repetition Data and Model Fits for Three Patients

Thirteen of the 21 patients originally tested in the naming experiment did a repetition test on the same words as the naming test. Two of these had greater than 15% nonresponses and so were not fit, leaving 11 patients. The predictions worked surprisingly well. The median RMSD was .024. Table 5 presents the data from two patients whose fit was near the median, JL and JF. Notice that the model not only predicts correctness, but also the absence of semantic errors and the relative patterning of nonwords and formals. There was only one really poor fit. This was for WR, and is also shown in the table. His naming was quite impaired and hence his repetition was predicted to be impaired as well (36% correct). However, the obtained repetition was 90% correct. This unusual case clearly falsifies the claim that repetition is always done by an error-free word recognition stage followed by a phonological encoding stage that is shared with naming. But, it is nonetheless quite interesting how far the assumption of perfect recognition can go. And the success at predicting repetition from the naming fits stands as further evidence for the value of the model.

5. Conclusions

We offer three conclusions and a final observation. The first conclusion is straightforward: We believe that the application of the model to aphasic naming deficits strengthens the case for an interactive two-step theory of lexical retrieval in production. Originally, this theory had garnered most of its support from studies of normal speech errors. Second, we conclude that the continuity thesis has been supported. The error patterns in patients reflect intermediate states between the normal error pattern and a pattern associated with random output on a given space of opportunities. These intermediate states result from simple quantitative alterations to normal processing parameters. Our third conclusion relates to the nature of the aphasic deficit. In addition to the large variation in severity among the patients, there is secondary variation due to the nature of the disruption. Patients vary in their ability to transmit activation from one processing level to another (which we tied to connection weights) and in their ability to maintain the integrity of a representation. The notion that these alterations affect the network globally, rather than locally within semantic, word, and phonological layers, is probably the most controversial of our conclusions.

Our final observation concerns the relation between the model and actual neural processes. The model is most definitely not a neural model in the sense that many of the models in this volume are. The structure of the network is motivated from the task at hand–lexical access–rather than from any particular brain structures. Moreover, the model accounts solely for behavioral data. There are no directly apparent predictions from it about heretofore undiscovered properties of brain anatomy or physiology.

The lack of direct predictions about neural implementation in our model is typical of models in its domain. At present, sophisticated models of linguistic knowledge and behavior–even those that employ connectionist or neural network principles–relate to the brain only indirectly. Language is a human skill and, hence, we are limited in the kinds of studies that can be ethically performed in the search for brain mechanisms. In addition, language involves multiple modalities and a great deal of learning and, hence, may be neurally represented in a manner that differs among individuals to a greater extent than that of simple sensory or motor skills. In sum, the neural mechanisms of language are not going to be easy to discover.

The absence of detailed neural models of language does not mean, though, that connections between existing models cannot be made with brain mechanisms. Our model of normal and impaired lexical access could, for example, be related to studies of lesion location and size. In addition, it could serve as a guide for interpreting the results of functional imaging studies, in particular, studies that have the capacity to map activation as a function of time. We would argue, though, that any model that guides the interpretation of clinical lesion analysis or imaging must first accord with the behavioral data. In the case of language and language breakdown, that data certainly must include the speech errors made by normal and aphasic speakers.

6. Acknowledgements

This research was supported by the National Institutes of Health (DC-00191 and DC-01924) and the National Science Foundation (SBR 93-19368). Further details are available in Dell et al. (1995) which can be obtained by contacting Gary Dell, Beckman Institute, University of Illinois, 405 North Mathews Avenue, Urbana, IL 61801 (gdell@s.psych.uiuc.edu).

7. References

1. T. Berg, *Die Abbildung des Sprachproduktionprozess in einem Aktivationsfluss modell* (Tuebingen: Max Niemeyer, 1988).

2. H. W. Buckingham, *Applied Psycholinguistics* **1** (1980) p. 199.

3. B. Butterworth, in *Lexical representation and process*, ed. W. Marslen-Wilson (MIT Press, Cambridge, MA, 1989)

4. G. S. Dell, *Psychological Review* **93** (1986) p. 283.

5. G. S. Dell and P. G. O'Seaghdha, *Psychological Review* **98** (1991) p. 604.

6. G. S. Dell, G. S. and P. A. Reich, *Journal of Verbal Learning and Verbal Behavior* **20** (1981) p. 611.

7. G. S. Dell, M. F. Schwartz, N. Martin, E. M. Saffran, and D. A. Gagnon, Lexical access in normal and aphasic speakers (1995) ms.

8. H.-J Eikmeyer and U. Schade, *Cognitive Systems* **3**(2) (1991) p. 128.

9. S. Freud, *Psychopathology of everyday life* (A. A. Brill, translator, New American Library, New York, 1958 (original work published 1901)).

10. V. A. Fromkin, *Language* **47** (1971) p. 27.

11 D. A. Gagnon, M. F. Schwartz, N. Martin, G. S. Dell, and E. M. Saffran, *Brain and Language* (in press).

12. M. F. Garrett, in *The psychology of learning and motivation*, ed. G. H. Bower (Academic Press, San Diego, 1975), p. 133.

13. T. A. Harley, *Cognitive Science* **8** (1984) p. 191.

14. G. Kempen and P. Huijbers, *Cognition* **14** (1983) p. 185.

15. S. E. Kohn and K. L. Smith, *Cognitive Neuropsychology* **7** (1990) p. 133.

16. W. J. M Levelt, H. Schriefers, D. Vorberg, A. S. Meyer, T. Pechmann, and J. Havinga, *Psychological Review* **98** (1991) p. 122.

17. D. G. MacKay, *The organization of perception and action: A theory for language and other cognitive skills* (Springer-Verlag, New York, 1987).

18. N. Martin, R. W. Weisberg, and E. M. Saffran, *Journal of Memory and Language* **28** (1989) p. 462.

19. A. S. Meyer and K. Bock, *Memory and Cognition* **20** (1992) p. 715.

20. M. Minsky and S. Papert, *Perceptrons.* (MIT Press, Cambridge, MA, 1969).

21. R. R. Peterson and P. Savoy, *Journal of Experimental Psychology: Learning, Memory & Cognition* (in press).

22. A. Roach, M. F. Schwartz, N. Martin, R. S. Grewal, and A. Brecher, *Clinical aphasiology* (in press).

23. A. Roelofs, *Cognition* **42** (1992) p. 107.

24. D. E. Rumelhart, G. E. Hinton, and R. J. Williams, in *Parallel distributed processing: Explorations in the microstructure of cognition, Vol 1*, ed. D. E. Rumelhart and J. L. McClelland (MIT Press, Cambridge, 1986), p. 318.

25. H. Schriefers, A. S. Meyer, and W. J. M. Levelt, *Journal of Memory and Language* **29** (1990) p. 86.

26. J. P. Stemberger, in *Progress in the psychology of language*, ed. W. W. Ellis (Erlbaum, Hillsdale, NJ, 1985).

CONNECTIONIST MODELING OF THE BREAKDOWN AND RECOVERY OF READING VIA MEANING

DAVID C. PLAUT

Department of Psychology, Carnegie Mellon University
and the Center for the Neural Basis of Cognition
Pittsburgh, PA 15213-3890, plaut@cmu.edu

At least two processing routes in the brain are involved in pronouncing written words: a *semantic* route that derives the pronunciation via meaning, and a *phonological* route that derives it via spelling-sound correspondences. Simulations involving partial damage to an isolated semantic route (Plaut & Shallice, 1993) provide a comprehensive account of the rather peculiar combination of symptoms exhibited by patients with *deep dyslexia*, including the occurrence of semantic errors (e.g., reading RIVER as "ocean"), their co-occurrence with visual errors, and influences of imageability or concreteness on correct and error performance. Furthermore, when a version of the model is retrained after damage (Plaut, 1996), the degree and variability of its recovery and generalization are qualitatively similar to the results of some cognitive rehabilitation studies. The results challenge traditional assumptions about the nature of the mechanisms subserving word reading, and illustrate the value of explicit computational simulations of normal and impaired cognitive processes. They also suggest that connectionist modeling can provide a framework for generating specific hypotheses about strategies for rehabilitation.

Cognitive neuropsychology attempts to relate the patterns of impaired and preserved abilities of brain-injured patients to models of normal cognitive functioning, with the goals of explaining the behavior of the patients in terms of the effects of damage in the model, and of informing the model based on the observed behavior of patients (Coltheart, 1985; Ellis & Young, 1988; Shallice, 1988). A major motivation for many researchers is that a more detailed analysis of the normal mechanism, and the way it is impaired in particular patients, should lead to the design of more effective therapy to remediate these impairments (Howard & Hatfield, 1987; Riddoch & Humphreys, 1994; Seron & Deloche, 1989). Moreover, the patterns of recovery exhibited by patients place additional constraints on models of normal and impaired cognitive processing. The purpose of this chapter is to illustrate in a particular domain—reading via meaning—how computational principles from connectionist or parallel distributed processing (PDP) research can provide insight into the nature of normal cognitive processes, how they can break down following brain damage, how they can recover, and how to design therapy to maximize this recovery.

Perhaps the most detailed attempts at relating the behavior of damaged connectionist networks to that of brain-injured patients has been in the domain of acquired reading disorders (see, e.g., Hinton & Shallice, 1991; Mozer & Behrmann, 1990; Patterson, Seidenberg, & McClelland, 1989; Plaut, McClelland, Seidenberg, & Patterson, 1996; Plaut & Shallice, 1993). This is in part because investigations of reading in both cognitive psychology and neuropsychology (Coltheart, 1987) have produced a rich and often counterintuitive set of empirical findings.

Prior to the late 1960's, the major distinction among acquired dyslexic patients was simply whether the reading deficit was accompanied by a deficit in writing—alexia with agraphia—or whether it occurred in isolation—alexia without agraphia, or *pure* alexia (Dejerine, 1892). Little attempt was made to distinguish among different types of reading deficits until Marshall and Newcombe (1966, 1973) identified a number of separate types of acquired dyslexia based on the typical patterns of errors that patients made in reading aloud. In particular, *surface* dyslexia involved phonological confusions in the procedure by which words are sounded-out based on typical spelling-sound correspondences (e.g., SEW → "sue"), whereas *deep* dyslexia involved semantic confusions, in which words were often misread as semantically related words (e.g., DINNER → "food").

Marshall and Newcombe (1973) explained the existence of these distinct types of dyslexia in terms of damage to a "dual-route" model of normal reading (also see Coltheart, 1978, 1985; Coltheart, Curtis, Atkins, & Haller, 1993; Meyer, Schvaneveldt, & Ruddy, 1974; Morton & Patterson, 1980; Paap & Noel, 1991). In Marshall and Newcombe's model, written words can be pronounced through either of two pathways. The first is a *phonological* pathway that translates from spelling to sound using grapheme-phoneme correspondence (GPC) rules. This pathway enables people to read word-like nonsense letter strings (e.g., MAVE) as well as so-called *regular* words that obey standard spelling-sound correspondences (e.g., GAVE). The second way of pronouncing words is via a *semantic* pathway in which a word is first recognized and assigned a meaning which is then used to access its pronunciation. The semantic pathway enables people to read so-called *exception* words that violate the standard GPC rules (e.g. HAVE). According to Marshall and Newcombe, surface dyslexic patients have a selective impairment of the semantic pathway, such that their errors reflect the isolated operation of the phonological pathway. Conversely, deep dyslexia reflects the isolated—and, according to more recent theories (see Shallice, 1988), partially impaired—operation of the semantic pathway following severe damage to the phonological pathway.

Considerable further research has examined the characteristics of both surface and deep dyslexia in more detail. The chapter by Patterson, Plaut, McClelland, Seidenberg, Behrmann, and Hodges (this volume) articulates and

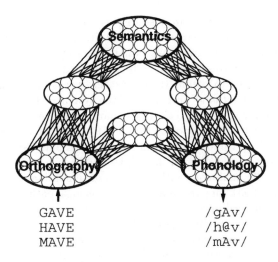

GAVE   /gAv/
HAVE   /h@v/
MAVE   /mAv/

Figure 1: A connectionist framework for lexical processing. Adapted from Seidenberg and McClelland (1989).

provides empirical support for an account of surface dyslexia based on connectionist implementations of the phonological pathway (Plaut et al., 1996). The current chapter focuses on deep dyslexia and, more generally, on the breakdown and recovery of the operation of the semantic pathway.

1 A Connectionist Framework for Lexical Processing

Seidenberg and McClelland (1989) presented a connectionist framework for lexical processing that has some similarities with—but also some important differences from—standard dual-route theory. Within the framework, depicted in Figure 1, orthographic, phonological, and semantic information is represented as distributed patterns of activity over groups of simple neuron-like processing units. Within each domain, similar words are represented by similar patterns of activity. Transformations among domains are accomplished via cooperative and competitive interactions among units, including intermediate or *hidden* units that mediate between the orthography, phonology, and semantics. In processing an input, units interact until the network as a whole settles into a stable pattern of activity—termed an *attractor*—corresponding to its interpretation of the input. Unit interactions are governed by weights on connections between them which collectively encode the system's knowledge and are learned through exposure to written words, spoken words, and their meanings.

Although this framework may seem reasonable at a general level, it actually reflects a radical departure from traditional theorizing about lexical processing, particularly in two ways. First, there is nothing in the structure of the system that corresponds to individual words *per se*, such as a lexical entry or "logogen" (Morton, 1969). Rather, words are distinguished from nonwords only by *functional* properties of the system—the way in which particular orthographic, phonological, and semantic patterns of activity interact (also see Van Orden, Pennington, & Stone, 1990). Second, although the system is composed of a phonological and a semantic pathway, these pathways operate according to very different principles and have very different functional properties than the analogous pathways in traditional dual-route models (e.g. Coltheart et al., 1993). In particular, the phonological pathway does not apply GPC rules that succeed only for regular words and nonwords. Rather, it learns to map orthography to phonology for all types of stimuli (including exception words) based on a sensitivity to spelling-sound *consistency* (Glushko, 1979). The degree of mastery achieved by the phonological route for items it finds most difficult—low-frequency exception words—will generally not be perfect and will depend on a number of factors, including the strength of contribution from the semantic during learning (see Patterson et al., this volume, and Plaut et al., 1996).

2 Impaired Reading Via Meaning in Deep Dyslexia

As suggested earlier, patients with deep dyslexia (see Coltheart, Patterson, & Marshall, 1980) seem to have a severe impairment of the phonological pathway. This is indicated, in part, by the fact that they are virtually unable to read pronounceable nonwords (e.g., MAVE). They also have impairments in reading words that suggest additional partial damage to the semantic pathway. In particular, deep dyslexics make *semantic* errors in oral reading (e.g., reading CAT as "dog"), along with pure *visual* errors (e.g., CAT → "cot"), mixed *visual-and-semantic* errors (e.g., CAT → "rat"), and even mediated *visual-then-semantic* errors (e.g., SYMPATHY → "orchestra", presumably via *symphony*). The likelihood that a word is read correctly depends on its part-of-speech (nouns > adjectives > verbs > function words) and its concreteness or imageability (concrete, imageable words > abstract, less imageable words). Performance on additional tests, such as auditory comprehension and picture-word matching, suggests that the secondary damage to the semantic pathway may occur before, within, or after semantics (Shallice & Warrington, 1980).

Hinton and Shallice (1991) reproduced the co-occurrence of semantic and

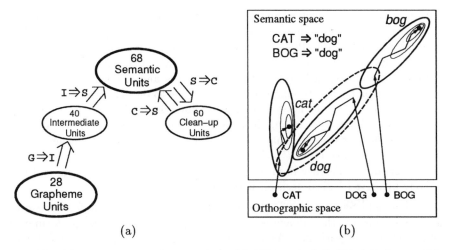

(a)   (b)

Figure 2: (a) A depiction of the network used by Hinton and Shallice (1991) to model deep dyslexia, corresponding to a portion of the semantic pathway of the Seidenberg and McClelland (1989) framework in Figure 1. Sets of connections are labeled by the initials of the connected groups of units (e.g., G⇒I for connections from the Grapheme units to the Intermediate units). (b) How damage to attractors (dashed oval) can cause both semantic and visual errors. The current patterns of activation in orthography and semantics are each represented as a point in a multi-dimensional *state space* in which the activation of each unit is coded along a separate dimension (for convenience, only two dimensions are depicted). Adapted from Hinton and Shallice (1991) and Plaut and Shallice (1993).

visual errors in deep dyslexia by damaging a network that mapped orthography to semantics (see Figure 2a). During training, the network learned to form attractors for word meanings (using a separate set of semantic "clean-up" units), such that patterns of semantic features that were similar to a known word meaning were pulled to that exact meaning over the course of settling. Following damage, the semantic activity caused by an input would occasionally fall within the attractor basin of a neighboring (related) word, giving rise to a semantic error. Visual errors also occurred due to the network's inherent bias towards similarity: visually similar words tend to produce similar initial semantic patterns which can lead to a visual error if the basins are distorted by damage (see Figure 2b).

Plaut and Shallice (1993) extended these initial findings in a number of ways. They established the generality of the co-occurrence of error types across a wide range of simulations, showing that it does not depend on specific char- acteristics of the network architecture, the learning procedure, or the way responses are generated from semantic activity. A particularly relevant simulation in this regard involved an implementation of the full semantic pathway—mapping orthography to phonology via semantics—using a deterministic Boltzmann Machine (Hinton, 1989; Peterson & Anderson, 1987). Lesions throughout the network gave rise to both visual and semantic errors, with lesions prior to semantics producing a bias towards visual errors and lesions after semantics producing a bias towards semantic errors (relative to the "chance" distribution; see Figure 3). Thus, the network replicated both the qualitative similarity and quantitative differences among deep dyslexic patients. The network also exhibited a number of other characteristics of deep dyslexia not considered by Hinton and Shallice (1991), including the occurrence of visual-then-semantic errors, greater confidence in visual as compared with semantic errors, and relatively preserved lexical decision with impaired naming.

Plaut and Shallice (1993, also see Plaut, 1995) carried out further simulations to address the influences of concreteness on the reading performance of deep dyslexic patients. As previously mentioned, deep dyslexic patients perform better at reading concrete, high-imageable words compared with abstract, low-imageable words. Strangely, the effects of concreteness—a semantic variable—interact with visual similarity in errors, such that abstract words are more likely than concrete words to produce visual errors, and the resulting responses tend to be more concrete than the stimulus (e.g., SCANDAL → "sandals" Barry & Richardson, 1988). These effects could not be addressed using the original Hinton and Shallice word set because it contains only concrete nouns.

Accordingly, Plaut and Shallice (1993) designed a version of the task of reading via meaning that would allow the effects of concreteness and visual similarity to be investigated directly. Twenty pairs of four-letter words were chosen such that one member of the pair was concrete, the other was abstract, and the two differed by only a single letter (e.g., ROPE and ROLE). The critical difference between the concrete and abstract words related to their semantic representations. Plaut and Shallice's approach to capturing this distinction was based in part on Jones' (1985) demonstration that words vary greatly in the ease with which predicates about them can be generated. For example, more predicates can be generated for basic-level words than for subordinate or superordinate words (Rosch, Mervis, Gray, Johnson, & Boyes-Braem, 1976). Jones showed that there is a very high correlation (0.88) between ease-of-predication ratings and imageability (which also correlates highly with concreteness), and that the relative difficulty of parts-of-speech in deep dyslexia maps perfectly onto their ordered mean ease-of-predication scores. He argued that the effects of both imageability and part-of-speech in deep dyslexia can be accounted for by assuming that the semantic pathway is sensitive to ease-of-predication. Plaut and Shallice instantiated this distinction by assigning

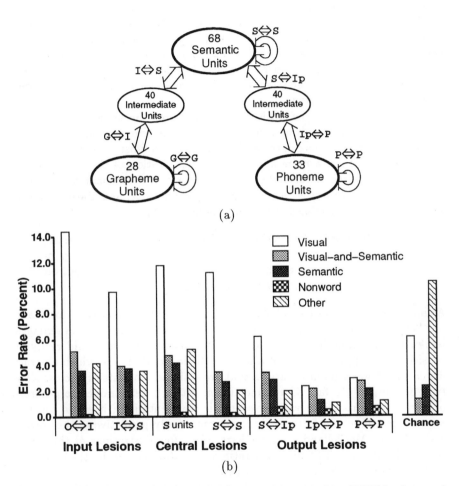

(a)

(b)

Figure 3: (a) The architecture of the deterministic Boltzmann Machine (DBM) implemented by Plaut and Shallice (1993). (b) Error rates produced by lesions to each main set of connections in the DBM network shown in (a). "Chance" is the distribution of error types if responses were chosen randomly from the word set. Its absolute height is set arbitrarily— only the relative rates are informative. Results are averaged over lesion densities which produced an overall correct response rate between approximately 20% and 80%. Adapted from Plaut and Shallice (1993).

concrete words more semantic features (predicates) than abstract words: an average of 18.2 versus 4.7 out of 98 possible features, respectively. The first 67 of the semantic features were based on those used by Hinton and Shallice (1991) and applied only to the concrete words; The remaining 31 features (e.g., *has-duration, relates-location, quality-difficulty*) applied primarily to abstract words but occasionally to concrete words as well. The ordering of the features and, in particular, the separation of concrete and abstract features, were irrelevant to the simulation.

Note that it would be misleading to interpret the assignment of more features to concrete words as a literal claim about semantic representations, given that abstract words can certainly make rich and substantial contributions to meaning. Rather, a more appropriate interpretation of the manipulation relates to the degree of *variability* across contexts in the semantics generated by different types of words. As Saffran, Bogyo, Schwartz, and Marin (1980, p. 400; see also Schwanenflugel, 1991) have pointed out,

> A concrete word—a reference term like "rose"—has a core meaning little altered by context (a rose *is* a rose) .... The meanings of abstract words, on the other hand, tend to be more dependent on the contexts in which they are embedded.

A similar contrast appears to hold among different parts-of-speech—for example, between nouns and verbs (Gentner, 1981). Thus, the use of fixed semantic representations containing fewer features for abstract words should really be considered an approximation of a more realistic simulation in which abstract words have fewer semantic features that are activated consistently across a variety of contexts. In fact, if a connectionist network were trained to generate pronunciations from such variable semantic representations, it would come to rely on just those few features that are consistently predictive of the correct response (see McClelland & Rumelhart, 1985, for illustrations of this property). The Plaut and Shallice semantic representations can be thought of as containing only these predictive features.

Plaut and Shallice (1993) trained a network with back-propagation through time (Rumelhart, Hinton, & Williams, 1986) to map orthography to phonology via these semantic representations. To enable the network to learn semantic attractors, the architecture included semantic "clean-up" units much like those in the Hinton and Shallice (1991) network (shown in Figure 2a). Because abstract words have far fewer semantic features, they are less able to engage this semantic clean-up mechanism effectively to form strong attractors during training. These words must therefore rely more heavily on the direct mapping from orthography to semantics, where visual influences are strongest. As a

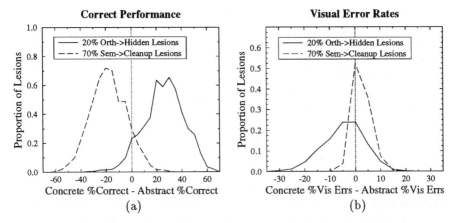

Figure 4: Differences between concrete and abstract words in (a) correct performance, and (b) visual error rates, after 1000 moderate lesions to the "direct" pathway from orthography to semantics (solid lines) in the Plaut and Shallice (1993) concrete/abstract network, and after 1000 severe lesions to the "clean-up" pathway that implemented the semantic attractors (dashed lines). Plotted values are differences (concrete−abstract); positive values (towards the right) reflect greater correct performance or visual error rates for concrete as compared with abstract words. The solid lines correspond to the pattern of deep dyslexia; the dashed lines correspond to the pattern of concrete word dyslexia. Adapted from Plaut (1995).

result, lesions to this pathway reproduce the effects of concreteness and their interaction with visual errors found in deep dyslexia: better correct performance for concrete over abstract words, a tendency for error responses to be more concrete than stimuli, and a higher proportion of visual errors in response to abstract compared with concrete words (see the solid lines in Figure 4).

Surprisingly, severe lesions to connections within the clean-up mechanism that implemented the semantic attractors produced the *opposite* effect: abstract words were now read better than concrete words, and concrete words produced more visual errors than did the abstract words (see the dashed lines in Figure 4). This reversal arises because, under this type of lesion, the processing of most concrete words is impaired but many abstract words can be read solely by the direct pathway. In fact, there is a single known exception to the advantage for concrete words shown by deep dyslexic patients: patient CAV with *concrete word dyslexia* (Warrington, 1981). CAV failed to read concrete words like MILK and TREE but succeeded at highly abstract words such as APPLAUSE, EVIDENCE, and INFERIOR. Overall, abstract words were more likely to be correctly read than concrete (55% vs. 36%). In complementary fashion, 63% of his visual error responses were more abstract than the stimulus. Furthermore, the hypothesis of severe damage to semantic attractors is consistent with other aspects of his performance: CAV's reading disorder was quite severe initially, and he also showed an advantage for abstract words in picture-word matching with auditory presentation, suggesting severe modality-independent damage at the level of the semantic system.

The double dissociation between reading concrete versus abstract words in patients was interpreted by Warrington and others (e.g., Morton & Patterson, 1980) as implying that concrete and abstract semantics are represented separately in the brain. The Plaut and Shallice (1993) simulation demonstrates that such a radical interpretation is unnecessary: the double dissociation can arise from damage to different parts of a distributed network, in which parts process both types of items but develop somewhat different functional specializations through learning (see Plaut, 1995, for further results and discussion).

Overall, the Plaut and Shallice (1993) simulations of deep dyslexia (and of the single, enigmatic case of concrete word dyslexia) provide strong support for characterizing the operation of the semantic pathway, and lexical semantic processing more generally, in terms of a distributed network like that in Figure 1, which learns to form attractors for word meanings. It should be pointed out, however, that it is possible to model analogous phenomena by using localist word units to implement the semantic attractors (see Martin, Dell, & Schwartz, 1994; Martin, Saffran, & Dell, 1996, and the chapter by Dell, Schwartz, Martin, Saffran, & Gagnon, this volume). The advantage of the fully distributed approach in the current context is that the properties of normal and impaired semantic processing arise out of the same computational principles that operate in the rest of the lexical system.

3 Rehabilitating Reading Via Meaning

A computationally explicit theory of normal and impaired cognitive processing should aid in attempts to remediate the impairments (Howard & Hatfield, 1987). In a complementary fashion, accounting for the patterns of recovery exhibited by brain-damaged patients undergoing specific treatment can provide a stringent test of cognitive theories. However, relatively few remediation studies have been based directly on cognitive analyses, and while these have been relatively successful, the specific contribution of the cognitive model—typically a box-and-arrow diagram—is often unclear (see Riddoch & Humphreys, 1994; Margolin, 1992; Seron & Deloche, 1989).

Coltheart and Byng (1989) undertook a series of remediation studies with a surface dyslexic patient, EE, with left temporal-parietal damage due to a fall. On the basis of a number of preliminary tests, they determined that EE had a specific deficit in deriving semantics from orthography. In one study, they gave EE 485 high-frequency words for oral reading and the 54 words he misread were divided in half randomly into treated and untreated sets. For words in the treated set, EE studied cards of the written words augmented with mnemonics for their meanings. As a result, his reading performance on the treated words improved from 44% to 100% correct. Surprisingly, the untreated words also improved, from 44% to 85% correct; that is, the improvement on untreated words was 73% as much as on treated words. This generalized improvement was specific to the intervention because EE's performance on the words was stable both before and after therapy. Two other studies with EE produced broadly similar results. Overall, Coltheart and Byng found excellent recovery of treated items and substantial generalization to untreated items (also see Weekes & Coltheart, in press).

Unfortunately, such promising results are not always found in rehabilitation studies, even those with very similar types of patients. Scott and Byng (1989) treated a surface dyslexic patient for homophone confusions in reading (e.g., TAIL/TALE) and produced improvement on treated items and, to a lesser extent, untreated items, but found no generalization to his writing of the same items (also see Behrmann, 1987). Behrmann and Lieberthal (1989) trained a globally aphasic patient with semantic impairments on a semantic category sorting task. They found improvement on untreated items only within some categories and minimal generalization to items in untreated categories. Finally, Hillis (1993) carried out an extensive rehabilitation program with a patient who had both orthographic and semantic impairments. The patient was able to learn trained tasks (e.g., lexical decision, naming) but showed virtually no generalization to untrained tasks.

Why some patients improve while others do not is not entirely clear. Furthermore, even in those patients who do improve and show generalization, the cause of this generalization—in terms of changes to the underlying cognitive mechanism induced by treatment—is unknown. An explanation of these findings should account not only for the occurrence of generalization in some patients and conditions, but also for its absence in others. As Hillis (1993) points out, what is needed is a theory of rehabilitation that provides a detailed specification of the impaired cognitive system, how it changes in response to treatment, and what factors are relevant to the efficacy of the treatment.

Early connectionist research (Hinton & Plaut, 1987; Hinton & Sejnowski, 1986) demonstrated that simple networks trained on unstructured tasks can, when retrained after damage, exhibit rapid recovery on treated items and generalization to untreated items. Plaut (1996) extended these findings to apply directly to understanding the basis and variability of recovery in patients, and

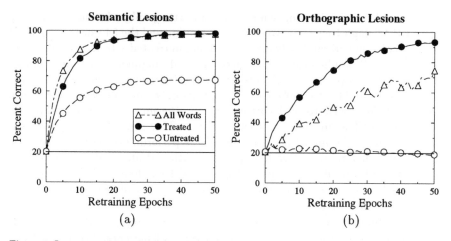

Figure 5: Improvement on treated and untreated items when retraining a network that maps orthography to semantics after (a) lesions within semantics (to the semantics-to-cleanup connections shown in Figure 2a), and after (b) lesions near orthography (to the grapheme-to-intermediate connections). Adapted from Plaut (1996).

to provide a platform for testing hypotheses on how to select items for treatment to maximize generalized recovery.

In one simulation, a replication of the Hinton and Shallice (1991) network shown in Figure 2a was subjected to damage either near orthography (to the grapheme-to-intermediate connections) or within semantics (to the semantics-to-cleanup connections) and retrained on half of the words. This retraining produced rapid improvement on treated words and substantial generalization to untreated words only after lesions within semantics; when retraining after lesions near orthography, improvement on treated words was erratic and there was no generalization to untreated words (see Figures 5a and b). This difference was due to the relative degree of *consistency* in the mapping performed at different levels of the network. Within semantics, similar words require similar interactions, so that the weight changes caused by retraining on some words will tend also to improve performance on other, related words (i.e., the optimal weight changes for words are mutually consistent). By contrast, similar orthographic patterns typically must generate very different semantic patterns. As a result, when retraining after lesions near orthography, the weight changes for treated items are unrelated to those that would improve the untreated items, and there is no generalization. These finding provide a basis for understanding the mechanisms of recovery and generalization in patients, and may help explain the observed variability in their recovery.

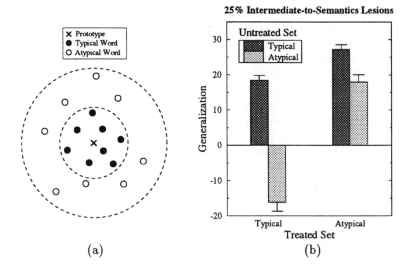

Figure 6: (a) A depiction of the relationship in semantic space between the prototype of a category and typical versus atypical exemplars in that category. (b) Generalization from retraining after lesions of 25% of the intermediate-to-semantics connections, as a function of the semantic typicality of the treated and untreated sets. Adapted from Plaut (1996).

In a second simulation, Plaut (1996) used an artificial version of the task of mapping orthography to semantics to investigate whether generalization was greater when retraining on typical versus atypical category exemplars (e.g., ROBIN vs. GOOSE). Somewhat surprisingly, although retraining on typical exemplars produced greater recovery on treated items, retraining on atypical exemplars produced greater generalization to untreated items (see Figure 6). These findings make sense given the adequacy with which sets of typical versus atypical exemplars approximate the range of semantic similarity among all of the words. Semantically typical words accurately estimate the central tendency of a category, but provide little information about the ways in which category members can *vary*. By contrast, each atypical word indicates many more ways in which members can differ from the prototype and yet still belong to the category. Thus, collectively, the semantic representations of atypical words cover more of the features needed by the entire set of words than do the representations of more typical words. At the same time, the average effects of retraining on atypical words provides a reasonable estimate of the central tendency of the category, yielding generalization to typical words (as found in human category learning by, e.g., Posner & Keele, 1968). In this way, the simulation generated a novel prediction about how to select items for treatment so as to maximize generalized recovery.

In a final simulation, Plaut (1996) used the *failure* of the network to replicate the error pattern of recovering deep dyslexic patients to constrain the
underlying theory: that the improvement of these patients must be due, at
least in part, to some recovery of function in the (unimplemented) phonological
pathway. The relevant empirical finding is that deep dyslexia can resolve into
phonological dyslexia (Beauvois & Derouesné, 1979). The defining characteristic of phonological dyslexic patients is that they have a selective impairment
in reading nonwords compared with reading words. Although such patients do
not make semantic errors, they can be quite similar to deep dyslexic patients
in other respects. In fact, Glosser and Friedman (1990, also see Newcombe &
Marshall, 1980) argued that deep and phonological dyslexic patients fall on
a continuum of severity of impairment, with deep dyslexia at the most severe end. Moreover, Friedman (1996, also see Klein, Behrmann, & Doctor,
1994) has argued that the symptoms in deep dyslexia resolve in a particular
order over the course of recovery, reflecting the continuum of impairment. The
occurrence of semantic errors is the first symptom to resolve, constituting a
somewhat arbitrary transition from deep to phonological dyslexia). The concreteness effect is the next symptom to resolve, followed by the part-of-speech
effect, then the visual and morphological errors, and only lastly, the impaired
nonword reading. A similar pattern of recovery has been documented in deep
dysphasic patients, who make semantic errors in repetition (see Martin, Dell, &
Schwartz, 1994; Martin, Saffran, & Dell, 1996, and Dell et al., this volume).

Plaut (1996) measured the changes in the distribution of error types brought
about by retraining an orthography-to-semantics network after damage. Rather
than semantic errors being the first to drop out, visual and unrelated errors
were eliminated earliest. Semantic and mixed visual-and-semantic errors were
eliminated only at the very end of retraining. Thus, the changes in the pattern of errors produced by the network in recovery to near normal levels of
correct performance failed to reproduce the transition from deep to phonological dyslexia observed in patients. This discrepancy between the behavior of
the network and that of patients can be understood if recovery in the patients
involves more than relearning in the semantic route alone. In particular, the
findings suggest that, within the current approach, the transition from deep to
phonological dyslexia must also involve some improvement in the operation of
the phonological pathway (or in phonology itself). Such improvement would
produce a greater reduction in semantic errors relative to other types of error because even partial correct phonological information about the stimulus
would be sufficient to rule out most semantic errors (Newcombe & Marshall,
1980).

One clear indicator of the operation of the phonological route is the ability to read pronounceable nonwords, as such items cannot be read via semantics. Thus, the above explanation is supported by the observation that, for many deep/phonological patients, as their rates of semantic errors dropped to near zero, their nonword reading performance improved. For example, on initial testing, patient GR (Glosser & Friedman, 1990) made 11% semantic errors and read correctly 5% (1/20) of nonwords. Seven months later, he made no purely semantic errors (although 3% were visual-and-semantic); concurrently, his nonword reading had improved to 44% (22/50). Similar results have been found with a number of other patients (e.g., DV, Glosser & Friedman, 1990; EG, Laine, Niemi, & Marttila, 1990; but see Plaut, 1996, for discussion of a possible exception: RL, Klein et al., 1994). Thus, while the behavior of the network on its own fails to account for the resolution of deep to phonological dyslexia, its performance is consistent with a more general account in which the phonological route also contributes to the nature of the recovery in these patients.

In summary, the Plaut (1996) simulations demonstrate that the investigation of relearning after damage in connectionist networks can provide insight into the basis and variability of recovery of the impairments of brain-damaged patients, can generate interesting hypotheses on how to design therapy to remediate these impairments, and can contribute valuable theoretical constraints on our understanding of normal and impaired cognitive processing.

4 Conclusions

The current work adopts a perspective on lexical processing in which distributed representations of orthographic, phonological, and semantic information interact and mutually constrain each other in the process of settling on the best interpretation and response for a given input. The success of connectionist implementations of the phonological pathway—from orthography to phonology—in modeling normal and impaired word reading (Plaut et al., 1996; Seidenberg & McClelland, 1989) stems in large part from the fact that connectionist networks are biased to give similar responses to similar inputs. For this very reason, though, mappings within the semantic pathway—from orthography to semantics to phonology—pose a particular challenge to such networks as there is no systematic relationship between the surface forms of (monomorphemic) words and their meanings.

Critically, even though very different problems are being solved within the phonological and semantic pathways, the same computational principles are effective for both. In particular, learning and processing in distributed connectionist networks are sensitive to the *frequency* with which particular items are presented for training, their *similarity* to other items within each domain, and the *consistency* of their mappings between domains with those of other items. Nonetheless, in meeting the different demands of the two pathways, the principles give rise to rather different functional properties. When applied within the phonological pathway, connectionist networks embodying these principles give rise to the empirical pattern of interaction between word frequency and spelling-sound consistency observed in the naming latencies of skilled readers and in the naming accuracy of surface dyslexic readers (see Patterson et al., this volume). When applied within the semantic pathway, networks learn to form *attractors* for familiar word meanings; under damage, these attractors give rise to semantic errors and their co-occurrence with visual errors, and effects of imageability/concreteness, as exhibited by deep dyslexic patients. Moreover, the degree of generalized recovery following retraining of the damaged semantic pathway depends on the degree of consistency of the optimal weight changes for treated and untreated items—which depend on the specific location of damage within the network and the items selected for treatment.

Taken together, the replication of the diverse set of empirical findings in both normal and impaired reading by networks embodying a common set of computational principles provides strong evidence that the same principles apply within the normal and impaired human reading system.

Acknowledgments

I would like to acknowledge Tim Shallice for his contributions to the research reported in this chapter. The research was supported by grants from the McDonnell-Pew Program in Cognitive Neuroscience (T89–01245–016), the National Science Foundation (ASC–9109215), and the National Institute of Mental Health (MH47566).

References

Barry, C., & Richardson, J. T. E. (1988). Accounts of oral reading in deep dyslexia. In H. A. Whitaker (Ed.), *Phonological processing and brain mechanisms* (pp. 118–171). New York: Springer-Verlag.

Beauvois, M.-F., & Derouesné, J. (1979). Phonological alexia: Three dissociations. *Journal of Neurology, Neurosurgery, and Psychiatry, 42*, 1115–1124.

Behrmann, M. (1987). The rites of righting writing: Homophone remediation in acquired dysgraphia. *Cognitive Neuropsychology, 4*, 365–384.

Behrmann, M., & Lieberthal, T. (1989). Category-specific treatment of a lexical semantic deficit: A single case study of global aphasia. *British Journal of Communication Disorders*, *24*, 281–299.

Coltheart, M. (1978). Lexical access in simple reading tasks. In G. Underwood (Ed.), *Strategies of information processing* (pp. 151–216). New York: Academic Press.

Coltheart, M. (1985). Cognitive neuropsychology and the study of reading. In M. I. Posner, & O. S. M. Marin (Eds.), *Attention and performance XI* (pp. 3–37). Hillsdale, NJ: Lawrence Erlbaum Associates.

Coltheart, M. (Ed.). (1987). *Attention and performance XII: The psychology of reading*. Hillsdale, NJ: Lawrence Erlbaum Associates.

Coltheart, M., & Byng, S. (1989). A treatment for surface dyslexia. In X. Seron, & G. Deloche (Eds.), *Cognitive approaches in neuropsychological rehabilitation* (pp. 159–174). Hillsdale, NJ: Lawrence Erlbaum Associates.

Coltheart, M., Curtis, B., Atkins, P., & Haller, M. (1993). Models of reading aloud: Dual-route and parallel-distributed-processing approaches. *Psychological Review*, *100*, 589–608.

Coltheart, M., Patterson, K., & Marshall, J. C. (Eds.). (1980). *Deep dyslexia*. London: Routledge & Kegan Paul, 2 edition.

Dejerine, J. (1892). Contribution à l'étude anatomoclinique et clinique des differentes variétés de cécité verbale. *Mémoires del la Société de Biologie*, *4*, 61–90.

Dell, G. S., Schwartz, M. F., Martin, N., Saffran, E. M., & Gagnon, D. A. (this volume). A connectionist model of naming errors in aphasia. In J. Reggia, R. Berndt, & E. Ruppin (Eds.), *Neural modeling of cognitive and brain disorders*. New York: World Scientific.

Ellis, A. W., & Young, A. W. (1988). *Human cognitive neuropsychology*. Hillsdale, NJ: Lawrence Erlbaum Associates.

Friedman, R. B. (1996). Recovery from deep alexia to phonological alexia. *Brain and Language*, *52*, 114–128.

Gentner, D. (1981). Some interesting differences between verbs and nouns. *Cognition and Brain Theory*, *4*, 161–178.

Glosser, G., & Friedman, R. B. (1990). The continuum of deep/phonological alexia. *Cortex*, *26*, 343–359.

Glushko, R. J. (1979). The organization and activation of orthographic knowledge in reading aloud. *Journal of Experimental Psychology: Human Perception and Performance*, *5*, 674–691.

Hillis, A. E. (1993). The role of models of language processing in rehabilitation of language impairments. *Aphasiology*, *7*, 5–26.

Hinton, G. E. (1989). Deterministic Boltzmann learning performs steepest descent in weight-space. *Neural Computation*, *1*, 143–150.

Hinton, G. E., & Plaut, D. C. (1987). Using fast weights to deblur old memories. In *Proceedings of the 9th Annual Conference of the Cognitive Science Society* (pp. 177–186). Hillsdale, NJ: Lawrence Erlbaum Associates.

Hinton, G. E., & Sejnowski, T. J. (1986). Learning and relearning in Boltzmann Machines. In D. E. Rumelhart, J. L. McClelland, & the PDP Research Group (Eds.), *Parallel distributed processing: Explorations in the microstructure of cognition. Volume 1: Foundations* (pp. 282–317). Cambridge, MA: MIT Press.

Hinton, G. E., & Shallice, T. (1991). Lesioning an attractor network: Investigations of acquired dyslexia. *Psychological Review, 98*, 74–95.

Howard, D., & Hatfield, F. M. (1987). *Aphasia therapy*. Hillsdale, NJ: Lawrence Erlbaum Associates.

Jones, G. V. (1985). Deep dyslexia, imageability, and ease of predication. *Brain and Language, 24*, 1–19.

Klein, D., Behrmann, M., & Doctor, E. (1994). The evolution of deep dyslexia: Evidence for the spontaneous recovery of the semantic reading route. *Cognitive Neuropsychology, 11*, 579–611.

Laine, M., Niemi, J., & Marttila, R. (1990). Changing error patterns during reading recovery: A case study. *Journal of Neurolinguistics, 5*, 75–81.

Margolin, D. (Ed.). (1992). *Cognitive neuropsychology in clinical practice*. Oxford: Oxford University Press.

Marshall, J. C., & Newcombe, F. (1966). Syntactic and semantic errors in paralexia. *Neuropsychologia, 4*, 169–176.

Marshall, J. C., & Newcombe, F. (1973). Patterns of paralexia: A psycholinguistic approach. *Journal of Psycholinguistic Research, 2*, 175–199.

Martin, N., Dell, G. S., & Schwartz, M. F. (1994). Origins of paraphasias in deep dysphasia: Testing the consequences of a decay impairment to an interactive spreading activation model of lexical retrieval. *Brain and Language, 47*, 609–660.

Martin, N., Saffran, E. M., & Dell, G. S. (1996). Recovery in deep dysphasia: Evidence for a relation between auditory-verbal-STM capacity and lexical errors in repetition. *Brain and Language, 52*, 83–113.

McClelland, J. L., & Rumelhart, D. E. (1985). Distributed memory and the representation of general and specific information. *Journal of Experimental Psychology: General, 114*, 159–188.

Meyer, D. E., Schvaneveldt, R. W., & Ruddy, M. G. (1974). Functions of graphemic and phonemic codes in visual word recognition. *Memory and Cognition, 2*, 309–321.

Morton, J. (1969). The interaction of information in word recognition. *Psychological Review, 76*, 165–178.

Morton, J., & Patterson, K. (1980). A new attempt at an interpretation, Or, an attempt at a new interpretation. In M. Coltheart, K. Patterson, & J. C. Marshall (Eds.), *Deep dyslexia* (pp. 91–118). London: Routledge & Kegan Paul.

Mozer, M. C., & Behrmann, M. (1990). On the interaction of selective attention and lexical knowledge: A connectionist account of neglect dyslexia. *Journal of Cognitive Neuroscience, 2,* 96–123.

Newcombe, F., & Marshall, J. C. (1980). Transcoding and lexical stabilization in deep dyslexia. In M. Coltheart, K. Patterson, & J. C. Marshall (Eds.), *Deep dyslexia* (pp. 176–188). London: Routledge & Kegan Paul.

Paap, K. R., & Noel, R. W. (1991). Dual route models of print to sound: Still a good horse race. *Psychological Research, 53,* 13–24.

Patterson, K., Plaut, D. C., McClelland, J. L., Seidenberg, M. S., Behrmann, M., & Hodges, J. R. (this volume). Connections and disconnections: A connectionist account of surface dyslexia. In J. Reggia, R. Berndt, & E. Ruppin (Eds.), *Neural modeling of cognitive and brain disorders.* New York: World Scientific.

Patterson, K., Seidenberg, M. S., & McClelland, J. L. (1989). Connections and disconnections: Acquired dyslexia in a computational model of reading processes. In R. G. M. Morris (Ed.), *Parallel distributed processing: Implications for psychology and neuroscience* (pp. 131–181). London: Oxford University Press.

Peterson, C., & Anderson, J. R. (1987). A mean field theory learning algorithm for neural nets. *Complex Systems, 1,* 995–1019.

Plaut, D. C. (1995). Double dissociation without modularity: Evidence from connectionist neuropsychology. *Journal of Clinical and Experimental Neuropsychology, 17,* 291–321.

Plaut, D. C. (1996). Relearning after damage in connectionist networks: Toward a theory of rehabilitation. *Brain and Language, 52,* 25–82.

Plaut, D. C., McClelland, J. L., Seidenberg, M. S., & Patterson, K. (1996). Understanding normal and impaired word reading: Computational principles in quasi-regular domains. *Psychological Review, 103,* 56–115.

Plaut, D. C., & Shallice, T. (1993). Deep dyslexia: A case study of connectionist neuropsychology. *Cognitive Neuropsychology, 10,* 377–500.

Posner, M. I., & Keele, S. W. (1968). On the genesis of abstract ideas. *Journal of Experimental Psychology, 77,* 353–363.

Riddoch, M. J., & Humphreys, G. W. (Eds.). (1994). *Cognitive neuropsychology and cognitive rehabilitation.* Hillsdale, NJ: Lawrence Erlbaum Associates.

Rosch, E., Mervis, C., Gray, W., Johnson, D., & Boyes-Braem, P. (1976). Basic objects in natural categories. *Cognitive Psychology, 8,* 382–439.

Rumelhart, D. E., Hinton, G. E., & Williams, R. J. (1986). Learning internal representations by error propagation. In D. E. Rumelhart, J. L. McClelland, & the PDP Research Group (Eds.), *Parallel distributed processing: Explorations in the microstructure of cognition. Volume 1: Foundations* (pp. 318–362). Cambridge, MA: MIT Press.

Saffran, E. M., Bogyo, L. C., Schwartz, M. F., & Marin, O. S. M. (1980). Does deep dyslexia reflect right-hemisphere reading? In M. Coltheart, K. Patterson, & J. C. Marshall (Eds.), *Deep dyslexia* (pp. 381–406). London: Routledge & Kegan Paul.

Schwanenflugel, P. J. (1991). Why are abstract concepts hard to understand? In P. J. Schwanenflugel (Ed.), *The psychology of word meanings*. Hillsdale, NJ: Lawrence Erlbaum Associates.

Scott, C., & Byng, S. (1989). Computer assisted remediation of a homophone comprehension disorder in surface dyslexia. *Aphasiology, 3*, 301–320.

Seidenberg, M. S., & McClelland, J. L. (1989). A distributed, developmental model of word recognition and naming. *Psychological Review, 96*, 523–568.

Seron, X., & Deloche, G. (Eds.). (1989). *Cognitive approaches in neuropsychological rehabilitation*. Hillsdale, NJ: Lawrence Erlbaum Associates.

Shallice, T. (1988). *From neuropsychology to mental structure*. Cambridge: Cambridge University Press.

Shallice, T., & Warrington, E. K. (1980). Single and multiple component central dyslexic syndromes. In M. Coltheart, K. Patterson, & J. C. Marshall (Eds.), *Deep dyslexia* (pp. 119–145). London: Routledge & Kegan Paul.

Van Orden, G. C., Pennington, B. F., & Stone, G. O. (1990). Word identification in reading and the promise of subsymbolic psycholinguistics. *Psychological Review, 97*, 488–522.

Warrington, E. K. (1981). Concrete word dyslexia. *British Journal of Psychology, 72*, 175–196.

Weekes, B., & Coltheart, M. (in press). Surface dyslexia and surface dysgraphia: Treatment studies and their theoretical implications. *Cognitive Neuropsychology*.

CONNECTIONS AND DISCONNECTIONS: A CONNECTIONIST ACCOUNT OF SURFACE DYSLEXIA

KARALYN PATTERSON
Medical Research Council Applied Psychology Unit
15 Chaucer Road, Cambridge CB2 2EF, UK, karalyn@mrc-apu.cam.ac.uk

DAVID C. PLAUT
JAMES L. MCCLELLAND
Department of Psychology, Carnegie Mellon University,
and the Center for the Neural Basis of Cognition, Pittsburgh, USA

MARK S. SEIDENBERG
Neuroscience Program, University of Southern California, Los Angeles, USA

MARLENE BEHRMANN
Department of Psychology, Carnegie Mellon University, Pittsburgh, USA

JOHN R. HODGES
Department of Neurology, University of Cambridge Clinical School, Cambridge, UK

The acquired reading disorder of surface dyslexia, in which lower-frequency words with atypical spelling-sound correspondences (e.g., PINT) become highly vulnerable to error, is presented in a framework based on interaction between distributed representations in a triangle of orthographic, phonological, and semantic domains. The framework suggests that low-frequency exception words are rather inefficiently processed in terms of orthographic-phonological constraints, because these words are neither sufficiently common to have much impact on learning in the network nor sufficiently consistent with the pronunciations of their orthographic neighbors to benefit from shared structure. For these words, then, the interaction between phonological and semantic representations may be especially important for settling on the correct pronunciation. It is therefore viewed as no coincidental association that all reported patients with marked surface dyslexia have also been profoundly anomic, suggesting reduced semantic-phonological activation. The chapter summarizes the simulation of surface dyslexia in the computational model of reading developed by Plaut, McClelland, Seidenberg, and Patterson (1996), and presents new data from three surface alexic patients. The graded consistency effects in the patients' reading performance are more compatible with the distributed connectionist framework than with dual-route models maintaining a strict dichotomy between regular and exception words.

1 Background

One of the main issues in reading research concerns the procedures that readers use to compute the pronunciation of written words. According to the dominant view, two different types of letter string in English demand two qualitatively different procedures: the ability of readers to pronounce letter strings that they have never seen before (for example, a nonsense word such as MAVE) requires a procedure based on rules for translating graphemes to phonemes; and the ability to pronounce familiar "irregular" words that break standard grapheme-phoneme correspondence rules (such as HAVE) requires a procedure in which the word's orthographic lexical entry activates its whole-word pronunciation. Considerable evidence—from normal adult readers, from adults with acquired disorders of reading, and from children with developmental dyslexia—has been interpreted as support for this dual-route model, mainly by Coltheart and his colleagues (Castles & Coltheart, 1993; Coltheart, 1985; Coltheart, Curtis, Atkins & Haller, 1993; Coltheart & Rastle, 1994) but by many other reading researchers as well (e.g., Baluch & Besner, 1991; Funnell, 1983; Paap & Noel, 1991). Dual-route theory, instantiated in computational models both by Coltheart et al. (1993) and by Reggia, Berndt and D'Autrechy (1994), is sufficiently well known and accessible in the literature to obviate the need for a full description here. Simply put, its basic premise is that no model of reading will succeed in explaining the known data unless it incorporates separate lexical and sub-lexical mechanisms for translating an orthographic string into a pronunciation (hereinafter O→P).

Despite the prominence and success of dual-route theory, it has had its critics and alternatives. For example, a number of reading researchers have argued that regular and exception words correspond to points on a consistency continuum rather than a dichotomy (Glushko, 1979; Seidenberg, Waters, Barnes & Tanenhaus, 1984; Shallice, Warrington & McCarthy, 1983). Others have claimed that nonword reading, instead of requiring a separate rule-based "non-lexical" system, could be accomplished by extracting and pooling knowledge from lexical representations for structurally similar words (Henderson, 1982; Humphreys & Evett, 1985; Kay & Marcel, 1981). In the last decade, the proposal that a single O→P mechanism is in fact capable of capturing both the generalizations and the exceptions in spelling- sound relationships has been developed in computational models of reading aloud, first by Sejnowski and Rosenberg (1987) and subsequently by Seidenberg and McClelland (1989). The Seidenberg and McClelland model, as a major theoretical statement about the acquisition and skilled performance of single-word reading, attracted considerable attention, much positive but some critical. For example, dual-route theorists (Besner, Twilley, McCann & Seergobin, 1990; Coltheart et al., 1993) contested the claim that Seidenberg and McClelland had demonstrated the adequacy of a single mechanism for reading both exception words and nonwords, because the original simulation achieved notably less success than most human readers do in generalizing its knowledge to the pronunciation of nonwords.

In the most recent phase of this debate, Plaut, McClelland, Seidenberg and Patterson (1996) presented four new simulations of the O→P computation in English. As one principal development on their predecessor (Seidenberg & Mc-Clelland, 1989), the networks in the Plaut et al. model employed orthographic and phonological representations designed to capture more successfully the similarities in orthographic and phonological space. This new design of representations enabled the model to attain accuracy in nonword reading well within the range of real adult readers. Three of the networks had a feedforward architecture; the fourth was an attractor network involving interactivity among the phonological output units and between the phonological units and the hidden-unit layer. Two of the simulations were trained using actual (Kucera & Francis, 1967) frequencies of the 3000 words in the corpus, while the others had some degree of frequency compression, either more or less severe (logarithmic and square-root, respectively). Detailed analyses of the results from these various simulations can be found in the original article; for present purposes, the important summary is the following. Given (a) orthographic and phonological representations that effectively capture spelling-sound consistencies, making the network appropriately sensitive to the range of consistencies in the training vocabulary, and (b) a training regime based on real or approximate word frequencies, making the performance of the network appropriately sensitive to the impact of word frequency, a network with a single O→P procedure can reproduce the pattern of accuracy and response times in naming regular words, exception words, and nonwords that is characteristic of real adult readers.

These results from the fully trained networks of Plaut et al. (1996) establish that a single mechanism, in addition to learning to pronounce both familiar regular words and exceptions, can generalize to novel words. Criticisms of Seidenberg and McClelland's (1989) model of reading, however, did not focus exclusively on its normal reading performance. Early attempts to simulate one prominent form of acquired reading disorder by damaging the Seidenberg and McClelland network had been acknowledged even by its authors as provocative but insufficient (Patterson, Seidenberg & McClelland, 1989); and Coltheart et al. (1993) argued that separate lexical and non-lexical routes are essential to account not only for the correct pronunciation of both nonwords and exception words by normal readers but also for the patterns of performance observed in neurologically acquired disorders of word naming. Another major component of the work by Plaut et al. (1996), therefore, was addressed to the issue of whether and how such disorders, in particular acquired surface dyslexia, might find an explanation in a model that dispenses with separate lexical and non-lexical procedures.

2 Surface Dyslexia

Surface dyslexia is one of the main forms of reading disorder observed when the previously competent reading ability of an adult is disrupted by brain injury or disease (Shallice & Warrington, 1980). This disorder was given its name by Marshall and Newcombe (1973) to convey the idea that, when surface dyslexic patients read a word aloud incorrectly, their errors typically reflect the "surface" structure of the word; the syndrome was contrasted with deep dyslexia, in which errors were construed as reflecting the word's "deep" structure. For the written word PINT, the typical surface dyslexic's error would be /pInt/ (i.e., pronounced like MINT and indeed every word with the spelling pattern -INT in English, except for PINT), whereas a deep dyslexic patient misreading pint would be likely to respond "quart" or possibly "beer" (at least in Britain, where beer in pubs is still served in pints). In describing the typical reading errors of surface dyslexia—often called *regularization* errors, because the irregular word pint is pronounced like its regular neighbors MINT, LINT, PRINT, etc.—Marshall and Newcombe (1973) had identified one of the most salient characteristics of the disorder. Further research (Behrmann & Bub, 1992; Bub, Cancelliere & Kertesz, 1985; McCarthy & Warrington, 1986; and Shallice, Warrington & McCarthy, 1983) established that, in its purest form, acquired surface dyslexia is characterized by reading performance on regular words and nonwords that is within normal limits of both accuracy and speed, and a deficit on irregular words that is strongly modulated by word frequency.

The account of surface dyslexia in Coltheart's DRC (Dual-Route Cascaded) model is as follows: the non-lexical grapheme-phoneme route, which can correctly compute O→P for regular words and nonwords, is intact; the lexical route, which is necessary for correct pronunciations of exception words, is damaged in a manner that still enables success on a high-frequency exception word like HAVE but fails on a less common word like PINT, forcing the patient to respond with the non-lexical route's output for this word, i.e., the regularization error /pInt/. As with the mainstream dual-route account of normal reading, this interpretation has been the leading, but not quite the only, bid on the surface dyslexic table. According to Marshall and Newcombe (1973, 1980)—and, with minor variations, to Hillis and Caramazza (1991) and Howard and Franklin (1988)—an adequate theory of O→P requires two routes, but not precisely the same two as proposed by Coltheart (1985; Coltheart et al., 1993). In these conceptions, the lexical route is a lexical semantic procedure; thus a written word can be translated to a phonological code either by sub-lexical correspondences or by activation of the word's meaning followed by the processes normally used, in object naming and spontaneous speech, to activate phonology from meaning. Surface dyslexic reading is thought to arise from a combination of intact sub-lexical procedure and damaged lexical-semantic route. The account of surface dyslexia offered by Plaut et al. (1996) differs somewhat from all of the above; as will be seen in a moment, however, in one crucial respect it is more akin to these alternative dual-route proposals than to Coltheart's view.

Before we explain our position, we should say that it is still evolving. We present our somewhat preliminary account here in the following spirit: McClelland (in his final discussion at the meeting that engendered this book) emphasized that, although all current models are bound to be wrong, they may nevertheless be groping their way towards some important, and even correct, underlying principles.

3   An Account of Surface Dyslexia in the Plaut et al. (1996) Framework

In the final empirical section of their paper, Plaut et al. turned their attention to surface dyslexia. While stopping short of agreeing with Coltheart's claim that damage to a single procedure never could, in principle, account for surface dyslexia, they acknowledged that the dramatic pattern of pure surface dyslexia (i.e., normal reading aloud of regular words and nonwords coupled with a severe, frequency-sensitive deficit on exception words) seems unlikely to arise from damage to the kind of single, direct $O \rightarrow P$ computation developed thus far. "Lesions" to the network sufficiently severe to reproduce the appropriate degree of impairment on exception words also disrupt the model's performance on regular and nonwords. The Plaut et al. model, however, like the Seidenberg and McClelland model before it, and also like the views of single-word processing proposed by Bullinaria (in press), Kawamoto and Zemblige (1992), and Van Orden and Goldinger (1994), has the broader "triangle" framework sketched in Figure 1. Therefore, despite the demonstration that a fully trained model of direct $O \rightarrow P$ translation is capable of learning to produce correct pronunciations for all sorts of letter strings, it may be that the typical human reader does not solve the $O \rightarrow P$ problem in precisely this way. In particular, the possibility remains that some aspects of skilled written word pronunciation might rely on access to semantic representations of words (S). This influence could occur on the basis of either $O \rightarrow S \rightarrow P$ activation or $O \rightarrow P \leftrightarrow S$ activation and interaction; in either case, the important component is the $S \rightarrow P$ link. The account developed in Plaut et al. is that communication from meaning to phonology is particularly critical for processing of words that are only weakly learned by direct $O \rightarrow P$, namely low-frequency words with atypical spelling-to-

182

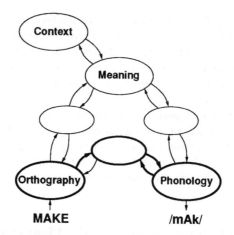

Figure 1: The "triangle" framework for single-word processing from Seidenberg and McClelland (1989) and Plaut, McClelland, Seidenberg and Patterson (1996).

sound correspondences, and that pure surface dyslexia is thus attributable to reduced activation from S→P. This is not a new idea: although the nature of the direct O→P translation in Plaut et al. differs from that in other theories of the reading process, recall that Hillis and Caramazza (1991), Howard and Franklin (1988), and Marshall and Newcombe (1973, 1980) all implicated word meaning in their accounts of surface dyslexia.

Before presenting the simulation work from Plaut et al. (1996) designed to explore this hypothesis, we shall briefly summarize existing evidence about human reading performance, both normal and abnormal, which supports the idea that semantic representations of words should be considered germane to the process of translating print to pronunciation.

(1) In the usual context for which reading skills are mobilized—text reading —few people would doubt that the pronunciation of written words must be open to semantic influences. For example, readers correctly pronounce heterophonic homographs (such as WIND, LEAD and BASS) when they are reading text aloud. Assuming that the human O→P direct computation has learned to activate both legitimate pronunciations of such words (like the networks in Plaut et al., which were trained on both), the pronunciation appropriate to a particular context (e.g., of the noun WIND, that blows, or the verb WIND, that one used to do to watches) can be selected via S→P activation.

(2) In a study of accuracy and response times (RTs) for single-word naming by normal adult readers, Strain, Patterson and Seidenberg (1995) manip-

ulated a semantic variable, imageability, in their selection of stimulus words. Hypothesizing that a significant impact of this variable on word naming should be observable mainly for words rather weakly supported by the direct O→P procedure, they also included the variables of word frequency and regularity. As predicted, a disadvantage in both accuracy and RT for words with low-imageability ratings was obtained primarily for lower-frequency words with atypical spelling-sound correspondences. This does not of course mean that, for words that are either commonly encountered or that fit the most common spelling-sound patterns, there is no automatic activation of word meaning; for such words, however, O→P activation on its own may be sufficient to achieve rapid and stable phonological representations. This computation is less effective for low-frequency inconsistent words; and then communication from S→P (which is stronger for imageable words with richer semantic representations) may detectably assist in settling on a pattern of phonological activation.

(3) If surface dyslexia is attributable to some disruption in communication between semantic and phonological representations, then patients with acquired surface dyslexia should be anomic, since naming of objects or concepts relies on the S→P link. As far as we know, there are no exceptions to this association; that is, all published cases of patients with acquired "pure" surface reading have also had a prominent anomia.

(4) It appears that the association between surface dyslexia and anomia may sometimes even respect category specificity: DRB (Franklin, Howard & Patterson, 1995), who was only measurably anomic for abstract words and concepts, was also significantly impaired in reading exception words only if they had abstract meanings.

(5) The entailment or prediction in this account is only for a disruption in communication from S→P. It should not matter, in principle, whether this difficulty arises from degraded semantic representations or from a reduced capacity for activating phonology from meaning. Although the majority of reported cases of pure surface dyslexia have had a profound impairment to semantic memory per se (e.g., Breedin, Saffran & Coslett, 1994; Bub et al., 1985; Funnell, in press; McCarthy & Warrington, 1986; Parkin, 1993; Patterson & Hodges, 1992), there are also surface dyslexic patients whose deficits in naming and reading have been assigned to the S→P link (Graham, Patterson & Hodges, 1995; Watt, Jokel & Behrmann, in press).

(6) In studies of patients whose surface dyslexia is attributed to degraded semantic memory, three separate groups of investigators have reported a significant concordance between reading aloud and comprehension: that is, with irregular words, the items that are named correctly (as opposed to regularized) tend significantly to be the same ones on which the patient succeeds in a

comprehension test such matching spoken words to pictures (Funnell, in press; Graham, Hodges & Patterson, 1994; Hillis & Caramazza, 1991).

Finally, it is important to note that surface alexia may sometimes be masked by additional deficits, especially at the level of speech production. One perspicacious question about our predicted association between impaired word comprehension and surface dyslexia has been: should one not then find a common association between surface dyslexia and Wernicke's aphasia, a language disorder standardly interpreted as a comprehension deficit? Our first response to this question is that speech production in Wernicke's aphasia is often so disturbed and distorted by phonological problems that it might be hard to observe an advantage in oral reading for regular over exception words. Our second response is that at least one Wernicke's aphasic patient without a profound phonological deficit has shown the frequency-by-regularity interaction in reading accuracy that is characteristic of surface alexia (Behrmann, unpublished data).

4 Simulation of Surface Dyslexia by Plaut et al. (1996)

The instantiation by Plaut et al. (1996) of the way in which word meaning might influence O→P translation did not attempt to provide a genuine representation of meaning; rather, the contribution of meaning was approximated by providing an extra source of input to the phoneme units to push them toward their correct activations. The simulation used a feedforward network with square-root compression of word frequency, plus a small weight decay factor; this biases the network to keep weights small and has the effect of preventing overlearning. The major change from the previous simulations performed without any semantic component was that, over the course of O→P training, the additional source of input to phoneme units (notional semantics) was gradually introduced. The basis for this graded procedure was the assumption that, because O→P mappings in an alphabetic orthography (even a quasi-regular one like English) are much more systematic than O→S mappings, beginning readers learn the former more rapidly than the latter. Furthermore, a larger additional input was provided for high- than for low-frequency words on the assumption that real O→S learning is stronger for frequently encountered words. The gradual and frequency-modulated additional input to phoneme units is illustrated in Figure 2, for a subset of the 2998 monosyllabic words in the training corpus, namely the high- and low-frequency words used in experiments by Taraban and McClelland (1987).

Performance during training is illustrated in Figure 3 for the sets of Taraban and McClelland (1987) words and Glushko (1979) nonwords. At early

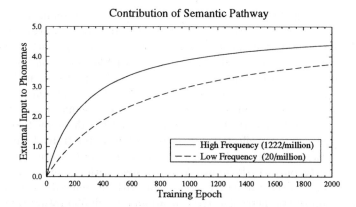

Figure 2: An illustration of the gradual addition of notional semantic input to the phoneme units during O→P training in the Plaut et al (1996) simulation of surface dyslexia; shown here for the Taraban and McClelland (1987) high- and low-frequency words.

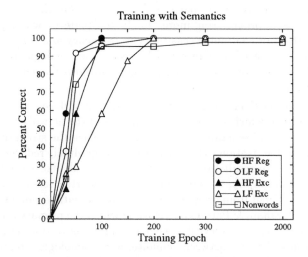

Figure 3: Performance of the Plaut et al (1996) O→P network trained with additional input (notional semantics) to the phoneme units, at various stages of training, on the Taraban and McClelland (1987) high-and low-frequency regular and exception words and the Glushko (1979) nonwords.

stages of training (epochs 50–100), adequacy of word pronunciations (percent correct, i.e., whether the correct phoneme unit at each segment of the monosyllable—onset, vowel, coda—is the most active unit) clearly varies as a function of both frequency and consistency; and performance on items which benefit from neither frequency nor consistency (LF Exc words in Figure 3) is still not perfect at epoch 150. By epoch 200, all word pronunciations are correct, and nonwords (which receive no additional "semantic" input) have achieved a level of 95% correct pronunciations. Although this network yields frequency and regularity effects characteristic of networks trained without notional semantics, the net with additional input naturally learns faster than simulations with only O→P input. A net trained with the identical learning parameters and initial random weights, but with no semantic contribution, reached asymptote on percent correct at around epoch 500 rather than 200.

From epoch 200 to 2000, when responses to the different word sets can no longer be distinguished by the percent correct measure (see Figure 3), a significant frequency-by-consistency interaction in the model's performance is still observable in the cross-entropy error score, a measure of the discrepancy between the pattern of activation over the phoneme units generated by the network and the precise target pattern of activation. On the assumption that output patterns approximating more closely to "perfect" will support more rapid responses, this continuing sensitivity to frequency and consistency in the model's fully trained performance can be seen as an analogue of the human skilled reader's response times to name high- and low-frequency regular and exception words.

The results particularly germane to modeling surface dyslexia are presented in Figure 4, which shows the performance of the network that had been trained with notional semantics for 2000 epochs, when the strength of this additional source of activation to the output units is gradually reduced. Although surface dyslexia can result from an abrupt brain insult like a cerebrovascular accident or a head injury, the great majority of reported cases of pure surface dyslexia have suffered from progressive brain disease: either semantic dementia (e.g., Hodges, Graham & Patterson, 1995), in which the primary impairment is apparently in conceptual knowledge itself, or a progressive aphasia which seems to affect mainly the link between semantic and phonological representations (e.g., Graham et al., 1995; Watt et al., in press). In both cases, we assume that there is a gradual reduction in the activation of phonology by semantics, and the simulation was intended to mimic this phenomenon by post-training withdrawal of the additional input to the phoneme units, leaving only orthographic input to phonology.

Although Figure 4 represents post-training performance, what it reveals is

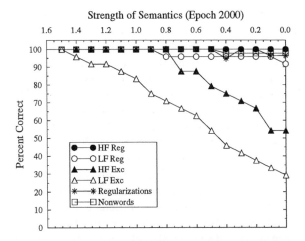

Figure 4: Performance of the Plaut et al (1996) O→P network trained with additional input (notional semantics) to the phoneme units for 2000 epochs, when the strength of the semantic input is gradually reduced; results are shown for percent correct on the Taraban and McClelland (1987) words and the Glushko (1979) words, and for percentage of errors to Exc words that are regularizations.

the effect of the notional semantic input during training. Because this second source of input pushes the activation of each output unit in the appropriate direction—up if it should be on for the target word, down if it should be off— the gradual increase in semantic input in the training phase reduces the amount of error in the network's responses, which in turn reduces pressure for further learning in the O→P computation. As error decreases, the weights become smaller (recall that this net was also trained with a tendency for weight decay). Larger weights are especially important for exception words, which must compete against the conspiracy of many smaller weights supporting typical spelling-sound correspondences. The impact of the additional semantic input during training is therefore an actual decline in O→P competence, first for LF Exc words and eventually, to some degree, even for HF Exc words. This effect is not observable in the model's accuracy during training because the incrementing semantic input keeps improving the net's performance. When, in the simulation of progressive brain disease, this additional input is gradually withdrawn, the underlying competence of O→P knowledge is revealed. As a function of decreasing strength of semantic input, accuracy of pronunciation (a) remains high for Reg words of any frequency and for nonwords, (b) declines steadily on LF Exc words, and (c) also declines on HF Exc words, though the vulnerability of these commonly encountered words is slower to emerge and always less dramatic.

There is one further curve in Figure 4, somewhat difficult to resolve visually from those indicating essentially ceiling accuracy on regular words and nonwords: the points represented by asterisks indicate the nature of the network's error responses to exception words. Essentially all of the errors were regularizations of the PINT → /pInt/ variety. In the purest cases of reported human surface dyslexia (e.g., Behrmann & Bub, 1992; McCarthy & Warrington, 1986), one also observes virtually perfect reading aloud of regular words and nonwords and almost exclusively regularization errors to exception words.

Although this is a preliminary and certainly incomplete account of surface dyslexia, the success of the simulation is considerable. The values of accuracy for the different word classes at various points along the abscissa in Figure 4 correspond reasonably well to those observed for genuine cases of surface alexia. For example, on similar (though not identical) sets of monosyllabic words, PB and KT (two of the progressive patients reported by Patterson & Hodges, 1992, Table 2, p. 1030) both scored 90–100% correct on high- and low-frequency regular words. PB's scores for the high- and low-frequency exception words were 86% and 48%, respectively, which is very close to the network's performance with "strength of semantics" reduced to 0.5; and KT's high- and low-frequency exception scores were 50% and 8%, respectively: not too far off the model's performance at the point where all putative semantic support has been withdrawn, though the patient's LF Exc value is clearly poorer than the net's. Critically, KT's comprehension loss was much more severe than PB's as measured by other tests such word-picture matching. We acknowledge that our framework (and perhaps those of others as well) is a long way from an understanding of individual differences in both normal and impaired reading skill. In particular, the ideas developed here have recently been challenged by reports of a few patients with deficits on semantic tests who are within the normal range of performance in reading exception words (Cipolotti & Warrington, 1995; Lambon-Ralph, Ellis & Franklin, 1995; Raymer & Berndt, 1994). Some possible interpretations of this dissociation, which is apparently incompatible with our prediction, are discussed in Plaut et al. (1996).

We conclude from this simulation work that, although the story is perhaps somewhat different from and more complicated than that originally envisioned, patterns of both normal and disordered reading can be understood in the framework proposed by Seidenberg and McClelland (depicted in Figure 1). Some, but not all, of the critique of this approach by Coltheart et al. (1993) was apposite. Contrary to their critique, the initial simulations of Plaut et al. (1996) demonstrate that a single mechanism for activating phonology from orthography is capable of acquiring knowledge that supports both pronouncing exceptions and generalizing to novel forms. In line with their critique, however, lesions to such networks do not reproduce the pattern of pure surface alexia. We therefore acknowledge that another "pathway" or, as we have character- ized it, another source of input to phonology appears to be necessary to model surface alexia. Perhaps an even better term is the one employed by Kawamoto and Zemblige (1992): source of constraint. They argue that their experimental results (which concern the precise time-course of normal skilled pronunciation of heterophonic homographs like bass and lead) can be explained by a dis- tributed perspective, but only if it provides two constraints on pronunciation, orthographic and semantic. On the basis of a quite different set of human and network results, we have reached the same conclusion.

Despite this new apparent similarity between dual-route and triangle per- spectives, some important differences remain. For one thing, and this is the reason that we prefer the phrase "source of input or constraint," we do not think in terms of two wholly separate pathways or routes. Unlike the DRC model of Coltheart et al. (1993), we assume that the same orthographic and phonological representations support both word and nonword reading. Al- though it has not been fully implemented, the triangle model of Figure 1 is meant to represent a genuinely interactive, recurrent system rather than the combination of two separate pathways, O→P and O→S→P. Secondly, it must be emphasized that the two sources of constraint in this approach do not divide the English language vocabulary neatly into rule-obeying and rule-infringing words as in the two routes of the DRC model. The orthographic source of constraint on pronunciation, even with additional semantic input, embodies considerable knowledge about the inconsistencies of O→P relationships, espe- cially derived from its experience with the more common exception patterns. This is why both the model and the patients still pronounce a fair number of exception words correctly even when all semantic support has been eliminated. Furthermore, as we shall argue below, performance on words with intermediate degrees of consistency—irregular by strict "rule," but with support from other similarly structured words—finds a more natural explanation in the triangle framework than in dual-route theories.

5   Further Observations on Surface Dyslexic Reading

In the final section of this chapter, we introduce some further data from our recent studies of surface dyslexic patients that seem especially compatible with the kind of framework presented here.

Table 1: Two sets of 12 exception words, showing—for each word—the Kucera-Francis frequency, the number of exemplars in the Body Neighborhood with Reg:Exc pronunciations, and the number of correct pronunciations (out of 3) for three surface alexic patients (MP, PB, AM); the lower part of the Table shows performance on the same sets of words by the Plaut et al. (1996) network with various degrees of reduced "semantic" input (as in Figure 4).

	Set A				Set B		
Word	Freq	Reg:Exc	+/3	Word	Freq	Reg:Exc	+/3
1a	464	9:1	3	1b	437	9:1	1
2a	37	15:3	3	2b	88	14:2	2
3a	3	10:3	3	3b	14	9:3	2
4a	4	4:1	3	4b	11	5:1	2
5a	760	4:1	3	5b	391	10:2	2
6a	11	3:1	3	6b	16	2:1	2
7a	67	3:2	3	7b	58	8:3	1
8a	5	12:1	2	8b	13	12:1	0
9a	81	9:1	2	9b	66	9:1	0
10a	2	5:1	2	10b	84	5:1	2
11a	94	2:1	2	11b	730	4:2	0
12a	4	4:1	1	12b	9	6:4	1
Mean	127.7	6.7:1.4	0.83		159.8	7.8:1.8	0.42

Network's proportion correct

semantic strength	= 0.6	1.00			0.67
	= 0.4	0.92			0.50
	= 0.2	0.83			0.42
	= 0.0	0.50			0.25

5.1 Sub-Regularities

Table 1 presents the performance of three surface alexic patients[a] on 24 monosyllabic exception words which have atypical pronunciations of the body/rime—words like PINT. The words in Set A were selected on a particular basis, to be explained in a moment, which led us to expect that surface alexic patients might attain an unusual degree of success in naming these particular exception words; the exception words in Set B were then chosen, from a larger list of words named by all of these patients, to match those in set a as closely as possible on two other measures known to affect performance:

[a]Descriptions of the general characteristics of the three patients in Table 1 can be found as follows: for MP: Behrmann and Bub (1992), Bub, Black, Hampson and Kertesz (1988) and Bub, Cancelliere and Kertesz (1985); for PB: Patterson and Hodges (1992); for AM: Hodges and Patterson (in press).

(i) Kucera and Francis (1967) written word frequency. Where it was not possible to find a Set B word with a precise frequency match to an a item, the bias was towards selecting a more frequent word for B, to work against our prediction of greater success in Set A. This bias is reflected in the mean frequencies for the two sets, which are close but favor Set B.

(ii) The ratio of regular:exception pronunciations within the set of monosyllabic words sharing that particular orthographic body. Word 8a, for example, is PINT; of the monosyllabic English words ending in -INT, 12 have regular pronunciations (HINT, LINT, PRINT, etc); PINT is the only exception. For each (unique) body represented in Table 1, the regular exemplars outnumber the exception exemplar(s), in most cases by a substantial number, as reflected in the means on this measure shown in the Table.

Although the numbers of items for this contrast are small, all three patients showed a reliable or nearly reliable advantage for Set A over B: MP, 9/12 vs. 4/12, $\chi^2(1)=4.2$, p=.04; PB, 10/12 vs. 4/12, $\chi^2(1)=6.2$, p=.01; AM, 11/12 vs. 7/12, $\chi^2(1)=3.6$, p=.059. Combining the three patients' data yields a highly reliable contrast, 30/36 vs. 15/36, $\chi^2(1)=13.3$, p<.001. No word in Set B was named correctly by all patients, whereas 7/12 Set A words were given correct pronunciations by all three. Virtually all of the errors by all three patients on both sets of words were regularizations: all three named PINT to rhyme with "hint" and GROSS to rhyme with "moss"; two of the three pronounced PUT to rhyme with "hut" and LOSE to rhyme with "nose"; and so on.

When the Plaut et al. (1996) network (where additional "semantic" input to the phoneme units during training is subsequently reduced in strength, as in Figure 4 described above) is tested on the same 24 words, it yields a similar advantage for Set A over B, as shown in the lower part of Table 1. As it happens, when the strength of additional input is at 0.2, the network's performance exactly matches the patients': 83% correct on Set A, 42% correct on Set B. All of the network's errors were regularizations.

What is it about Set A words that makes them relatively (though clearly not altogether) immune to regularization, by both patients and network? The answer, in our view, is that these words enjoy a kind of sub-regularity, based not on the body/rime but on the combination of the initial consonant and vowel. Almost all (10/12) of the words in set a begin either WA- or WO-, and the remaining two (SWAMP and QUART) have the same character.[b] Leaving aside

---

[b] In view of demonstrations that at least normal readers' pronunciations of words and nonwords may be subject to priming or biasing effects from other similar items in the list context (Kay & Marcel, 1981; Seidenberg et al., 1984), it should be noted that the patients were not asked to read the 12 W-words as a block; these items were embedded in, and well distributed throughout, a much larger list of words and nonwords (total $N = 198$) . Furthermore, as this list contained both regular words and nonwords with the same bodies

words such as WAKE or WOKE where the pronunciation of the vowel is signalled by the final -E, a substantial majority of WA- words are pronounced not in accordance with the usual pronunciation of the vowel and body (as in CASH or CART) but rather like WASH or WART. Likewise, a great majority of WO-words are pronounced not with the vowel in NORTH but rather like WORTH. As discussed by Seidenberg (1992), in quasi-regular systems like spelling-sound correspondence and past-tense verb formation in English, a number of patterns that do not follow the most general rule are nonetheless characterized by this sort of shared irregularity, thus forming a sub-regularity. Spelling-sound knowledge apparently reflects this sub-regularity; as a result, compared to other exception words with similar familiarity levels and body neighborhoods, "W-words" depend less on the additional source of constraint on pronunciation and so are less vulnerable to its removal.

Dual-route models like that of Coltheart et al. (1993) can, of course, account for the relative invulnerability of W-words, but only by complicating the rule system.

5.2   The Fate of Regular Words in Progressive Surface Dyslexia

Over the past five years or so, various authors of this chapter have carried out detailed investigations of around a dozen patients with acquired surface dyslexia. All of these cases have had either a moderate-to-severe impairment of semantic memory (e.g., Behrmann & Bub, 1992; Patterson & Hodges, 1992) or at least a profound impairment in activation of phonology by semantics, as revealed for example by severe anomia (e.g., Graham, Patterson & Hodges, 1995; Watt, Jokel & Behrmann, 1996). All but one of the cases has suffered from a neuro-degenerative disease[c] characterized behaviorally as semantic dementia or progressive aphasia (see Hodges, Patterson, Oxbury & Funnell, 1992, for further description); the one exception is MP, who sustained a major head injury resulting in unusually focal damage to the left temporal lobe (Behrmann & Bub, 1992; Patterson & Behrmann, submitted). With a number of the progressive patients, we have been able to perform longitudinal assessments of reading performance, some of which are still in progress. On initial assessment,

---

as the W-words (e.g., FORK and LORK as well as WORK, FARM and DARM as well as WARM; words sharing bodies as well as onsets were well separated throughout the set), any biasing effect from the pronunciation of other W-words should have been offset by effects of these items with the same body but discrepant pronunciations.

[c]For readers interested in the underlying pathology of these conditions: three of the patients reported in Patterson and Hodges (1992) have come to post-mortem analysis. Two had Pick's disease. The third had Alzheimer pathology but in a highly atypical distribution: the profound focal left temporal atrophy and severe neuronal loss in this region was more characteristic of semantic dementia due to Pick's disease than of AD.

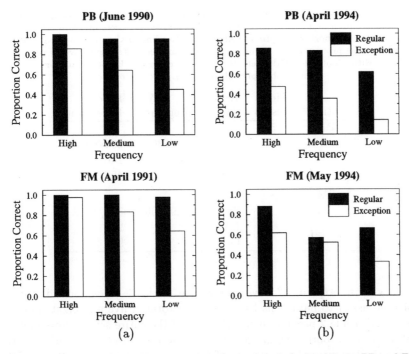

Figure 5: Reading performance by two progressive surface dyslexic patients, PB and FM, (a) at their initial assessment, on the Patterson and Hodges (1992) high-, medium- and low-frequency regular and exception words; and (b) about 4 (PB) and 3 (FM) years later.

virtually all of the patients could be described as having a pattern of pure surface dyslexia, in the sense that their accuracy of word naming was notably outside normal limits for exception words but within normal range for regular words. This is illustrated in Figure 5 for PB and FM, two of the cases from the Patterson and Hodges (1992) study. These data are from the list of words employed in that study, which consists of 126 pairs of monosyllabic regular and exception words (e.g., PINE and PINT, BLACK and BLOOD, etc) matched for frequency, length and initial phoneme, in three frequency bands. Figure 5 also shows the two patients' performance on the same list approximately three (FM) or four (PB) years later. Although there is still a highly reliable advantage for regular over exception words for both patients at this stage, regular words now yield both errors and a degree of frequency sensitivity (with a slight reversal for FM between medium- and low-frequency regular words).

What is the nature of these emerging errors on regular words, and how

Table 2: Error data from multiple administrations of the surface list to PB and FM, showing each patient's total numbers of errors and the classification of these into two broad classes: (1) LARC errors (short for Legitimate Alternative Reading of Components), e.g., PINT (an exception word) pronounced to rhyme with "mint" and HOOT (a regular word) pronounced to rhyme with "foot"; (2) Other errors (variously described by other authors as visual, orthographic, phonological), e.g., ONCE→"ounce."

Patient	Times Tested	Error Type	Word Type Regular	Exception
PB	5			
		Total	71/630	291/630
		LARC	34	246
		Other	37	45
FM	8			
		Total	129/1008	337/1008
		LARC	41	243
		Other	88	94

are they to be explained? Over the course of the 3–4 year period, PB and FM were asked to name this list of words a total of five and eight times, respectively. Table 2 provides a classification of the entire set of errors made by each patient, on both regular and exception words, into two broad categories. Taking the less interesting category of "Other" errors first, both PB and FM— like virtually all patients with surface alexia (see for example Coltheart et al., 1983), and indeed like virtually all patients with any kind of reading disorder— make a certain number of errors where the response bears a relationship to the target word that is neither "surface" nor "deep" but simply resembles it orthographically and/or phonologically. FM in particular has become more prone to "Other" errors as her reading disorder has worsened; for example, she now makes a number of the letter confusion errors, mainly between visually similar letters (e.g., PRAY→"bray"), that are more characteristic of "pure than of surface alexia. Most, though not all, of the "Other" errors are substitutions of an orthographically/phonologically similar real word for the target, as in ONCE→"ounce," THROAT→"trout," etc. Both PB and FM produced roughly equal numbers of "Other" errors to regular and exception words. This is as we would expect, provided that the regular and exception words are reasonably well matched in orthographic and phonological characteristics (such as similarity to other words in their neighborhoods), and differ only in the predictability of the relationship between spelling and sound.

The error category germane to the present discussion is what we have dubbed *LARC* errors (a term first used by Patterson, Suzuki, Wydell & Sasanuma, 1995), short for Legitimate Alternative Reading of Components. LARC means that the incorrect response reflects a legitimate pronunciation of each component of the word, in the sense that the orthographic component takes that pronunciation in other English words. The "Other" response THROAT→"trout" cannot be classed as a LARC error because there are no English words (at least in the dialect of English spoken by PB and FM), in which TH is pronounced /t/, and there are also no words in which OA is pronounced /au/ as in "trout." The quintessential LARC error is a regularization like PINT→/pInt/; but there are other types of such errors as well. First of all, exception words can and do yield LARC errors which are not pure regularizations. For example, the regularization of BLOOD would rhyme with "food," but PB pronounced it like "good"; the regularization of SWEAT would rhyme with "treat" but he pronounced it like "great"; and so on. Secondly, of even greater interest, regular words also yield LARC errors: PB named HOOT to rhyme with "foot," YEAST like "breast," HEAR like "bear"; FM pronounced BROWN with the body/rime of "blown," HEAT like "threat," COST like "post"; and so on. Not surprisingly, since the very definition of an exception word is that at least one of its components has a different, legitimate, and indeed more common, pronunciation, both PB and FM made far more LARC errors to exception words than to regular words. The important observation is that while errors to regular and exception words may differ in quantity, they do not differ in nature and therefore do not require a different kind of account.

Many of the regular words yielding LARC errors are, of course, the type of word known (since Glushko, 1979) as *regular inconsistent*. A regular inconsistent word (like HOOT) takes the pronunciation that is most typical of its body neighborhood; but one or more words with the same body have a conflicting pronunciation (e.g., FOOT). According to the framework and simulations in Plaut et al. (1996), such regular inconsistent words—rather akin to the W-words— represent an intermediate case between words with completely predictable components and true exceptions. The relatively infrequent but illuminating reading errors of surface dyslexic patients to these words strike us as another significant match between the triangle model and real data. As with the decreased vulnerability of W-words in surface dyslexia, the slightly increased vulnerability of regular inconsistent words is a direct prediction of the triangle framework. No doubt these data can also be given an explanation in a dual-route framework. In the DRC model, this would presumably involve interaction between the phoneme system (which is activated by the GPC rule system, and should support correct reading of a regular word like hoot) and the phonological output lexicon. If presentation of HOOT partially activates the lexical representations for orthographically similar words like FOOT and SOOT, the rule-based pronunciation of HOOT might occasionally succumb to this influence and be ir-regularized. As suggested by Sasanuma, Itoh, Patterson and Itoh (in press), to the extent that such interactive influences between lexical and non-lexical systems provide a major explanatory principle in the DRC model, the differences between the two approaches become less critical.

We conclude with an observation which, in the context of this book, may constitute preaching to the converted: that both components of the book's topic are proving important in the effort to understand the human brain and its capabilities. Not only must we build computational models whose predictions can be tested; the data against which the models are tested must include disordered as well as normal functioning.

Acknowledgments

The work reported here was supported in part by grants from the NIMH (USA) to J. L. McClelland and colleagues, and from the MRC (UK) to J. R. Hodges and colleagues. We are grateful to Naida Graham and Eamon Strain for research assistance.

References

Baluch, B., & Besner, D. (1991). Visual word recognition: Evidence for strategic control of lexical and nonlexical routines in oral reading. *Journal of Experimental Psychology: Learning, Memory and Cognition, 17*, 644–652.

Behrmann, M., & Bub, D. (1992). Surface dyslexia and dysgraphia: Dual routes, single lexicon. *Cognitive Neuropsychology, 9*, 209–251.

Besner, D., Twilley, L., McCann, R. S., & Seergobin, K. (1990). On the connection between connectionism and data: Are a few words necessary? *Psychological Review, 97*, 432–446.

Breedin, S. D., Saffran, E. M., & Coslett, H. B. (1994). Reversal of the concreteness effect in a patient with semantic dementia. *Cognitive Neuropsychology, 11*, 617–660.

Bub, D., Black, S., Hampson, E and Kertesz, A. (1988). Semantic encoding of pictures and words: Some neuropsychological observations. *Cognitive Neuropsychology, 5*, 27–66.

Bub, D., Cancelliere, A., & Kertesz, A. (1985). Whole-word and analytic translation of spelling to sound in a nonsemantic reader. In K. Patterson, J. C. Marshall & M. Coltheart (Eds.), *Surface dyslexia* (pp. 15–34). London: Erlbaum.

Bullinaria, J. A. (in press). Connectionist models of reading: Incorporating semantics. In *Proceedings of the 18th Annual Conference of the Cognitive Science Society*. Hillsdale, NJ: Erlbaum.

Castles, A., & Coltheart, M. (1993). Varieties of developmental dyslexia. *Cognition, 47*, 149–180.

Cipolotti, L., & Warrington, E. K. (1995). Semantic memory and reading abilities: A case report. *Journal of the International Neuropsychological Society, 1*, 104–110.

Coltheart, M. (1985). Cognitive neuropsychology and the study of reading. In M. I. Posner and O. S. M. Marin (Eds.), *Attention and performance XI* (pp. 3- 37). Hillsdale, NJ: Erlbaum.

Coltheart, M., Curtis, B., Atkins, P., & Haller, M. (1993). Models of reading aloud: Dual-route and parallel-distributed-processing approaches. *Psychological Review, 100*, 589–608.

Coltheart, M., Masterson, J., Byng, S., Prior, M., & Riddoch, J. (1983). Surface dyslexia. *Quarterly Journal of Experimental Psychology, 35A*, 469–495.

Coltheart, M., & Rastle, K. (1994). Serial processing in reading aloud: Evidence for dual-route models of reading. *Journal of Experimental Psychology: Human Perception and Performance, 20*, 1197–1211.

Franklin, S., Howard, D., & Patterson, K. (1995). Abstract word anomia. *Cognitive Neuropsychology, 12*, 549–566.

Funnell, E. (1983). Phonological processing in reading: New evidence from acquired dyslexia. *British Journal of Psychology, 74*, 159–180.

Funnell, E. (in press). Response biases in oral reading: An account of the co-occurrence of surface dyslexia and semantic dementia. *Quarterly Journal of Experimental Psychology*.

Glushko, R. J. (1979). The organization and activation of orthographic knowledge in reading aloud. *Journal of Experimental Psychology: Human Perception and Performance, 5*, 674–691.

Graham, K. S., Hodges, J. R., & Patterson, K. (1994). The relationship between comprehension and oral reading in progressive fluent aphasia. *Neuropsychologia, 32*, 299–316.

Graham, K. S., Patterson, K., & Hodges, J. R. (1995). Progressive pure anomia: Insufficient activation of phonology by meaning. *Neurocase, 1*, 25–38.

Henderson, L. (1982). *Orthography and Word Recognition in Reading*. London: Academic Press.

Hillis, A. E., & Caramazza, A. (1991). Mechanisms for accessing lexical representations for output: Evidence from a category specific semantic deficit. *Brain and Language, 40*, 106–144.

Hodges, J. R., Graham, N., & Patterson, K. (1995). Charting the progression in semantic dementia: Implications for the organisation of semantic memory. *Memory, 3*, 463–495.

Hodges, J. R., & Patterson, K. (in press). Non-fluent progressive aphasia and semantic dementia: A comparative neuropsychological study. *Journal of the International Neuropsychological Society.*

Hodges, J. R., Patterson, K., Oxbury, S., & Funnell, E. (1992). Semantic dementia: Progressive fluent aphasia with temporal lobe atrophy. *Brain, 115*, 1783–1806.

Howard, D., & Franklin, S. (1988). *Missing the meaning?* Cambridge, Mass: MIT Press.

Humphreys, G. W., & Evett, L. J. (1985). Are there independent lexical and nonlexical routes in word processing? An evaluation of the dual-route theory of reading. *Behavioral and Brain Sciences, 8*, 689–740.

Kawamoto, A. H., & Zemblige, J. H. (1992). Pronunciation of homographs. *Journal of Memory and Language, 31*, 349–374.

Kay, J., & Marcel, A. J. (1981). One process, not two, in reading aloud: Lexical analogies do the work of nonlexical rules. *Quarterly Journal of Experimental Psychology, 33A*, 397–414.

Kucera, H., & Francis, W. N. (1967). *Computational analysis of present-day American English.* Providence, RI: Brown University Press.

Lambon-Ralph, M., Ellis, A. W., & Franklin, S. (1996). Semantic loss without surface dyslexia. *Neurocase, 1*, 363–369.

Marshall, J. C., & Newcombe, F. (1973). Patterns of paralexia: A psycholinguistic approach. *Journal of Psycholinguistic Research, 2*, 175–199.

Newcombe, F., & Marshall, J. C. (1980). Transcoding and lexical stabilization in deep dyslexia. In M. Coltheart, K. Patterson & J. C. Marshall (Eds.), *Deep dyslexia* (pp. 176–188). London: Routledge.

McCarthy, R., & Warrington, E. K. (1986). Phonological reading: Phenomena and paradoxes. *Cortex, 22*, 359–380.

Paap, K. R., & Noel, R. W. (1991). Dual route models of print to sound: still a good horse race. *Psycholinguistic Research, 53*, 13–24.

Parkin, A. J. (1993). Progressive aphasia without dementia due to focal left temporo-frontal hypometabolism—A clinical and cognitive analysis. *Brain and Language, 44*, 201–220.

Patterson, K., & Behrmann, M. (1996). Frequency and consistency effects in a pure surface dyslexic patient. Submitted to *Journal of Experimental Psychology: Human Perception and Performance.*

Patterson, K., & Hodges, J. R. (1992). Deterioration of word meaning: Implications for reading. *Neuropsychologia, 30*, 1025–1040.

Patterson, K., Seidenberg, M. S., & McClelland, J. L. (1989). Connections and disconnections: Acquired dyslexia in a computational model of reading. In R. G. M. Morris (Ed.), *Parallel distributed processing: Implications for psychology and neuroscience* (pp. 131–181). Oxford: OUP.

Patterson, K., Suzuki, T., Wydell, T., & Sasanuma, S. (1995). Progressive aphasia and surface alexia in Japanese. Neurocase, 1, 155–165.

Plaut, D. C., McClelland, J. L., Seidenberg, M. S., & Patterson, K. (1996). Understanding normal and impaired word reading: Computational principles in quasi-regular domains. *Psychological Review, 103*, 56–115.

Raymer, A. M., & Berndt, R. S. (1994). Models of word reading: Evidence from Alzheimer's disease. *Brain and Language, 47*, 479–482.

Reggia, J. A., Berndt, R. S., & D'Autrechy, C. L. (1994). Connectionist models in neuropsychology. In F. Boller & J. Grafman (Eds.), *Handbook of Neuropsychology, Vol. 9* (pp 297–33). North Holland, Elsevier.

Sasanuma, S., Itoh, H., Patterson, K., & Itoh, T. (in press). Phonological alexia in Japanese: A case study. *Cognitive Neuropsychology.*

Seidenberg, M. S. (1992). Connectionism without tears. In S. Davis (Ed.), *Connectionism: Advances in theory and practice* (pp 84–137). Oxford: OUP.

Seidenberg, M. S., & McClelland, J. L. (1989). A distributed, developmental model of word recognition and naming. *Psychological Review, 96*, 523–568.

Seidenberg, M. S., Waters, G. S., Barnes, M. A., & Tanenhaus, M. K. (1984). When does irregular spelling or pronunciation influence word recognition? *Journal of Verbal Learning and Verbal Behavior, 23*, 383–404.

Sejnowski, T. J., & Rosenberg, C. R. (1987). Parallel networks that learn to pronounce English text. *Complex Systems, 1*, 145–168.

Shallice, T., & Warrington, E. K. (1980). Single and multiple component central dyslexic syndromes. In M. Coltheart, K. Patterson & J. C. Marshall (Eds.), *Deep dyslexia* (pp. 119–145). London: Routledge.

Shallice, T., Warrington, E. K., & McCarthy, R.(1983). Reading without semantics. *Quarterly Journal of Experimental Psychology, 35A*, 111–138.

Strain, E., Patterson, K., & Seidenberg, M. S. (1995). Semantic effects in single word naming. *Journal of Experimental Psychology: Learning, Memory and Cognition, 21*, 1140–1154.

Taraban, R., & McClelland, J. L. (1987). Conspiracy effects in word recognition. *Journal of Memory and Language, 26*, 608–631.

Van Orden, G. C., & Goldinger, S. D. (1994). Interdependence of form and function in cognitive systems explains perception of printed words. *Journal of Experimental Psychology: Human Perception and Performance, 20*, 1269–1291.

Watt, S., Jokel, R., & Behrmann, M. (in press). Surface dyslexia in non-fluent progressive aphasia. *Brain and Language.*

SIMULATION OF NEUROGENIC READING DISORDERS WITH A DUAL-ROUTE CONNECTIONIST MODEL

Carol S. Whitney
Department of Neurology, University of Maryland School of Medicine
22 S. Greene St., Baltimore, Md. 21201, USA
E-mail: cwhitney@cs.umd.edu

Rita S. Berndt
Department of Neurology, University of Maryland School of Medicine
E-mail: rberndt@umabnet.ab.umd.edu

James A. Reggia
Department of Computer Science, University of Maryland
A.V. Williams Building, College Park, Md. 20742, USA
E-mail: reggia@cs.umd.edu

ABSTRACT

Computational models of oral reading have succeeded in simulating the general patterns of lexical and non-lexical reading disorders that occur secondary to focal brain injury. This study describes the simulation of more detailed aspects of the performance of dyslexic patients using a connectionist, dual-route model that employs competitive distribution of activation to control interaction among the model's components. Distinct simulated "lesions" are inflicted on the model to reproduce the interaction of orthographic regularity and frequency found in the word reading of Surface Dyslexics, and to model two patterns of sensitivity to the structural characteristics of non-lexical letter strings found in patients with Phonological Dyslexia. Study of the model's performance when lesioned provides a valuable source of information about how degraded information of different types combines to produce correct and incorrect reading responses.

1 Introduction

One of the most common and most devastating effects of focal brain damage is impairment of the ability to read. Neurological classification schemes for the "acquired" (as distinct from developmental) dyslexias have stressed their co-occurrence with other symptoms such as agraphia and aphasia. More recently, acquired dyslexias have been the subject of cognitively-oriented analyses of print-to-sound transcoding, and the symptoms found among patients with reading disorders secondary to brain injury have provided an important source of constraint on the elaboration of models of normal oral reading (see Coltheart 1986, for review). One fact about acquired reading disorders that has motivated this interest from cognitive psychologists is that two contrasting patterns of disorder, apparently reflecting quite different functional sources of impairment, have been described. These patterns can be found when the nature of the material to be read is carefully manipulated as to its structure and meaningfulness.

Patients with "Surface Dyslexia" (Patterson, Marshall & Coltheart 1985) can read aloud unfamiliar letter strings ("non-words") and real words with regular spelling/sound correspondences, but they have difficulty pronouncing words with exceptional (irregular) correspondences. Errors tend to be "regularizations", e.g., reading PINT as if it rhymes with MINT. A contrasting pattern is found among patients with "Deep" and "Phonological" Dyslexia, who read real words without regard to the regularity of their spelling but have great difficulty "sounding out" unfamiliar letter strings (e.g., TOK) (Beauvois & Derousne 1979; Coltheart, Patterson & Marshall 1980).

This contrasting pattern among patients with acquired dyslexia is one of the primary sources of data supporting models of normal reading that incorporate distinct processing routines for the transcoding of non-words and of real words (some of which have irregular spelling/sound correspondences). Such models are typically referred to as "dual route" models (even though more than two routes may be hypothesized to exist), and they postulate separate processes for 1) accessing stored word pronunciations from familiar letter strings via their meanings; and 2) assembling phonological forms from sub-lexical segments generated from letters and letter clusters. Considerable controversy has surrounded many of the assumptions and assertions made by proponents of dual-route models, and there remains much debate concerning the independence of the hypothesized routes, the nature of the processes responsible for sub-lexical transcoding (rules vs. associations), and the size of the sub-lexical segments involved in non-word reading (see, for example, Humphreys & Evett 1985; Kay & Bishop 1987; Patterson & Coltheart 1987). Nonetheless, models that explicitly postulate distinct processing routines for known and unknown words can naturally accommodate pathogenic conditions that appear to affect selectively the reading of known vs. unknown words.

A number of computational models of oral reading have been constructed to simulate single word oral reading (Coltheart, Curtis, Atkins & Haller 1993; Seidenberg & McClelland 1989; Norris 1985; Plaut & Shallice 1993; Reggia, Marsland & Berndt 1988), and they have been "lesioned" in an attempt to reproduce patterns found in acquired dyslexia. Not surprisingly, computational models that do not incorporate a dual-route architecture have had some difficulty simulating these dyslexic patterns. For example, Patterson, Seidenberg and McClelland (1989) lesioned their completely distributed, single route model in an attempt to simulate the regular word advantage in Surface Dyslexia, but have encountered some problems reproducing several aspects of patient behavior, including regularization errors (see Coltheart, Curtis, Atkins & Haller 1993, for critique). Patterson *et al.* have not to date attempted to simulate Phonological Dyslexia; in fact, their unlesioned model has considerable difficulty pronouncing non-words (Besner, Twilley, McCann & Seergobin 1990).

Coltheart *et al.* (1993) and Reggia *et al.* (1988), working with dual-route computational models, have simulated the regular word advantage in Surface Dyslexia, as well as the tendency for responses to exception words to be regularized in their pronunciation. These models can be given a different "lesion" to simulate the non-word reading deficit found in Phonological and Deep Dyslexia. The dual-route architecture of these models requires a local representation of information, and thus these models differ from the fully distributed models in many important ways. In fact, this brief description of existing computational models of single word oral reading fails to capture the level of interest and controversy that has surrounded their development. Not only have such models provided a framework for elementary debate about the number and nature of distinct procedures that are needed to support normal oral reading, but they have raised new issues — both clinical and cognitive — that can be explored in experimental study. For example, Plaut (1996) has studied patterns of recovery from "lesions" in his connectionist model of Deep Dyslexia (Plaut & Shallice 1993). These simulations have led to non-obvious (and testable) predictions about the potential efficacy of specific rehabilitation strategies. Coltheart and Rastle (1995) have refined claims about the processing characteristics of non-lexical print-to-sound conversion on the basis of their model's behavior, and have tested their ideas in studies with normal subjects. Examples such as these suggest that investigations of the performance of computational models can play an important role in a program of research aimed at understanding cognitive processes and their neurogenic impairment.

Despite these and other undeniable contributions from computational models, it is clear that the simulations of acquired dyslexia that have been reported to date considerably simplify complicated symptom patterns that occur among actual patients with these reading disorders. The idealized "mirror image" pattern contrasting Surface and Phonological Dyslexia virtually never occurs in pure form. For example, detailed studies of the reading abilities of patients with Surface Dyslexia have found evidence both for impairments within the (hypothetically spared) non-lexical route (Newcombe & Marshall 1985), and considerable sparing of (hypothetically impaired) lexical reading of words with exceptional spellings (e.g., Behrmann & Bub 1992). Similarly, some Phonological Dyslexic patients have obvious difficulty reading abstract words using their (hypothetically spared) lexical route (Sartori, Barry & Job 1984), and they frequently demonstrate considerable knowledge of grapheme/phoneme associations when reading via the (hypothetically impaired) non-lexical route (Derouesne & Beauvois 1985). It is likely that the marked heterogeneity among patients who demonstrate the general characteristics of these types of reading disorders reflects the combined effects of multiple functional lesions, of varying severity, to distinct reading routines. To date, no attempts have been made to model these types of combined effects.

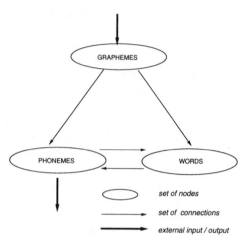

Figure 1: Overview of the network structure. The lexical route is along the grapheme to word to phoneme connections. The non-lexical route is along the grapheme to phoneme connections.

This chapter describes such an attempt to simulate actual patterns of dyslexic symptoms, including patients' sensitivity to the characteristics of the input stimuli as well as their production of different types of errors. A modified version of a previously-described "dual-route" connectionist model of print-to-sound transformation (Reggia et al. 1988; Goodall, Reggia, Peng & Berndt 1990) is used. The model encompasses two distinct processes or "routes" for obtaining a pronunciation from print. The lexical route models the process of mapping character strings onto words via the visual word recognition system, followed by mapping of the words onto their phonemic representations. It is important to note that, at this time, lexical activation is accomplished without semantic mediation, as in other dual-route computational models (Coltheart et al. 1993). The non-lexical route models direct translation from character strings to phonemes. The input to the model is in the form of character strings segmented into graphemes (one or more letters that correspond to a single phoneme). A simplified characterization of the model is presented in Figure 1.

2 Model Description

The print-to-sound network uses a local representation of information with nodes representing graphemes, words, and phonemes. Connections between the nodes represent associations between those entities. Input is supplied to the grapheme nodes. The activations of the phoneme nodes, accomplished via one of two different pathways or routes, represent the network's output. The lexical route is composed of connections from grapheme nodes (an input string) to 3,500 word nodes[a], and connections from word nodes to phoneme nodes (representing a pronunciation). Grapheme and phoneme nodes are position specific. Each grapheme node is connected to all word nodes having that grapheme in that position (there are 148 potential grapheme nodes per position). Each word node has connections to the corresponding phonemes in the appropriate positions (there are 48 phonemes per position). Activation flows from the grapheme nodes to the word nodes to the phoneme nodes, as well as from the phoneme nodes back to the word nodes, allowing feedback within the lexical route and interaction between the routes.

The non-lexical route associates input character strings to their phonemic correspondents by weighted links connecting grapheme nodes directly to phoneme nodes. Unlike the characterization of this route as governed by abstract linguistic principles (e.g., Venezky 1970) and implemented computationally as rules (as in Coltheart *et al.* 1993), our model's non-lexical route assigns weights to grapheme/phoneme links on the basis of probabilities of association between graphemes and phonemes that were calculated from a large number of English words (Berndt, Reggia & Mitchum 1987). Thus, although the model does not incorporate mechanisms for the learning of these associations, the grapheme/phoneme probabilities that serve as the basis for the non-lexical route are assumed to be comparable to a set of association weights that would emerge from experience in mapping a large number of printed words to their pronunciations. This characteristic of non-lexical translation in the model is consistent with evidence that sub-lexical associations, rather than explicit rules, constitute the basis for phonological assembly in skilled readers (Patterson & Coltheart 1987).

The network is built specifically for each word being simulated. For each grapheme in the word, there exists a grapheme node representing the grapheme in that position, and a set of 48 phoneme nodes representing all possible phonemes of English. Each grapheme node is connected to its phonemes in its corresponding phoneme set (i.e., all phonemes that could possibly be the pronunciation of that grapheme). Each grapheme node is also connected to every word node representing a word whose

---

[a]The word corpus consists of all monosyllabic words from the NETTalk corpus (Sejnowski & Rosenberg 1987), modified as described in Berndt, D'Autrechy & Reggia (1994).

spelling has that grapheme in that position. Similarly, each phoneme node is connected to every word whose pronunciation has that phoneme in that position. In general, each word node is connected to one phoneme in each position-specific phoneme set in order to represent the pronunciation of that word. However, if the word represented by a word node is shorter than the word being simulated, then there are no connections to the phoneme sets in positions beyond the length of the target word. Also, a word can be connected to two phonemes in one set if the word has two alternative pronunciations (such as the word WIND, where the I grapheme is connected to both the /ih/ and /ai/ phonemes[b]).

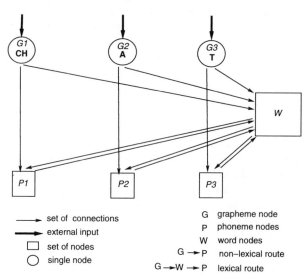

Figure 2: Example network for the word CHAT. The non-lexical and lexical routes each consist of three position-specific paths.

For example, for the word CHAT, there would be three position-specific paths in the network (see Figure 2). On the first path, the grapheme node would represent the grapheme CH and would be connected to all words having CH as the first grapheme (e.g., the word nodes for CHAT, CHECK, CHIP, etc.). The first grapheme node would also be connected to all phonemes in the first position-specific set which could be spelled with a CH grapheme (e.g., /tch/ as in CHAT, /k/ as in CHOIR, and

---

[b]Throughout this chapter, written character strings to be pronounced are printed in uppercase; phoneme pronunciations are expressed as keyboard-compatible equivalents of the International Phonetic Alphabet, printed in lowercase and bounded by slashes. These phonetic equivalents are relatively transparently pronounceable; they are listed with example words in Table 1 of Berndt *et al.* (1994).

/sh/ as in CHEF). Similarly, on the second path, the grapheme node would represent A, and have suitable connections to word and phoneme nodes, and so forth for all remaining graphemes in the input string.

2.1 Competitive Distribution of Activation

The functioning of many networks, including our print-to-sound network, depends on competition between nodes representing alternative possibilities. Such competition has been widely viewed as important in the activation and learning rules of many computational models of cognitive processes (e.g., McClelland & Rumelhart 1981; Waltz & Pollack 1985; Hanson & Gluck 1991). In most models, competition between nodes is implemented by having negatively weighted connections between nodes. However, the number of connections required can be very large when inhibitory links are used to achieve the desired interactions. This issue of scale is extremely important when modeling reading, when the number of separate word nodes needed for a realistic simulation is known to be very large.

An alternative to explicit inhibitory connections, adopted here, is to introduce competition into the mechanism by which the spread of activation is controlled (Reggia 1987; Reggia, D'Autrechy, Sutton & Weinrich 1992). In such a model, a node can be thought of as having a fixed amount of activation to distribute to the nodes to which it is connected. A receiving node gets its share of this activation based on its current activation level and the activation levels of all the other receiving nodes. More formally, consider a source node j with activation level a_j. Node j sends activation of amount out_{ij} to each node i to which it is connected, where

$$out_{ij} = c_{ij}a_j \quad \text{and} \quad \sum_i c_{ij} = 1 \quad \text{and} \quad c_{ij} \geq 0. \tag{1}$$

The weighting factor, c, is a function of the levels of activation of all the receiving nodes, and of the positive connection weights, w_{ij}, from the source node to the receiving nodes. A typical selection for c is

$$c_{mj} = \frac{w_{mj}a_j}{\sum_i w_{ij}a_i} \tag{2}$$

where i ranges over all the nodes to which node j is connected, and m is the node for which c is being computed. Note that in the usual, non-competitive distribution models, the amount of activation going to a receiving node is independent of the amount going to the other receiving nodes. Here, that is not the case, as the weighting factor, c, depends on the activations of all the other receiving nodes. Thus, in essence, the receiving nodes have to compete with each other to get activation from the source node.

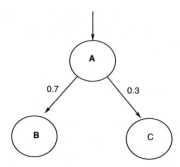

Figure 3: Network for competitive distribution of activation example. Nodes B and C compete without lateral inhibitory links. The numbers specify the connection weights.

Table 1: Node activations for the competitive distribution of activation example showing that node B inhibits node C.

Iteration	A	B	C
0	0	0	0
5	.344	.022	.007
10	.613	.216	.013
20	.865	.596	.011
40	.984	.937	.004
60	.998	.992	.001
100	1.000	1.000	.000

For example, consider the network in Figure 3 where all nodes start with zero activation and a constant external input of 1.0 is applied to node A. Each node uses the competitive distribution mechanism specified by Eqs. (1) – (2). The activation of a node is specified as a differential equation where the change in the activation value is specified as a function of the current activation and the incoming input:

$$\dot{a}_i = [in_i - a_i(1 - in_i)](1 - a_i) \tag{3}$$

where i ranges over A, B and C, $in_i = out_{Ai}$ for $i = $ A and B, and $in_i = 1.0$ for $i = $ C. The first factor causes a_i to rise when $in_i > a_i(1 - in_i)$ and to decrease when $in_i < a_i(1 - in_i)$ and insures that $a_i \geq 0$. The second factor insures that a_i has a maximum value of 1.0. The activation values over time for the example network are given in Table 1. The network displays a winner-takes-all behavior where one of the receiving nodes, B, is fully activated and the others are totally inactive (in this case, just one node, C). Thus the network behaves as if nodes B and C have mutually inhibitory connections, when there are no connections between nodes B and C.

It is also possible to obtain other outcomes, rather than winner-takes-all, with competitive distribution of activation. Suppose, in the above example, node C also receives activation from some node D, in addition to activation from node A. If node D were to provide non-zero input to node C, then node A would continue to send activation to node C, since the activation of node C would not fall to 0. This could lead to an equilibrium where nodes B and C are both active.

Competitive distribution of activation is used to implement competition in the print-to-sound network. Grapheme-to-word connections are competitive; since only one of the words corresponds to the input graphemes, these connections implement winner-takes-all behavior. Similarly, phoneme-to-word connections are winner-takes-all competitive. Grapheme-to-phoneme connections are also winner-takes-all competitive, since only one phoneme can be correct in each position. Word-to-phoneme connections are not competitive, since the pronunciation of the word is represented by all the connections. An example of the functioning of competitive distribution in the network will be given in Section 3.

2.2 Route Interaction

In the early stages of development of this model, the two routes were only weakly interactive with each other. (Some route interaction occurred due to the competitive distribution of activation, as discussed in Reggia *et al.* 1988.) There is evidence that lexical and non-lexical processing mechanisms are interactive to a degree not easily captured in the earlier model (see Humphreys & Evett 1985, for arguments). In order to model this degree of interaction between the lexical and non-lexical routes, we have added phoneme-to-word connections. In addition, we have implemented a mechanism to vary the relative importance of the two routes automatically based on the activations of the word nodes and the phoneme nodes.

Conceptually, competition occurs in two stages on the outgoing connections from the grapheme nodes. First, competition between the routes occurs, where a grapheme node's outgoing activation is divided between the lexical and non-lexical routes. Then competition occurs within the routes. The portion of activation going to the lexical route is distributed to the word nodes, and the portion of activation going to the non-lexical route is distributed among the phoneme nodes. Thus, the two routes compete with each other for activation, and elements within the routes compete among each other for activation.[c]

---

[c]This two-stage competition on the grapheme-to-phoneme connections and the grapheme-to-word connections is implemented by the addition of intermediate nodes on those connections. For each position-specific path, a grapheme node is connected to the word nodes via an intermediate node (graphemeW), and each grapheme node is connected

For simulations of normal reading (where both routes are intact), the competition between the routes does not yield winner-takes-all behavior; the distribution of activation between the routes works out to be about equal by the end of a simulation. For simulations of dyslexic performance (where one of the routes is degraded), most of the activation shifts to the undamaged route.

2.3   Summary

Conceptually, there are three types of nodes in the network: grapheme, word, and phoneme. There is one grapheme node for each grapheme position in the word being simulated, one set of word nodes, and one set of 48 phoneme nodes for each grapheme node. There are four different types of connections among the nodes in the network:

Outgoing two-stage competitive connections from grapheme nodes:

- A connection from a grapheme node to its position-specific set of phoneme nodes. (Determines the activation going to the non-lexical route, and distributes that activation between all phonemes associated with that grapheme.)

- A connection from a grapheme node to the set of word nodes. (Determines the activation going to the lexical route, and distributes that activation among the words having that grapheme in that position.)

Connections involving phoneme nodes and word nodes:

- Non-competitive connections from a word node to all of the sets of phoneme nodes. (A word node is connected to one phoneme in each set, corresponding to the phoneme that is pronounced in that position.)

- Competitive connections from a phoneme node to the set of word nodes. (Distributes activation to all words having that phoneme in that position.)

The activation equations for all node types are described in Appendix B.

---

to the phonemes via an intermediate node (graphemeP). Route competition occurs between the grapheme-to-graphemeW and the grapheme-to-graphemeP connections. There are feedback connections from the word nodes and the phoneme nodes, allowing this competition to be influenced by the activations of those nodes. See Appendix A for a diagram of the network structure.

3 Normal Reading

Before attempting to model dyslexic performance, it is necessary to demonstrate that the intact model can simulate some of the effects from normal subjects that have been used to support the dual-route model. Three such effects are relevant. First, a pervasive finding from studies of normal print/sound transcoding is that words are pronounced faster than non-words (Forster & Chambers 1973). This "lexicality effect" can be generalized to the finding that familiar words are pronounced more quickly than unfamiliar words. Second, the word frequency advantage for familiar words has been shown to interact with spelling regularity, such that less frequent words are pronounced faster if they have regular spelling-to-sound correspondences (e.g., Seidenberg, Waters, Barnes & Tanenhaus 1984). This "frequency-by-regularity interaction" has been taken as evidence that the two routes of a dual route model have a differing time course, with the effects of the (slower) non-lexical route not being felt unless direct lexical access is also slow (for low frequency words) (e.g., Paap & Noel 1991). A third finding of interest in normal readers is that non-words that "sound like" words when they are sounded out (e.g., BRANE) produce faster naming times and fewer errors than control non-words (McCann & Besner 1987). This "pseudohomophone effect" has been interpreted as an indication of substantial lexical involvement in the reading of non-words.

These effects are typically manifested in subjects' Reaction Times (RTs). In our simulation studies of the same phenomena, RT is simulated by the number of iterations that are necessary for the network to settle into a state where, for each phoneme set, only one of the phonemes has an activation > 0.9, and all of the rest have an activation < 0.1.

We have simulated the lexicality effect, the frequency-by-regularity interaction, and the pseudohomophone advantage. These simulations used published experimental test stimuli as inputs. For the frequency-by-regularity simulations, the test words (N=13/condition) were from experiment 3 of Seidenberg et al. (1984). For the pseudohomophone simulations, stimuli were 24 pseudohomophones and 24 control non-words derived from high frequency words by Taft and Russell (1992)[d]. Both sets of stimuli can be used to evaluate the model's relative performance with words and non-words.

---

[d]Six pairs from the original set were not used because they were not pseudohomophones in American English (e.g., LARST), or because the grapheme-phoneme weights used by the model did not generate the correct vowel to yield a pseudohomophone. Both the pseudohomophone and its control non-word were deleted from the stimulus set

212

Normal Reading – Experimental Data   Normal Reading – Simulation Results

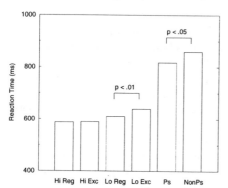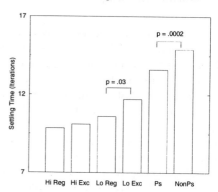

Figure 4: Experimental and simulation results for normal reading. Hi – high frequency, Lo – low frequency, Reg – regular, Exc – exception, Ps – pseudohomophones, and NonPs – non-pseudohomophone control non-words.

As shown in Figure 4, the relative sizes of the simulated effects are in line with the experimental evidence presented in the published studies. In general, the network takes longer to settle when producing pronunciations for non-words compared to words. It may seem surprising that this lexicality effect is produced, since the model's non-lexical route is shorter than the lexical route. However, the output takes many iterations to settle; thus, the relative length of the routes is less important than how activation combines in the network. The lexicality effect arises because the phonemes of words receive activation from both the non-lexical and lexical routes, while non-word phonemes virtually only receive activation from the non-lexical route. (There is minimal activation from the lexical route secondary to partial matching with words.)

There was no difference[e] in settling times for the high frequency regular (mean = 9.85) and exception (mean = 10.1) words ($t(12) < 1$), but there was a significant difference for the low frequency regular (mean = 10.6) and exception (mean = 11.7) words ($t(12) = 2.188$, $p = .03$, two-tailed). Low frequency irregular words took longer to settle than low frequency regular words because of conflicting information from the non-lexical and lexical routes in the paths corresponding to the irregularities. For high frequency irregular words, there is less delay in settling time because information from the lexical route arrives quickly enough to dominate and minimize conflict.

---

[e]To avoid making distributional assumptions about settling times in the simulation data, we calculated the probability that differences in the settling times for the different stimulus sets occurred by chance using randomization tests (Edgington 1987). Thus, the p-values reflect the the number of times a difference as large as that obtained in the simulation would arise in all possible random permutations of the data.

Table 2: Activations for the phoneme nodes /ih/ and /ai/ and the relevant word nodes during the simulation of MINT (subscript M) and PINT (subscript P). The symbol '.' represents an activation $< .01$. No activations are given for iterations > 9 for MINT because the simulation had completed.

Iteration	$/ih/_M$	$/ai/_M$	$MINT_M$	$/ih/_P$	$/ai/_P$	$PINT_P$
5	.01	.	.	.01	.	.
6	.03	.	.02	.03	.	.02
7	.11	.	.04	.06	.	.04
8	.33	.	.14	.13	.	.07
9	.95	.	1.00	.25	.	.18
10				.29	.07	.51
11				.29	.99	1.00
12				.	1.00	1.00

Table 3: Activations for the phoneme nodes /ay/ and /ae/ and the relevant word nodes during the simulation of TAKE (subscript T) and HAVE (subscript H).

Iteration	$/ay/_T$	$/ae/_T$	$TAKE_T$	$/ay/_H$	$/ae/_H$	$HAVE_H$
5	.	.	.01	.	.	.01
6	.03	.	.05	.02	.	.06
7	.18	.	.23	.05	.	.29
8	.98	.	1.00	.01	.58	1.00
9				.	1.00	1.00

For example, consider the activations of the /ih/ and /ai/ phonemes for the low frequency words MINT (regular) and PINT (irregular) given in Table 2. Since /ih/ is the most probable phoneme corresponding to the grapheme I, and lexical information has not yet reached the phonemes, /ih/ starts rising initially for both MINT and PINT. However, when the word node PINT becomes activated, it sends conflicting information as it activates the /ai/ phoneme. The /ai/ phoneme then draws the activation away from the /ih/ phoneme. This process takes time, causing the network to take longer to settle for PINT than for MINT. (Note: the reason that the activation of the word node MINT rose much more quickly than the node for PINT in iterations 8-9 is not due to differences in frequency between the words. Rather, it is due to the phoneme-to-word connections. Since the correct phonemes for MINT were partially activated from graphemes via the non-lexical route, they helped to raise the activation of the MINT node quickly.)

Now consider the activations of the /ae/ and /ay/ phonemes for the high frequency words TAKE (regular) and HAVE (irregular) given in Table 3. For HAVE, the incorrect, but more likely, phoneme /ay/ never becomes very active because the correct phoneme /ae/ receives lexical support relatively early in the simulation. Thus, there is little difference in the settling times as a function of regularity for the high frequency words.

Figure 4 also shows that the settling times for pseudohomophones (mean = 13.6) were significantly shorter than those for the control non-words (mean = 14.9) (t(23)= 3.706, p = .0002, two-tailed). This pseudohomophone effect arose in the simulations from the feedback connections from the phonemes to the words. When the phonemes of a pseudohomophone were partially active, these feedback connections led to activation of the base word node, which in turn more quickly activated the phonemes.

4 Impaired Reading

As noted in the Introduction, the dual-route architecture of our model should provide a straightforward means of simulating the general impairments to non-word versus irregular word reading found in Surface and Phonological Dyslexia. The "pure" patterns can be relatively easily reproduced by degrading each of the routes. By disabling the non-lexical route, we have simulated pure Phonological Dyslexia, i.e., the complete inability to read non-words, with preserved ability to read words including exception words. With no input from the non-lexical route, the network produces no response, or an incorrect response, for a non-word. Similarly, by disabling the lexical route, we have simulated pure Surface Dyslexia, i.e., the complete inability to read exception words with the preserved ability to read regular words and non-words. With no lexical input, the network produces regularizations for all exception words (see also Reggia et al. 1988).

However, it is well known that most patients with acquired dyslexia do not show pure forms of these disorders. Patients with Phonological or Surface Dyslexia often retain the ability to read some non-words or exception words, respectively. That is, the affected reading route is not abolished, but functions abnormally. We were interested to see if the model could reproduce the error patterns involved in these partial degradations of reading ability.

4.1   Surface Dyslexia — Partial "Lesioning" of the Lexical Route

Patients with Surface Dyslexia, with putative impairment of the lexical reading route, frequently provide evidence that that route is partially functional. Often, preservation of the ability to read exception words is correlated with the words' frequencies (Bub, Cancelliere & Kertesz 1985; Behrmann & Bub 1994). A larger percentage of high frequency exception words is read correctly compared to low frequency exception words. For example, patient MP (Bub *et al.* 1985) displayed the ability to pronounce approximately 80% of high frequency (> 300 per million)[f] exception words, versus 40% of low frequency exception words (< 25 per million). We have simulated this type of error pattern by degrading the lexical route in the model. The test word sets were those used in the frequency-by-regularity simulations.

The model was "lesioned" by reducing the activations of word nodes. The activation of each word node was calculated in the normal manner, and then multiplied by a constant < 1.0. This new value was then used as the node's activation. Using a reduction constant of 0.3, 100% of the high frequency exception words were correct, versus 38% of the low frequency exception words. Using a value of 0.2, 62% of the high frequency words were correct, versus 15% of the low frequency. Incorrect responses were regularizations of the test words.

This pattern arises in the simulations for the same reason that low frequency exception words take longer to process than high frequency words, namely, the rate at which activation rises is a function of word frequency. When the activations of word nodes are degraded (as in the Surface Dyslexia simulations), low frequency words do not become active fast enough to dominate input from the non-lexical route, and regularization errors result. However, high frequency words become active much more quickly, and can overcome competing activation from the non-lexical route.

4.2   Phonological Dyslexia — Partial "Lesioning" of the Non-Lexical Route

We have studied a group of patients with Phonological and Deep Dyslexia to investigate the effect of various non-word attributes on correct pronunciation ability in patients with assumed impairment to the non-lexical route. Two sets of stimuli used in those studies are relevant here (see also Berndt, Haendiges & Mitchum, in preparation). Two sets of non-word stimuli were constructed with simple consonant-vowel-consonant (CVC) structure that differed in the probability that their graphemes corresponded to a specific set of phonemes. Non-words with high grapheme-phoneme correspondence (high GPC) probability (N = 33) are letter strings with extremely

---

[f] Frequencies as given in Kucera & Frances (1967).

predictable pronunciations (e.g., NEEP). Non-words with low grapheme-phoneme correspondence (low GPC) probability (N = 20) consist of graphemes with more variable phonemic pronunciations (e.g., CEACH), although twelve adult control subjects were consistent in their pronunciations of these non-words. Additional non-words included a set of twenty pseudohomophones (e.g., WEHPON) and twenty orthographic control non-words (e.g., WEEPON) which were derived pairwise from the same set of base words by letter changes in the same position. These non-word stimuli were part of a large battery of tasks assessing word and non-word reading, phonological analysis and manipulation skills, grapheme- phoneme knowledge, etc., which were administered to patients in weekly sessions over a period of three months.

Eleven pre-morbidly literate adult patients have completed testing with the battery. All patients were previously right-handed victims of left hemisphere cerebrovascular accident. Although all patients had some difficulty pronouncing the CVC non-words, they varied widely in the extent of this problem, as well as in the general characteristics of their language impairments. Only three of the eleven patients produced non-negligible rates of semantic errors (>20%) in word reading, qualifying them for classification as Deep Dyslexic.

We have selected two patients who did not produce semantic errors and have simulated their non-word reading performance. These patients differ markedly in the degree to which their non-word reading is impaired. Patient WE displays moderately impaired non-word reading, with greater ability to read high GPC non-words (85% correct) than low GPC non-words (41% correct) (χ^2 = 9.67, p = .002). WE shows no improved ability to read pseudohomophones relative to their non-word controls (60% correct for both pseudohomophones and their controls). In contrast, patient MVB shows almost no ability to read non-words (6% correct for high GPC, and 9% correct for low GPC), except for pseudohomophones (30% correct versus 10% correct for control non-words) (Fisher's exact test = 5.50, p = .02).

To simulate a lesion to the non-lexical route, the incoming connections to phoneme nodes were degraded. There are two components to this lesioning: a reduction in the amount of activity reaching a phoneme node, and the addition of noise to the incoming activity. These two components can be varied independently of each other. For simplicity, the incoming activation to a phoneme node is calculated as usual, and then passed through a lesioning function, les. The lesioned incoming activation, $lesin_i$, of a phoneme node, i, is given by

$$lesin_i = les(in_{GP}) + in_W \qquad (4)$$

where in_{GP} and in_W are as in the activation function for a phoneme node given by Eq. (12), and

$$les(in_{GP}) = A \, in_{GP} + N(R - O) \qquad (5)$$

where A, N, and O are constants between 0 and 1, and R is a uniformly distributed random number on $[0,1]$. A new value for R is chosen each time that les is invoked. The first term of les specifies the reduction of activity, and the second term specifies the noise. The constant O is used in the noise term to allow noise with negative values. Passing in_{GP} through the lesioning function is the only change from the normal model; all other parameters are retained. The quantity $lesin_i$ is then used in place of the normal incoming activation, in_i, in Eq. (12) for calculating the activation of the phoneme node. The parameters A, N, and O are held constant across simulation trials when simulating a single subject. By varying A, N and O, different error patterns are created, corresponding to the different error patterns observed between subjects. The lesion parameters were determined by iterating through various combinations in order to find the settings that best matched the experimental data.

The settling criterion was more liberal in the patient simulations than in simulations of normal reading. This different criterion corresponds to the fact that patients were encouraged to give some response, even if they were unsure of it, and they typically did so. If the network failed to settle according to the normal criterion, then the simulation was stopped after 40 iterations. For each position, the most active phoneme with an activation of at least 0.05 was chosen. If no phoneme had this minimum activation, then that position was ignored, unless it corresponded to a vowel. In that case, the position was assigned a value of /uh/. For the high/low GPC simulations, the input non-words were a subset of those seen by the patients. For the pseudohomophone simulations, this was not possible because the experimental test data included two-syllable pseudohomophones whose base words are not in the model corpus. Instead, the pseudohomophones and their controls derived from low frequency words by Taft and Russell (1992) were used.

The actual and simulated data for patient WE are given in Figure 5. Patient WE, with a relatively mild impairment of non-word reading, showed considerable sensitivity to the grapheme-phoneme associations of non-words, but little sensitivity to whether non-words sounded like words when correctly "sounded out". This pattern was reproduced in the simulation of his data: 81% of the high GPC non-words were correct, versus 30% of the low GPC non-words ($\chi^2 = 9.47$, p = .002). There was no significant difference in the simulation's performance with pseudohomophones (66%) versus the control non-words (50%)($\chi^2 = 1.37$, p = .38). In the simulations, this GPC effect arose from the noise added to the grapheme-to-word connections. For connections with a high connection weight (corresponding to having a high probability of G-P association), the addition of noise had less influence than on connections with a low connection weight.

Patient MVB was much more severely impaired in non-word reading than was WE, showing no effect of grapheme-phoneme probability but a high degree of sensitivity to pseudohomophony. In the simulation of MVB's performance, shown in Figure 6, 9% of the high GPC and 5% of the low GPC non-words were correct ($\chi^2 < 1$). In contrast, simulated performance with pseudohomophones (41%) was much better than performance with the matched controls (8%) ($\chi^2 = 5.44$, p = .002).

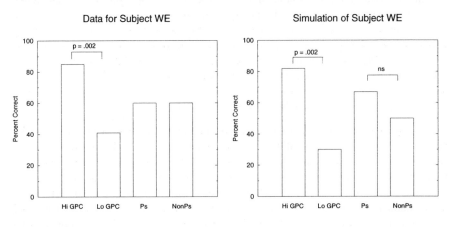

Figure 5: Experimental and simulation results for non-word reading for patient WE. The lesion parameters were $A = .7$, $N = .25$, and $O = .5$.

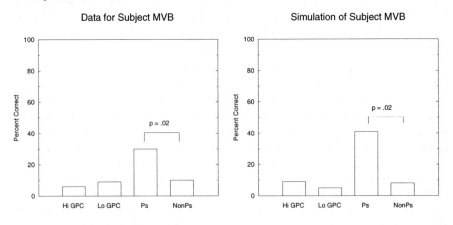

Figure 6: Experimental and simulation results for non-word reading for patient MVB. The lesion parameters were $A = .3$, $N = .25$, and $O = .6$.

In these simulations of MVB's more severely impaired performance, there was no effect of G-P probability because the grapheme-to-phoneme connections were so degraded that the noise overwhelmed even connections with high weights. Further, the MVB simulations suggest that the pseudohomophone effect in impaired subjects is not based solely on orthographic similarity, even for subjects with virtually no ability to read non-words. In the simulations, the pseudohomophone effect arose because of feedback from phoneme-to-word connections. When these connections were removed, the effect disappeared, indicating that it was not attributable to stronger orthographic similarity of pseudohomophones to words (i.e., the grapheme-to-word connections). How could this be the case when the simulated responses to the non-pseudohomophone non-words were almost all incorrect, indicating severe degradation of the ability to generate the correct phonemes? The answer depends on the fact that during the course of the simulation, many of the possible phonemes become partially active for each position. If the non-word is a pseudohomophone, partial activation of the correct phonemes can lead to additional activation from the base word node via the phoneme-to-word connections. This additional activation can make the difference between a correct and an incorrect response. However, the WE simulations showed no pseudohomophone effect, since the additional activation from base word nodes in pseudohomophones was small compared to the activations from the mildly-impaired grapheme-to-phoneme connections.

This analysis of the pseudohomophone effect in patients with impairment of non-lexical reading differs from other possible explanations of the effect. For example, Patterson & Marcel (1992) and Derouesne & Beauvois (1985) have suggested that the pseudohomophone advantage in at least some patients with Phonological Dyslexia is attributable to difficulty synthesizing ("assembling") sub-lexical sound segments into a unified whole for articulation. Pseudohomophones by-pass this assembly step to the extent that patients can gain access to stored phonological representations for words from the pseudohomophones' orthography. These earlier accounts of the pseudohomophone effect suggests that the extent of the pseudohomophone advantage should be negatively correlated with patients' ability to "blend" phonemes or other sound segments into a unified word-like unit. We evaluated this prediction with the data from our group of eleven patients with non-lexical reading impairment, who were also given a variety of phonological manipulation tasks including phoneme blending (e.g., "put together the sounds /k/, /ae/, /t/ to make a word"). The rank order correlation between pseudohomophone reading and performance on the phoneme blending task was quite low ($\rho = .46$, p $= .16$). The "blending" account of the pseudohomophone advantage would also seem to predict that pseudohomophone reading should be correlated with a high rate of lexicalization errors to non-words. This prediction was likewise not supported by correlational analysis of our group data in that pseudohomophone performance was negatively correlated with lexicalization rate for non-words ($\rho = -.39$, p $= .22$).

The explanation of the pseudohomophone advantage that is suggested by our modeling results requires that patients have relatively severe difficulty activating phonemes from graphemes non-lexically; however, this ability must not be completely abolished. Some minimal phoneme activation must be generated from graphemes in order to trigger the rise of activation in related word nodes. Our group patient data provide some weak support for this analysis: the correlation between pseudohomophone reading and knowledge of grapheme-phoneme associations (tested in written/spoken non-word matching) was moderate ($\rho = .53$, p = .09). For example, patient MVB, with very little ability to pronounce non-words, was considerably above chance (.78) in matching a spoken non-word to one of two written non-words (z = 4.27, p < .001). These preliminary investigations of potential sources of the model's results provide an example of the utility of computational modeling for the generation of hypotheses that can be tested using data from patients.

One advantage of our model compared to other models of oral reading is that errors are produced that can be compared to the errors produced by patients. The network generated three different types of errors that are similar to those produced by patients: lexicalizations (giving an orthographically similar word, e.g., NEED for NEEP), truncations (leaving out one or more phonemes, e.g., /l uh+/ for LUN), and substitutions (replacing a phoneme with a related one, e.g., /z er n/ for ZUN). Lexicalizations arose in the simulations when the lexical route came to dominate the input to the phonemes. Due to the competition between the routes, activation can shift to the lexical route, causing a partially matched word to drive the response. Truncations arose when no phoneme became sufficiently active in some position. Substitutions arose when noise caused an incorrect phoneme to become the most active.

One interesting aspect of the patients' errors when reading non-words is that they were more likely to produce the correct phoneme for the initial grapheme of the non-word than for graphemes in other positions (e.g., for high/low GPC non-words, the first consonant was correct in 58% of errors, while the last consonant was correct in only 11% of errors). The simulations also produced this result, somewhat less dramatically, despite the lack of any explicit seriality in the model. For the two patients simulated, the first consonant in the high/low GPC non-words was reproduced in 77% of errors, and the second consonant in 46% of errors. Coltheart and Rastle (1995) have argued that left-to-right seriality is a processing characteristic that distinguishes the lexical and non-lexical route, adding support to the argument that these routes are distinct. Coltheart's dual route computational model incorporates explicit coding of seriality in the non-lexical route to accomplish the types of serial effects found in patient data and, arguably, in normal non-word pronunciation tasks. Our model shows a tendency to produce correct phonemes at the beginnings of input strings when the non-lexical route is degraded, without explicit serial coding. If the non-lexical route is partially damaged, and a non-word with four graphemes is presented, the activation of the initial phoneme rises more rapidly than that of the final phoneme. This is due to activation coming from word nodes that are partially matched. Since all words have a first phoneme, but not all words have a fourth phoneme, there is more activation going to the first phoneme in the output. It is not yet clear that this effect will be sufficient to simulate serial effects in longer non-words. Nonetheless, it is important to note that it emanates in the model from an interaction of the two routes.

5 Discussion

The simulation results presented here demonstrate the feasibility and utility of modeling actual data gathered from individual dyslexic patients. Contemporary cognitive neuropsychological investigations of neurogenic language disorders are increasingly focused on the analysis of results from single cases, since even patients who are similar in the general characteristics of their impairment can demonstrate important differences in performance (see, for example, Miceli, Silveri, Romani & Caramazza (1989); Sartori *et al.* 1984).

Information processing ("box and arrow") models that have been developed to account for the complex patterns of impairments found among patients have proven to be very useful in motivating general characterizations of underlying cognitive deficits. However, they are quite limited in their ability to accommodate performance that results from different degrees of partial degradation to independent components of the model. For example, Caramazza and colleagues have developed a model of the interaction between non-lexically derived phonological information and semantic activation in a dual-route model to explain patients' ability to read aloud irregular words that they do not understand (Miceli, Capasso & Caramazza 1994; Hillis & Caramazza 1995). This "Summation Hypothesis" holds that partial information about a word's meaning can "summate" with partial non-lexically derived information about its pronunciation to yield a correct response. Hillis and Caramazza (1995, Figure 2) have generated a series of box-and-arrow models to represent the outcome of various combinations of impairment to these two systems. However, their assumptions about how much information of each type needs to be available before a particular response is produced are purely hypothetical. An implemented computational model of this interaction could prove to be very useful in fleshing out the details about how partial information from different sources could be combined.

Our simulations have demonstrated how these kinds of interactions can be modeled to produce outcomes that are not always predictable. Interactions between lexical and non-lexical information flow, apportioned through competitive interaction, reproduced replicable behavioral phenomena such as lexicality effects, the frequency-by-regularity interaction and the pseudohomophone advantage shown by normal readers.

Analysis of the model's behavior allowed us to attribute these effects to specific sources of activity within the model, e.g., the pseudohomophone advantage clearly arose in the model because of feedback from phoneme-to-word connections rather than from orthographic similarity among the word nodes.

Simulations of data from dyslexic patients using the computational model were informative because the aspects of the model that we "lesioned" were transparently representative of hypothesized cognitive constructs. That is, a "lesion" to the model's non-lexical route is interpretable as a degradation of the information base and processes that associate letters and letter clusters with sound segments. Moreover, the mechanisms for producing computational "lesions", although clearly not comparable to actual structural lesions, are intended to degrade information flow in a manner that is consistent with what has been hypothesized about "functional" lesions. In our simulations of Phonological Dyslexia, two separate approaches were taken to degrading information flow in the non-lexical route — reduction in activation from grapheme nodes, and the addition of noise. Although the lesion parameters that were employed here were determined by data fitting rather than by an analysis of our patients' underlying impairments, we believe that these lesion mechanisms are consistent with the functional deficits that have been hypothesized for patients with Phonological Dyslexia. For example, Bub, Black, Howell & Kertesz (1987) describe a Phonological Dyslexic patient who made the same types of errors when reading or repeating non-words, but was able to repeat and read real words with considerable success. The explanation given to this pattern by the authors is that abnormal noise or interference within a memory buffer preferentially degrades less familiar (presumably less strongly represented) non-lexical phonological strings. In contrast, we reported data from a Deep/Phonological Dyslexic patient whose repetition of non-words was significantly better than her reading of non-words (Berndt 1992). In this case, noise that preferentially interferes with unfamiliar phonological strings is unlikely to be the primary type of impairment. Rather, insufficient activation of non-lexical phonological information from print would be a more likely explanation of this pattern. For many patients, both types of functional disruption of information transmission may be working to degrade performance, as in our simulations.

Further development of this model will need to incorporate changes to address several critical but difficult issues that we have thus far ignored. First is the question of how incoming letter strings are segmented into units of the size needed to provide input to non-lexical translation procedures. We have predicated our model on the grapheme-phoneme unit because we believe that this unit size will ultimately prove to be most valuable in simulating results with multi-syllabic words. A bottom-up procedure for segmenting strings into graphemes will need to deal with the fact that most letter clusters that can function as a grapheme (i.e., can correspond to a single phoneme) actually do so only in some subset of their total occurrences (Berndt *et al.* 1994). This aspect of non-lexical reading clearly contributes importantly to the determination of a word's "regularity"; at least one patient has been described whose primary deficit involved the inability to segment letter strings into clusters for pronunciation (Newcombe & Marshall 1985).

Other difficult issues to be addressed include the addition of a semantic component — the ultimate goal of all lexical reading is to activate meanings — and the addition of mechanisms for phonological processes that will support the modeling of multi-syllabic words. The existing dual-route architecture will provide a base for the development of these new components, since it seems clear that the modeling of normal and dyslexic pronunciation of printed letter strings requires distinct lexical and non-lexical mapping procedures.

Acknowledgements

This research was supported by research grant number 5 RO1 DC00699 from the National Institute on Deafness and Other Communication Disorders, National Institutes of Health.

References

Beauvois M-F., & Derouesne, J. (1979), *Journal of Neurology, Neurosurgery & Psychiatry* **42**, 1115.

Behrmann, M., & Bub, D. (1992), *Cognitive Neuropsychology* **9**(3), 209.

Berndt, R.S. (1992), in *Aphasia Treatment: Current Approaches and Research Opportunities* ed. J. Cooper (NIH Publication No. 93-3424), 47.

Berndt, R.S., Reggia, J.A., & Mitchum, C.C. (1987), *Behavior Research Methods, Instruments and Computers* **19**, 1.

Besner, D., Twilley, L., McCann, R.S., & Seergobin, K. (1990), *Psychological Review* **97**, 432.

Bub, D., Cancelliere, A., & Kersetz, A. (1985), in *Surface Dyslexia: Neuropsychological and Cognitive Studies of Phonological Reading*, eds. K.E. Patterson, J.C. Marshall & M.Coltheart (Lawrence Erlbaum Associates, London), 15.

Bub, D., Black, S., Howell, J. & Kertesz, A. (1987) in *The Cognitive Neuropsychology of Language* eds. M. Coltheart, G. Sartori and R. Job (LEA, London), 79.

Coltheart, M., Patterson, K. & Marshall, J. C. (1980), *Deep Dyslexia* (Routledge and Kegan Paul, London).

Coltheart, M. (1986), in *Attention and Performance XI*, eds. M. Posner, & O.S.M. Marin (Lawrence Erlbaum Associates, Hillsdale, NJ), 3.

Coltheart, M., Curtis, B., Atkins, P., & Haller, M. (1993), *Psychological Review* **100**(4), 589.

Coltheart, M., & Rastle, K. (1995), *Journal of Experimental Psychology: Human Perception and Performance* **20**(6), 1197.

Derouesne, J., & Beauvois, M.-F. (1985), in *Surface Dyslexia: Neuropsychological and Cognitive Studies of Phonological Reading*, eds. K.E. Patterson, J.C. Marshall & M. Coltheart (Lawrence Erlbaum Associates, London), 399.

Edgington, E. S. (1987), *Randomization Tests* (M. Dekker, New York).

Forster, K. I., & Chambers, S. M. (1973), *Journal of Verbal Learning and Verbal Behavior*, **12**, 627.

Goodall, S., Reggia, J.A., Peng, Y., & Berndt, R.S. (1990), *Proceedings from 14th Symposium on Computer Applications in Medical Care* (Washington, D.C.), 294.

Hanson, J., & Gluck, M. (1991), *Advances in Neural Information Processing Systems 3*, 656.

Hillis, A. E., & Caramazza, A. (1995), *Cognitive Neuropsychology* **12**, 187.

Humphreys, G. W., & Evett, L.J. (1985), *The Behavioral & Brain Sciences* **8**, 689.

Kay, J., & Bishop, D. (1987), in *Attention and Performance XII: The Psychology of Reading*, ed. M. Coltheart (Lawrence Erlbaum Associates, London), 449.

Kucera, H. & Francis W. N. (1967), *Computational Analysis of Present-day American English* (Brown University Press, Providence, RI).

McCann, R. S., & Besner, D. (1987), *Journal of Experimental Psychology: Human Perception & Performance* **13**, 14.

McClelland, J., & Rumelhart, D. (1981), *Psychological Review* **88**, 375.

Miceli, G., Capasso, R., & Caramazza, A. (1994), *Neuropsychologia* **32**, 317.

Miceli, G., Silveri, M., Romani, C., & Caramazza, A. (1989), *Brain and Language* **36**, 447.

Newcombe, F., & Marshall, J.C. (1985), in *Surface Dyslexia: Neuropsychological and Cognitive Studies of Phonological Reading*, eds. K.E. Patterson, J.C. Marshall & M.Coltheart (Lawrence Erlbaum Associates, London), 35.

Norris, D. (1985), *Journal of Experimental Psychology: Human Perception and Performance* **20**(6), 1212.

Paap, K. R., & Noel, R. W. (1991) *Psychological Research* **53**, 13.

Patterson, K., & Coltheart, V. (1987), in *Attention and Performance XII: The Psychology of Reading*, ed. M. Coltheart (Lawrence Erlbaum Associates, London), 421.

Patterson, K., & Marcel, A. (1992), in *Analytic Approaches to Human Cognition*, eds. J. Alegria, D. Holender, J. Junca de Morais, & M. Radeau (Elsevier Science Publishers B.V., North Holland), 259.

Patterson, K., Marshall, J.C., & Coltheart, M. (1985), *Surface Dyslexia: Neuropsychological and Cognitive Studies of Phonological Reading* (Lawrence Erlbaum Associates, London).

Patterson, K., Seidenberg, M.S., & McClelland, J.L. (1989), in *Parallel Distributed Processing: Implications for Psychology and Neurobiology*, ed. R.G.M. Morris (Clarendon Press, Oxford), 131.

Plaut, D.C. (1996), *Brain and Language* **52**(1), 25.

Plaut, D.C., & Shallice, T. (1993), *Cognitive Neuropsychology* **10**(5), 377.

Reggia, J. (1987), in *Proceedings of the First International Conference on Neural Networks Vol. II* (San Diego, CA), 131.

Reggia, J.A., Marsland, P., & Berndt, R.S. (1988), *Complex Systems* **2**, 509.

Reggia, J., D'Autrechy, C., Sutton, G., & Weinrich, M. (1992), *Neural Computation* **4**, 287.

Sartori, G., Barry, C., & Job, R. (1984), in *Dyslexia: A Global Issue*, eds. R.N. Malatesha, & H.A. Whitaker (Martinus Nijhoff, The Hague), 339.

Seidenberg, M.S., & McClelland, J.L. (1989), *Psychological Review* **96**(4), 523.

Seidenberg, M.S., Waters, G.S., Barnes, M.A., & Tanenhaus, M. (1984), *Journal of Verbal Learning and Verbal Behavior* **23**, 383.

Sejnowski, T.J., & Rosenberg, C.R. (1987), *Complex Systems* **1**, 145.

Taft, M., & Russell, B. (1992), *The Quarterly Journal of Experimental Psychology* **45A**(1), 51.

Waltz, D., & Pollack, J. (1985), *Cognitive Science* **9**, 51.

Venezky, R.L. (1970), *The Structure of English Orthography* (Mouton, The Hague).

APPENDIX A — Network diagram

Network structure including intermediate nodes on the outgoing grapheme connections. Nodes are shown for one position-specific path only.

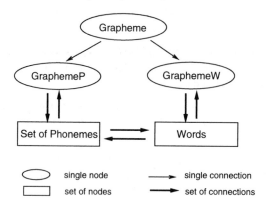

APPENDIX B — Activation Rules

Most of the activation rules are given in terms of a first order differential equation, where the change in the activation level of node i is specified as a function of the current activation level of the node, a_i, and the incoming activation to the node, in_i. The weight on a connection into node i from node j is denoted as w_{ij}. The weights for all connection types are set to 1.0, with the following exceptions. The connection from a graphemeW node to a word node has weight $1/n$, where n is the total number of word nodes to which the graphemeW node is connected. Similarly, the connection from a phoneme node to a word node has weight $1/m$, where m is the total number of word nodes to which the phoneme is connected. The connection from a graphemeP node to a phoneme node has a weight corresponding to the conditional probability that the grapheme will be pronounced as that phoneme (Berndt et al. 1987). Correspondingly, the sum of the weights over all connections emanating from a single graphemeP node is 1.

For a node j which distributes its activation competitively, we denote the output from j to node i as out_{ij}. For a grapheme node, the output function is

$$out_{ij} = a_j \frac{w_{ij} a_i}{\sum_m w_{mj} a_m} \qquad (6)$$

where m ranges over all nodes to which node j is connected (in this case a graphemeP node and a graphemeW node). For the other types of nodes which use competitive connections, the output function is

$$out_{ij} = a_j \frac{w_{ij} a_i^2}{\sum_m w_{mj} a_m^2}. \qquad (7)$$

Squaring a_i makes the competition stronger, leading quickly to a winner-takes-all outcome.

Grapheme Nodes

The activation rule for a grapheme node is

$$\dot{a}_i = 0.05 in_i(1.0 - a_i) \tag{8}$$

where in_i is externally supplied input to the network and is equal to 1.0.

GraphemeP and GraphemeW Nodes

The activation rule for either a GraphemeP or GraphemeW node is

$$\dot{a}_i = 0.5(in_i - a_i) \tag{9}$$

with

$$in_i = in_G + in_F \tag{10}$$

where $in_G = out_{iG}$ for corresponding grapheme node, G, and in_F denotes feedback activation from either the word nodes or the phoneme nodes, depending on the type of node
i. If node i is a graphemeP node, then $in_F = 0.01 \sum_{j \in P} a_j$, where P denotes the set of all
phoneme nodes. If node i is a graphemeW node, then $in_F = 0$ if $S_W < 0.06$, and $in_F = S_W$
otherwise, where $S_W = \sum_{j \in W} a_j$, and W denotes the set of all word nodes.

Phoneme Nodes

In order to accelerate simulations, the activation rule for a phoneme node is a sigmoid rule,
rather than a differential equation, given by

$$a_i = \frac{1}{1 + e^{-15(in_i - 0.5)}} \tag{11}$$

with

$$in_i = 1.8(in_W + in_{GP}) \tag{12}$$

where $in_{GP} = \sum_{j \in GP} out_{ij}$ for graphemeP nodes GP, and $in_W = \sum_{j \in W} a_j$ for word nodes
W.

Word Nodes

The activation rule for a word node is

$$\dot{a}_i = 0.5 in_i(1.0 - a_i) \tag{13}$$

with

$$in_i = in_{GW} + in_P \tag{14}$$

where in_{GW} denotes the inputs from the graphemeW nodes, GW, and in_P denotes the
inputs from the phoneme nodes, P. The equations for in_{GW} and in_P have the same form.
The equation for in_{GW} is given below; the equation for in_P is the same, but with P
substituted for GW.

$$in_{GW} = inavg_{GW} - 3.0a_i(1.0 - 12.0k_i - inmin_{GW}) \tag{15}$$

where $inavg_{GW}$ is the average of the path-specific inputs to the ith word node from GW, and $inmin_{GW}$ is the minimum of the path-specific inputs to the ith word node from GW, and k_i is a logarithmic function of the ith word's prior probability, p_i, given by $k_i = 0.45 \log(10^6 p_i)$. (For low frequency words, k_i lies around 1.0, and for high frequency words, it lies between 2.0 and 3.5.) The average of the path specific inputs is calculated taking the sum of the activations over all the paths, and dividing by the length of the ith word. The minimum is calculated by choosing the minimum of the activations over all the paths. If the ith word is longer than the word being simulated, then this minimum is 0.

COVERT RECOGNITION IN A CONNECTIONIST MODEL OF PURE ALEXIA

KATE MAYALL

and

GLYN W HUMPHREYS

School of Psychology, University of Birmingham, Edgbaston, Birmingham, B29 6SA, UK.
E-mail: k.a.mayall@bham.ac.uk

ABSTRACT

Covert recognition, apparent knowledge without consciousness, has been described in several cognitive disorders, including pure alexia. Patients have been documented who cannot name briefly presented words, but can make semantic categorisation and lexical decisions to a degree of accuracy above chance. Here, we describe a simple connectionist model which, when lesioned, demonstrates many of the performance characteristics of pure alexia, including covert recognition. It is concluded that covert recognition can be explained in terms of the functioning of a damaged processing system, and it is not necessary to assume a disconnection of a normally functioning system from conscious expression.

1. Covert Recognition

In many areas of Cognitive Neuropsychology, there have been reports of patients with an apparent loss of conscious awareness in a particular cognitive domain (see Schacter et al. [1] and Young & De Haan [2] for reviews). For example, patients have been described who appear, and claim, not to be able to see or to process visual stimuli fully, but who show knowledge of the stimulus when information is tapped covertly. Examples of disorders in which covert recognition has occurred include blindsight, prosopagnosia, alexia, hemineglect, amnesia and aphasia. In some, but not all, patients suffering from these impairments, covert tests can demonstrate existence of knowledge which is not apparent when the knowledge is tested overtly. We shall briefly review all of the above impairments, then describe in more detail the covert abilities which have been demonstrated in prosopagnosia and pure alexia, for which explanations have been offered in terms of connectionist models. Other interpretations of patterns of overt and covert ability will be discussed at the end of this section.

229

1.1. Blindsight and Visual Attention Disorders

Investigations of blindsight constituted the first systematic studies of apparent loss of conscious awareness of perception or cognitive processing in neurological patients [3, 4]. The term "blindsight" was first used by Weiskrantz et al. [4] to describe the apparently unconscious awareness of stimuli within an area of cortical blindness or "scotoma". Pöppel et al. [3] tested ex-servicemen who were suffering from visual field defects. When a brief flash of light was presented within an area of scotoma, patients reported that they could not see it. However, when they were told to guess at its position, their eye movements tended to be towards the position of the flash. Weiskrantz and his colleagues [4, 5, 6, 7] studied in depth a patient, DB, who could point relatively accurately to the position of a flash of light presented within his scotoma, despite claiming he was unable to see it. He could distinguish static from moving light, and could make simple orientation and shape discriminations.

Similar findings have been reported concerning neuropsychological patients demonstrating spatial "extinction". These patients are able to detect a single stimulus presented anywhere within their field of vision. However, if two stimuli are presented simultaneously, one in the left and one in the right visual field, they tend to ignore the stimulus presented in the visual field contralateral to their brain lesion. Volpe et al. [8] described four patients who demonstrated spatial extinction when presented with two stimuli, but, when asked if the two stimuli presented were the same or different, patients were remarkably accurate.

Covert processing has also been demonstrated in visual neglect, with patients showing knowledge of items presented on the left which they cannot report when requested to do so directly [9, 10]. For example, Marshall and Halligan [9] documented a patient who reported that she could see no difference between pictures of a plain house and pictures of the same house with flames coming from its left-hand side. Despite this, when asked which house she would prefer to live in, she consistently chose the house which was not on fire.

These three types of patient have in common the fact that they appear on the face of things to be unable to see, or attend to, particular visual stimuli or parts of stimuli. However, in each case, stimuli have been shown to have been processed at least to some extent. (See Milner [11] for a discussion of covert recognition in the domain of vision.)

1.2. Loss of Conscious Awareness in Non-visual Impairments

Covert recognition has also been reported in non-visual impairments. Examples have been found in both amnesia and aphasia. Some amnesic patients have been shown to recover memories when tested implicitly, but not when tested explicitly [12, 13]. In early cases, the amnesic patients tested by Warrington and Weiskrantz [12, 13] were facilitated at a fragmented picture and word identification task the second time they attempted it. This occurred despite the patients claiming to have no memory of attempting the task before.

There have also been reports of covert recognition in both Broca's and Wernicke's aphasia. Broca's aphasics produce slow effortful speech, and function words in sentences are often omitted, producing a "telegraphic" style of speaking. Wernicke's aphasics, in contrast, produce relatively fluent speech, but it tends to be full of lexical selection and grammatical errors. Andrewsky and Seron [14] asked a Broca's aphasic to read or complete sentences with words which could be read as either content words or function words, depending on the context. When the words appeared as function words they tended to be omitted. But when the same words appeared as content words they tended to be included in the aphasic's sentences. Tyler [15] reported a similar patient who, despite having a syntactic processing deficit which was apparent in free speech, was slower to respond to a target word embedded in a syntactically disrupted sentence than to the same word within acceptable, or semantically disrupted, sentences. Both of these patients appear to have some residual implicit knowledge of grammar.

Wernicke's aphasics, tested by Milberg and Blumstein [16], performed poorly on a semantic relatedness judgement task, which overtly tested semantic knowledge. However, when tested on a lexical decision task, the aphasic patients were facilitated on word judgements if the word followed a semantically related prime. This suggests an implicit knowledge of the semantics of the words on which they were tested.

One further example of loss of conscious awareness is anosagnosia, the denial of suffering from a disability. This impairment is slightly different from the others discussed, since there are no covert tests to indicate that knowledge does in fact exist. However, it certainly reflects a form of lack of conscious awareness, and reviewers have tended to group it with the other deficits [2]. An example of anosagnosia is the existence of patients who suffer from both hemiplegia and hemianopia, but are aware of only one of the disorders [17]. Bisiach et al. [17] described a patient who claimed to move his left arm, for example, when in fact the left side of his body was completely paralysed.

1.3. Covert Recognition in Prosopagnosia

Prosopagnosia is the inability to recognise faces which were once familiar, e.g. those of family, friends and famous celebrities. Prosopagnosic patients can generally perceive and describe facial features, but cannot recognise people from the features, and rely on other cues, such as voice, for recognition. However, evidence exists for covert knowledge of face identity in some patients. Several different experiments have been reported in the literature and are described below.

Firstly, psychophysiological indications of face identity knowledge has been demonstrated in prosopagnosics [18, 19, 20]. Bauer [18] used the "Guilty Knowledge Test" to demonstrate that, for pictures of faces which could not be named by his prosopagnosic patient, skin conductance responses were greater when the picture was presented with the correct name as opposed to an incorrect name. Tranel and Damasio [19, 20] further showed that skin conductance responses were greater when familiar faces were presented to prosopagnosic patients, as opposed to unfamiliar faces.

Using indirect behavioural assessments of face identity knowledge, De Haan et al. [21, 22] demonstrated that, in a test of whether two faces were the same or different, their prosopagnosic patient, PH, was faster at responding to familiar faces. Further, he was slower to classify names (as politicians or actors) if the name was accompanied by an incorrect picture. PH's response time was slightly faster if, for example, the name of a politician was accompanied by another politician rather than by a picture of an actor. PH also demonstrated associative priming effects from pictures he could not name, on the task of classifying a written name as famous or non-famous [23]. For example, he was faster to respond to the name "Diana Spencer" if it followed a picture of Prince Charles than if it followed a picture of an unrelated person.

In summary, a variety of tasks presented to certain prosopagnosic patients all appear to have generated the same findings. When tested indirectly these patients indicate knowledge of face identities, which, when tested directly, they cannot recognise.

1.4. Covert Recognition in Pure Alexia

The final area for which a significant amount of evidence has been provided for covert recognition is pure alexia. The most notable characteristic of this disorder is that reading can be literally "letter-by-letter": the word CAT may be read, either silently or aloud, "C..A..T..cat". The argument for letter-by-letter reading is supported by evidence that reading latencies increase linearly with word length [24] and are abnormally long.

Landis et al. [25] described the first case of covert word recognition in alexia. Their patient could correctly point to objects corresponding to briefly presented words he could not name. A number of pure alexic patients have been reported subsequently who are able to make correct lexical decision and semantic categorisation judgements on words presented too briefly to be named overtly [26, 27, 28, 29]. For example, the pure alexic patient, ML [26], performed significantly above chance when asked to answer questions such as "Is it an author or a politician?" or "Is it pleasant or unpleasant?" for briefly presented words he could not read. All four patients reported by Coslett and Saffran [27] were able to report, to a proficiency above chance level, whether a briefly presented word was an "animal" or not, or whether it was a "food" or not. Further, Coslett and Saffran [28] showed that their patient could match a briefly presented word to one of two pictures with an accuracy rate above chance.

1.5. Theories of Covert Recognition

There are three main groups of theories of covert recognition. The first is that the particular information processing module being tapped is undamaged, but is no longer linked to higher cognitive processes which support consciousness [1, 2]. The second is that there are (at least) two separable systems capable of achieving the task in question [6, 18, 26, 27, 28]. One of these, which is connected to consciousness, is damaged and cannot be used. A second system, which does not have an output to consciousness, is undamaged and is used by the patient. The third set of theories suggest that individual modules are damaged, but that indirect tasks can tap the residual processing of the module [30, 31].

Young and De Haan [2] argue that the dissociation between overt and covert face recognition in prosopagnosia is caused by a disconnection of output from an adequately functioning face processing system to processes which support awareness of recognition. They also explain the other disorders mentioned above as a disconnection from consciousness. Schacter et al. [1] agree that covert recognition is caused by a disconnection of a processing module from a conscious mechanism, although they do concede that "some of these phenomena may turn out to be related to one another only superficially" (p.243).

Bauer [18], in discussing prosopagnosia, suggested that there may be two neural systems for face recognition, only one of which is linked to consciousness. It is suggested that both ventral and dorsal visual areas are capable of face recognition, but only processing by the ventral system can lead to conscious expression. The dorsal system, which is relied on by those prosopagnosics who demonstrate covert recognition, normally mediates affective responses to faces. Further evidence is provided by Tranel et al. [32] who report the opposite dissociation following frontal lobe damage. Weiskrantz [6] provided a similar interpretation for blindsight. He suggested that the disorder could be explained by use, not of the geniculo-striate pathway, but of one of the other branches of the optic nerve which project to the midbrain or subcortical areas.

Interpretations of covert recognition in pure alexia have included suggestions of a disconnection of a normally functioning word recognition system from consciousness, but also of right hemisphere reading [26, 27, 28]. This is comparable to the explanations of blindsight and covert recognition in prosopagnosia which suggest that there are two functionally and anatomically separate systems involved, one used for overt and one for covert recognition [6, 18].

Finally, covert recognition may reflect residual processing in a damaged system. Farah et al. [30] and Mayall and Humphreys [31] suggest that covert recognition in prosopagnosia and pure alexia, respectively, can be explained in this way. They provide simple connectionist models which suggest that covert effects can be found in a single system without recourse to a disconnection from consciousness or the use of second processing system.

2. Farah et al.'s Model of Covert Recognition in Prosopagnosia

Farah et al. [30] have suggested that covert recognition in prosopagnosia can be explained in terms of residual processing in a damaged face processing system. The support they provided for this argument included the fact that prosopagnosics who display covert recognition can score above chance on overt tasks (though not as highly as on covert tasks), thus suggesting that the face recognition system is not completely obliterated. In order to demonstrate that covert recognition can emerge from a damaged system, Farah et al. developed a connectionist model of the face processing system, which when lesioned could perform better on "covert" than on "overt" tasks.

2.1 The Model

Farah et al's [30] model consisted of a set of face units, a set of name units and a set of semantic units. Both the face units and the name units were connected to the semantic units via a set of hidden units specific to the type of input. The network was recurrent, and the output of each set of units fed back into itself. Representations of names and faces were random and distributed. Representations of semantics were also distributed and random, except for 2 units, one of which referred to the occupation "actor" and one to the occupation "politician". The model was trained on five "actors", five "politicians" and twenty "other people" using the contrastive Hebbian learning algorithm. Training consisted of 320 epochs on the set, with each epoch consisting of one of the three representations (name, face or semantics) being presented and associations with the other two being learned. The model was lesioned by removing varying numbers of face input units or hidden units from the visual input to the semantic units.

2.2 The Simulations

Three main sets of simulations with lesioned versions of the model were conducted to compare performance with that of prosopagnosic patients who display covert recognition. Firstly, the lesioned model's ability to relearn face-name pairs was examined. After damage, the number of correct names produced for faces was reduced. Relearning was tested by giving the model 10 learning epochs, in one condition with correct face-name pairs and in a second condition with incorrect face-name pairs. For all types and size of lesion, the model was better at relearning the correct pairings than at learning the incorrect pairings.

In the second simulation, Farah et al. tested whether visual analysis of a face pattern proceeded more quickly if the face was familiar than if it was not. After lesioning, the face representations of the five "actors" and five "politicians" taught to the network, plus another five "actors" and five "politicians", were presented to the model. The number of iterations for the visual units to settle was recorded for each face. On the whole, the lesioned models needed fewer cycles to settle for familiar than for unfamiliar faces. If it is assumed that number of iterations is comparable with reaction times, the lesioned model shows the same pattern as the prosopagnosic patient studied by De Haan et al. [22] who was faster at classifying familiar faces as same or different, than unfamiliar faces.

The third simulation considered semantic priming on occupation decisions. Names were presented in three conditions: individually, paired with different faces from the same occupation category, and paired with different faces from the other occupation category. The number of cycles for one of the occupation units to attain a positive activation value was recorded. Fewer cycles were required when the face accompanying the name was from the same category compared to when it was from the other category. This suggests that the model possessed covert semantic knowledge, as faces from the incorrect category produced interference.

Farah et al. concluded from their modelling work that it is possible for a damaged face recognition system to exhibit covert recognition. A disconnection from conscious expression is thus not the only possible interpretation of the results found with these prosopagnosic patients. It was suggested that, while this was not necessarily the case with covert recognition in all disorders, covert recognition in prosopagnosia could reflect residual processing in a damaged system.

3. A Connectionist Model of Pure Alexia

We [31] have developed and lesioned a simple model of word recognition in an attempt to demonstrate that covert recognition in pure alexia could result from residual processing in a damaged word recognition system, and so also does not necessarily need to be explained in terms of a disconnection of the word recognition system from conscious expression. In this section we will describe the model and the experiments performed with simulated lesions.

3.1. General Framework of Model

The Mayall and Humphreys [31] model does not stand as an attempt to model all aspects of word recognition and identification, but was developed to study covert recognition in word naming and to test two assumptions: (1) that there are separable routes to access phonology and semantics; and (2) that words resemble each other more than do letters, and that both are represented within the same visual recognition system. It is intended that the model simulates lexical processing, and, when lesioned, it simulates residual word recognition rather than the use of any compensatory letter-by-letter reading strategy. This is a simple exploratory model, and as such, was only tested with one set of initial weights and one type of lesion (the complete removal of processing units). As a previous smaller model with the same general architecture produced similar results, and as dissociations within the current model were robust over lesion sizes, we argue that the pattern of results is not simply an artefact of an overly small network (see Bullinaria & Chater [33]).

3.2. Specific Architecture

The model is of the form shown in Figure 1. Input units represent orthography, and output units represent phonology and semantics. The input units and the hidden units are fully interconnected, however, only half of the hidden units are connected to the phonological output units and half are connected to the semantic output units. Evidence from neuropsychology suggests that phonological or semantic information can be retrieved in isolation [26, 27, 34, 35, 36]. We recognise that, in a more complete model, semantic and phonological units would also be connected to allow spontaneous speech to occur.

The tasks we used to examine the model included not only naming and semantic categorisation, but also lexical decision. This is of interest as some pure alexic patients have demonstrated a level of performance above chance on lexical decision when words are presented too briefly to be named overtly. Besner and McCann [37] argued that lexical decisions involve a familiarity check in which the orthographic familiarity of a string contributes to decision making. Seidenberg and McClelland [38] used a similar assumption in their connectionist model of word recognition. Lexical decisions were carried out in their model by a form of auto-association in which the orthographic description of a string was reconstructed by feedback from hidden units. A familiar string was judged to be one where the reconstructed orthographic representation was similar to the original input representation; an unfamiliar string was taken as one for which the reconstructed representation was dissimilar to the input. We incorporated a similar procedure here. Orthographic input values were mapped through the two sets of hidden units (phonological and semantic) to a set of "orthographic lexical" units, which during the training phase had values matching the input units (and so led to auto-associative learning of input values). Lexical decision could then be based on comparing activation values over the orthographic

238

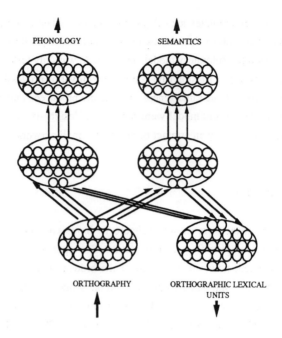

Figure 1. Architecture of the Mayall and Humphreys [31] Model.

lexical units for words and nonwords. (The criterion for a word response was taken as the error score where the two distributions crossed.)

Seidenberg and McClelland's model has been criticised for the way in which it simulates lexical decision, as performance by the unlesioned model is not as good as that by normal humans [39]. However, in our unlesioned model there is no overlap in the distributions of orthographic lexical errors scores for words and nonwords. Therefore the unlesioned model performs "lexical decision" perfectly. Secondly, we do not claim that an orthographic familiarity check is the only process involved in lexical decision. Phonological and semantic information influences the orthographic lexical units through the hidden units.

Hidden units in the model can be thought of as lexical units from which phonology and semantics are derived. The orthographic lexical units can then be assumed to constitute an orthographic output lexicon, which can be used to produce orthographic outputs from other input modalities, or as a familiarity check for use in lexical decision.

The model consisted of 16 input units, 90 hidden units (45 phonological and 45 semantic) and 74 output units (29 phonological, 29 semantic and 16 orthographic lexical). It was trained on 69 words and 10 letters.

3.3. Representations

Orthography, phonology and semantics in the model were represented by distributed patterns of 1's and 0's. There was no representation of constituent letters within words. Our intention here was not to capture details of how orthography is presented in skilled readers, but only of how similarity influences performance in a damaged system. Letters and words were represented over the same set of input units, as representations of single letters, having specific pronunciations, may only differ from those of words in terms of semantics (see Arguin & Bub [43]). The same number of units were used to represent letters and words, as the model was intended to be of a lexical system which processes words as single wholes.

The difference between letters and words was represented in terms of the similarity of orthographic representations, with words having more similar representations than letters. In modelling orthography in this way we made the following assumptions. Printed letters are, visually, relatively simple representations; there are only 52 different lower and upper case forms and these are made up of distinguishing stroke features. Words, on the other hand, are more complicated being made up of several letters. There are many more words than letters, and many contain letters in the same positions making them visually more similar to one another. Many studies of word processing have shown interference between multiple letters presented in words (e.g. Bouma [44]), whilst we know of no comparable evidence indicating interference between multiple features presented in letters.

Phonology was represented by a 29-bit vector pattern of 14 1's and 15 0's. The phonology of letters and words was of identical construct, as the spoken form of words and letters is fundamentally the same (indeed, some letters and words are homophones, e.g. b and bee; c and sea; t and tea).

Semantic representations were subdivided into two sets of units: "category units", which were identical for words within the same category (e.g. all animals), and "individuating units" which differed between each word. Of the 29 semantic units, 14 represented the super-ordinate category, whilst the remaining 15 differentiated the word from others in the same category. All semantic units of letters had activation values of 0, based on the assumption that individual letters hold negligible semantic information. Word imageability was also represented within the semantic units. (See Mayall & Humphreys [31] for discussion of imageability representations and effects.)

3.4. Training and Testing the Network

All weights in the model initially were assigned random values of between -0.1 and 0.1. To ascertain whether a particular representation over output units (e.g. a phonological representation) was correct firstly a "thresholding" procedure was undertaken where units below 0.2 were rounded down to 0, and units above 0.8 were rounded up to 1. Output units with a value of between 0.2 and 0.8 were taken as "undetermined". Using the values which were determined, the response was taken as the word (or letter) whose target output had the greatest overlap in activation values with the actual output. Whilst our model does not include feedback loops, the process by which an output is assessed includes a simple notion of "attraction" [40, 41, 42], as responses are taken as the word or letter with the closest known representation. An advantage of using our procedure is that exact responses can be generated so that we can measure when the system fails to produce a response and when it produces a correct response.

The model was trained via standard back propagation [45]. During training, the model was run through 50 000 iterations of the training set. The number of occurrences of a word within the training set was a function of its Kucera and Francis [46] word frequency. Items were divided into four relative frequency bands, and the number of occurrences of the word in the training set were 4:3:2:1 across the four frequency bands. (See Mayall & Humphreys [28] for a discussion of frequency effects in the model.)

Having been trained to near perfect performance on all stimuli, the model was lesioned to varying degrees of severity. Four different lesions of 33%, 50% and 67% of the hidden units were undertaken. (Input unit lesions were also investigated but are not discussed here, see Mayall & Humphreys [31].) The lesions were designed to overlap as little as possible. (Throughout this chapter the four lesions of the same size are referred to as A, B, C, and D. For example, the 50% lesions are referred to as 50A, 50B etc.)

Here we will discuss three simulations with lesioned versions of the model: a comparison of word and letter naming, which is crucial to modelling pure alexia, and comparisons of semantic categorisation and lexical decision with word naming, which are of interest in terms of covert recognition. Further simulations using the model are described by Mayall and Humphreys [31].

3.5. Simulation 1 - Letter and Word Naming

Alexic patients are usually not perfect at letter naming, but their performance at letter naming is substantially superior to that of word naming; hence they may adopt a letter-by-letter reading strategy. Figure 2 shows the percentage of letters and words correctly named by the model. At the 33% and 67% lesions, there was superior letter naming over word naming performance [33% lesions - 75% (30/40) correct letter naming vs. 49.61% (127/256)[1] correct word naming, $\chi^2 = 7.96$, df=1, p<0.01; 67% lesions - 27.5% (11/40) correct letter naming vs. 12.5% (32/256) correct word naming, $\chi^2 = 5.12$, df=1, p<0.05]. When lesion 50A was removed from the calculations, there was also superior letter naming over word naming for the 50% lesions [40% (12/30) correct letter naming vs. 27.60% (53/192) correct word naming, $\chi^2 = 6.86$, df =1, p<0.01]. Lesion 50A shows the reverse effect with better word naming than letter naming [10% (1/10) correct letter naming vs. 42.19% (27/64) correct word naming]. Interestingly, there has been a deep dyslexic patient reported in the literature who, similarly, is surprisingly good at word naming whilst performing poorly a letter matching [47]. This apparent double dissociation in the model is discussed in detail by Mayall and Humphreys [31].

As the number of hidden units was reduced, the model became less capable of discriminating between input patterns. As inputs for words were more similar to each other than those for letters, words became indiscriminable first after damage. When the activations of hidden units were studied it was noted that letters had more hidden units highly activated than words (mean number of hidden units with activation values greater than 0.8: Letters - 10.7, Words - 8.56). This difference is likely to render letters more robust to damage than words, as a random lesion is less likely to remove the necessary proportion of highly activated units to produce the correct output. It is possible that the greater visual distinctiveness of letters compared to words similarly leads to the superior

---

[1]Only 64 words were tested for each lesion, as 5 word phonologies were not "learned" during training.

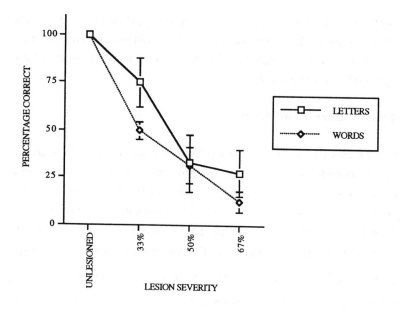

Figure 2. Percentage of Letters and Words Correctly "Named" by the Model.

performance of pure alexic patients on letter naming compared to word naming.

3.6. Simulation 2 - Word Naming vs. Semantic Categorisation

Several pure alexic patients have been described who are able to perform above chance on forced choice semantic categorisation tasks, when words are presented too briefly to be named overtly [26, 27, 28, 29]. A comparison between these tasks was therefore made for the model. More correct responses over semantic category units than over phonology units were produced by the model for all lesion severities (see Figure 3).

It must be taken into consideration, however, that as there are 79 phonological representations known to the model but only 14 semantic categories, the level of chance

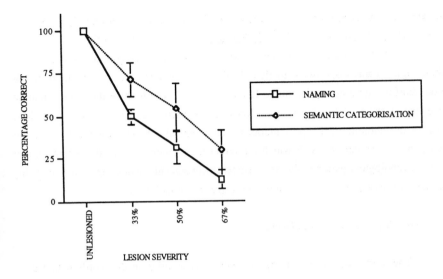

Figure 3. Percentage of Words Correctly Named and Categorised.

report is greater for semantic categorisation than for naming (7.14% vs. 1.27%). Guesses were corrected by assuming that the network either "knew" the correct response or "guessed". Thus:

$$p(correct) = p(know) + (1-p(know)) \times p(guess)$$

so: $$p(know) = \frac{p(correct) - p(guess)}{1-p(guess)}$$

where p(correct) is the observed correct performance across equivalent conditions (lesion instances), p(know) is the probability that the network knows the correct response, and p(guess) is the chance correct rate. Comparing across the lesion instances, p(know) for semantic categorisation was reliably higher than p(know) for naming (33% lesions - t(3)=14.49; 50% lesions - t(3)=5.53; 67% lesions - t(3)=5.07, all p<0.05).

The fact that the model produced more correct semantic categorisations than correct phonological name responses is likely to be due to the semantic category units receiving more reinforcement during learning. In most cases five words share the same semantic category, so the model received more exposure to the semantic category representations than to the phonological representations. There are also fewer alternative semantic category representations with which the target must compete. As applied to human neuropsychological patients, this is consistent with semantic categorisation benefitting because it is based on a reduced number of response alternatives [26].

3.7. Word Naming vs. Lexical Decision

The model was tested on 20 "nonwords" in addition to the words it had been taught. Nonwords had orthographic and phonological representations of similar structure to the known words, but the semantic units were all assigned 0's. As lesion severity increased, so the distributions of orthographic lexical error scores for words and nonwords overlapped further, reducing lexical decision ability. Measures of d' were calculated for the results of each lesion. d' provides a measure of discrimination sensitivity and has been used to quantify the lexical decision ability of neuropsychological patients. At the 33% lesion level performance was significantly above chance, but after 50% and 67% lesions the difference was not significant. [33% lesions - 69.38% (247/356) correct, χ^2=26.99, df=1, p<0.001; 50% lesions - 54.49% (194/356) correct, χ^2=1.267, df=1, NS; 67% lesions - 52.53% (187/356) correct, χ^2=0.360, df=1, NS.]

It should be noted that at the 33% lesion level word naming was also relatively good (49.61% correct word naming vs. 69.38% correct lexical decision). As chance level for lexical decision is 50%, lexical decision performance is not greatly superior to word naming performance. We suggest that this may be because the orthographic lexical units, whose activation values are used in lexical decision, receive equal input from both phonological and semantic hidden units. If lexical decision in the lesioned model was based only on input from semantic hidden units, performance may improve (as semantic categorisation performance is superior to word naming performance following lesions). If pure alexic patients have difficulty in retrieving phonology from briefly presented words, their lexical decisions under these conditions are more likely to be based on visual and semantic information than phonological information.

4. General Discussion

We have described a very simple model of the word recognition system. When lesioned, it is intended that the model simulates residual word recognition capabilities, as opposed to any letter-by-letter reading strategies, which may be resorted to by pure alexic patients. The model produces significantly better performance on a "semantic categorisation" task than on a "word naming" task, as is found with patients who demonstrate covert recognition [26, 27, 28, 29]. It also performs lexical decisions at an accuracy level above chance, at least after 33% hidden unit lesions, and we have suggested how this performance in the lesioned model could be improved.

In addition to the simulations described above, the Mayall and Humphreys [31] model successfully simulated several other performance characteristics of pure alexia, e.g. frequency effects, imageability effects, the production of mainly visual errors plus a few semantic errors and a case mixing x task interaction. Further, predictions were made for super vs. sub-ordinate categorisation, category specificity effects and the naming of category headings compared to category members.

Two important points to note about the model are, firstly, that a single network has simulated many different performance characteristics of pure alexia, and, secondly, that it models aspects of covert recognition. Correct semantic categorisations, and to some extent, lexical decisions, have been made by the model even when naming is incorrect. The model provides an existence proof that it is possible to explain the dissociation in the reading of pure alexic patients in terms of architecture and processes. Hence, as argued by Farah et al. [30] with regard to prosopagnosia, it is not necessary to conclude that covert recognition is a manifestation of a disconnection of consciousness from a normally functioning reading system. Neither is it necessary to argue that covert recognition reflects right hemisphere reading. The present model has no representations that can easily be linked to right as opposed to left hemisphere processing.

In conclusion, the above model has provided more weight to the argument that covert recognition does not necessarily have to be explained in terms of undamaged processing modules that have been disconnected from consciousness, or even in terms of two separable systems capable of the same processing. The Farah et al. [30] and Mayall and

246

Humphreys [31] models both provide examples of processing systems which, when lesioned, can demonstrate "covert" without "overt" recognition. The fact that not all prosopagnosic or pure alexic patients demonstrate covert recognition may suggest that the type or size of the lesion may influence whether covert recognition occurs or not. While it appears possible to explain covert recognition in pure alexia and prosopagnosia in terms of damage to the relevant processing system itself, we would not wish to claim that this extends to all disorders which display covert recognition. Nevertheless, it is plausible that at least some other examples of covert recognition, for instance those in amnesia and aphasia, could similarly be explained in terms of damage to a normal processing system, and could be simulated in connectionist terms, as we have described above.

5. References

1. D. L. Schacter, M. P. McAndrews and M. Moscovitch, in *Thought Without Language*, ed. L. Weiskrantz (Oxford University Press, Oxford, 1988).

2. A. W. Young and E. H. F. De Haan, *Mind and Language* 5 (1990) 29-48.

3. E. Pöppel, R. Held and D. Frost, *Nature* 243 (1973) 295-296.

4. L. Weiskrantz, E. K. Warrington, M. D. Sanders and J. Marshall, *Brain* 97 (1974) 709-728.

5. L. Weiskrantz, *Quarterly Journal of Experimental Psychology* 32 (1980) 365-386.

6. L. Weiskrantz, *Blindsight: A Case Study and Implications* (Oxford University Press, Oxford, 1986).

7. L. Weiskrantz, *Brain* 110 (1987) 77-92.

8. B. T. Volpe, J. E. Ledoux and M. S. Gazzaniga, *Nature* 282 (1979) 722-724.

9. J. C. Marshall and P. W. Halligan, *Nature* 336 (1988) 766-767.

10. A. Berti and G. Rizzolatti, *Journal of Cognitive Neuroscience* 4 (1992) 345-351.

11. A. D. Milner, *Neuropsychologia* 33 (1995) 1117-1130.

12. E. K. Warrington and L. Weiskrantz, *Nature* 217 (1968) 972-974.

13. E. K. Warrington and L. Weiskrantz, *Nature* 228 (1970) 628-630.

14. E. L. Andrewsky and X. Seron, *Cortex* 11 (1975) 379-390.

15. L. K. Tyler, *Cognitive Neuropsychology* 6 (1989) 333-356.

16. W. Milberg and S. E. Blumstein, *Brain and Language* 14 (1981) 371-385.

17. E. Bisiach, G. Vallar, D. Perani, C. Papagno and A. Berti, *Neuropsychologia* **24** (1986) 471-482.

18. R. M. Bauer, *Neuropsychologia* **22** (1984) 457-469.

19. D. Tranel and A. R. Damasio, *Science* **228** (1985) 1453-1454.

20. D. Tranel and A. R. Damasio, *Behavioral Brain Research* **30** (1988) 235-249.

21. E. H. F. De Haan, A. W. Young and F. Newcombe, *Cortex* **23** (1987a) 309-316.

22. E. H. F. De Haan, A. W. Young and F. Newcombe, *Cognitive Neuropsychology* **4** (1987b) 385-415.

23. A. W. Young, D. Hellawell and E. H. F. De Haan, *Quarterly Journal of Experimental Psychology* **38A** (1988) 297-318.

24. E. K. Warrington and T. Shallice, *Brain* **103** (1980) 99-112.

25. T. Landis, M. Regard and A. Serrat, *Brain and Language* **11** (1980) 45-53.

26. T. Shallice and E. M. Saffran, *Cognitive Neuropsychology* **3** (1986) 429-458.

27. H. B. Coslett and E. M. Saffran, *Brain* **112** (1989) 327-359.

28. H. B. Coslett and E. M. Saffran, *Brain and Language* **43** (1992) 148-161.

29. H. B. Coslett, E. M. Saffran, S. Greenbaum and H. Schwartz, *Brain* **116** (1993) 21-37.

30. M. J. Farah, R. C. O'Reilly and S. P. Vecera, *Psychological Review* **100** (1993) 571-588.

31. K. A. Mayall and G. W. Humphreys, *British Journal of Psychology* (in press).

32. D. Tranel, H. Damasio and A. R. Damasio, *Journal of Cognitive Neuroscience* **7** (1995) 425-432.

33. J. A. Bullinaria and N. Chater, *Language and Cognitive Processes* **10** (1995) 227-264.

34. M. Coltheart, in *Deep Dyslexia*, eds. M. Coltheart, K. E. Patterson and J. C. Marshall (Routledge and Kegan Paul, London, 1980).

35. E. K. Warrington and T. Shallice, *Brain* **102** (1979) 43-63.

36. M. F. Schwartz, E. M. Saffran and O. S. M. Marin, in *Deep Dyslexia*, eds. M. Coltheart, K. E. Patterson and J. C. Marshall (Routledge and Kegan Paul, London, 1980).

37. D. Besner and R. S. McCann, in *Attention and Performance, XII*, ed. M. Coltheart (Erlbaum, London, 1987).

38. M. S. Seidenberg and J. L. McClelland, *Psychological Review* **96** (1989) 523-568.

39. D. Besner, L. Twilley, R. S. McCann and K. Seergobin, *Psychological Review* **97** (1990) 432-446.

40. G. E. Hinton and T. Shallice, *Psychological Review* **98** (1991) 74-95.

41. D. C. Plaut and T. Shallice, *Cognitive Neuropsychology* **5** (1993) 377-500.

42. D. C. Plaut and J. L. McClelland, in *Proceedings of the 15th Annual Conference of the Cognitive Science Society* (Erlbaum, Hillsdale NJ, 1993).

43. M. Arguin and D. N. Bub, in *The Neuropsychology of High-level Vision*, eds. M. Farah and G. Ratcliffe (Erlbaum, Hillsdale NJ, 1994).

44. H. Bouma, *Vision Research* **11** (1971) 459-474.

45. D. E. Rumelhart, G. E. Hinton and R. J. Williams, in *Parallel Distributed Processing*, eds. J. L. McClelland and D. E. Rumelhart (MIT Press, Cambridge, Massachusetts, 1986).

46. H. Kucera and W. N. Francis, *Computational Analysis of Present-day American English* (Brown University Press, Providence, Rhode Island, 1967).

47. D. Howard, in *The Cognitive Neuropsychology of Language*, eds. M. Coltheart, G. Sartori and R. Job (Erlbaum, London, 1987).

NEUROLOGICAL
DISORDERS

COMPUTATIONAL APPROACHES TO NEUROLOGICAL DISEASE

Howard Crystal
Department of Neurology, Albert Einstein College of Medicine, Bronx, NY
E-mail: crystal@aecom.yu.edu
and
Leif H. Finkel
Department of Bioengineering and Institute of Neurological Sciences,
University of Pennsylvania, Philadelphia, PA

Abstract

Computational models have contributed to current understanding of normal brain function, and can offer new insights into the pathophysiology of neurological disease. We define some of the outstanding clinical questions in stroke, CNS injury, Alzheimer's disease, Parkinson's disease, and epilepsy from a neurologist's perspective, and discuss the potential impact of computational neurology on computational neuroscience. We consider representative examples of models constructed at several different levels of biological detail--from detailed membrane-level simulations to connectionist networks. We focus on what has been learned from several generations of models concerned with the after-effects of neural injury. In particular, we discuss how model assumptions, sometimes of ancillary importance, have constrained the ability to predict subsequent experimental results.

1. Introduction

Computational modeling is not the first approach one might consider in seeking to understand neurological disease. First, there is the complexity of the problem: brain function, which is poorly understood under normal conditions, is further complicated in situations of dysfunction. And the major neurological conditions: stroke, Alzheimer's disease, Parkinsonism, epilepsy, and CNS injury are multifarious in their expression and protean in their manifestations. There is also the complexity of the solution: any framework proposed for explaining functional loss must take account of processes at multiple levels of organization--from the molecular to the behavioral. And it is difficult to see how a computational model can translate into rehabilitation or treatment strategies aimed at these various levels. Finally, in contrast to computational simulations, molecular biology offers both a reductionistic approach, and the potential for treatment and cure.

251

There are, however, several compelling reasons for attempting to develop models and simulations of disease--not as a replacement for other approaches, but as a means of new insight into pathogenesis and treatment. In some sense, the function of the brain is computation, thus the underlying computational processes must be uncovered to understand the basis of disease. Alzheimer's disease cannot be understood outside of the context of a model of memory consolidation and storage, and Parkinsonism requires an understanding of how the extrapyramidal system controls voluntary movement. The development of such models is made richer and more robust by consideration of clinical data, just as pathology has always enriched the understanding of physiology.

Secondly, the nervous system is sufficiently complex that understanding its function requires detailed simulation. How can one weigh the importance of calcium concentration, local recurrent excitation, loss of cell numbers, slowing of conduction velocities, and normal aging processes in assessing functional behavior in an Alzheimer's patient? Simulations provide a means of thinking about complex systems, particularly those with rich interactions between levels. Despite the fact that the principles of aerodynamics are well understood, no one would build a modern aircraft without extensive CAD-CAM simulations. How then can we hope to understand neural function, and perturbations to normal function, without detailed simulations. And how else can we hope to arrive at the neural equivalent of "aerodynamics", the underlying computational principles of brain function, without a process of building increasingly more complex approximations to real neural circuits.

Finally, disease may do more for computational neuroscience than modeling does for disease. Models have always considered how function breaks down as a result of various structural degradations, but it has only recently become possible to incorporate sufficient detail at the appropriate levels of organization to make use of the troves of clinical knowledge about the brain.

In this overview, we will consider some of these issues in the context of what would be useful to clinical neurology and what can be achieved by computational methods. We will define those clinical conditions which, from our perspective, appear most amenable to computational study. We will discuss some representative examples of promising approaches in this area, and try to draw lessons from some attempts in the past. And we will try to elucidate what strategies and techniques might be most successful in developing this new arena, particularly, how computational techniques may be combined with imaging and signal analysis.

The spectrum of neurological disease is wide and ravaging. From a public health perspective, it represents a multi-billion dollar a year problem, and from the patient's perspective it usually represents a diagnosis without much hope. Despite advances in anatomical imaging and molecular analysis, the major neurological diseases remain poorly understood. In what follows, we attempt to define how computational approaches may be of use in several of the major neurological conditions.

2. Alzheimer's Disease

Alzheimer's disease (AD) is a degenerative brain disorder that affects 3-4 million Americans, and accounts for over 70% of all cases of dementia (Katzman, 1986). After age 60, the prevalence of AD doubles every 5.5 years, and between 10-40% of Americans over the of age 80 suffer from AD (Evans et al, 1991). The disease is slowly progressive; rates of progression from initial symptoms to end stage dementia range from 2 to 25 years, with most patients in the 8 to 12 year range. AD may have a very long preclinical course of 20 or more years with biochemical and pathological changes preceding clinical symptoms.

Pathologically, AD is characterized by degenerating neurites, abnormal accumulations of amyloid protein in so-called "senile plaques", and intracytoplasmic "neurofibrillary tangles". There is specificity to both the anatomical distribution of these lesions and the resulting clinical symptomatology. The first lesions of AD probably occur in entorhinal cortex and then "spread" to involve areas CA1, CA3, and the subiculum of the hippocampus. In later stages, the disease involves polymodal association cortex in the superior temporal and inferior parietal lobes and association cortex in the frontal lobe (Braak et al, 1991. However, even in severe disease, at most 40-60% of pyramidal cells are lost (Katzman, 1986). Immunological methods have demonstrated a substantial decrease in the concentration of specific synapse associated proteins in AD (Terry et al, 1991; Honer et al, 1992). In some studies, these measures were inversely correlated with global measures of cognitive function (Terry et al, 1991). Concomitant with these changes is severe "retraction of dendritic arbor" of the pyramidal cells (Scheibel et al, 1978). It is important to emphasize that some brain regions are spared even in end stage patients. Thus pyramidal cells within primary cortex such as Brodmann areas 1,2, 3, 4, 17, and 41 are rarely affected.

In the mid 1970s, two different observations led to the "cholinergic hypothesis" of AD. College students given the anti-muscarinic drug scopolamine showed memory impairment somewhat similar to that seen in AD (Drachman et al, 1974). Post mortem studies of AD brains showed that although many neurotransmitter systems are impaired in AD, deficiencies in the cholinergic system are usually the most severe (Davies et al, 1976; Perry et al, 1978). These observations led to numerous studies to treat memory impairment in AD with drugs that modulate the cholinergic system. The acetylcholinesterase inhibitor, tacrine (or tetrahydroaminoacridine) is currently the only drug approved by the FDA specifically for treatment of AD (Summers et al; 1991; Davis et al, 1992); unfortunately, its efficacy is frequently marginal.

In the past 15 years, extensive studies of the biochemistry and genetics of AD have shown that the amyloid protein found in the cores of senile plaques results from abnormal processing of a larger protein, called amyloid precursor protein (APP). Mutations in the amyloid precursor gene are associated with some cases of autosomal dominant presenile AD. It has also been shown that late onset AD (starting after age 65) is associated with the apolipoprotein e4 genotype (Saunders et al, 1993). It is estimated that 40% of cases of late onset AD are due to this gene.

The challenge in understanding Alzheimer's disease is to be able to map what is known about biochemical and cellular pathology to the abnormal behaviors characteristic of the disease. To date, clinicopathological studies have taken a "black box" approach by correlating specific pathological markers with global measures of cognitive function. The choice of pathological marker is usually not made by an assessment of what structures are needed for specific cognitive functions, but rather with the underlying assumption that any widespread pathology probably interferes with cognitive function. Some of the most important studies of AD have taken this approach. Thus the seminal studies of Blessed, Tomlinson, and Roth (1968) that demonstrated that AD and not vascular disease was the most important cause of dementia in the elderly were based on demonstrating that cognitive impairment was correlated with quantitative measures of AD pathology. Two decades later, a similar approach was taken in the important studies of Terry and Masliah (1991) that showed significant correlations between global measures of cognitive function and immunological estimates of the concentration of synapse associated proteins.

Ruppin and colleagues (Horn and Ruppin, 1993; 1995; Ruppin and Reggia, 1995) have investigated the consequences of changes in synaptic connection densities in a series of network models. AD leads to decreases in the number of functioning synaptic connections, but several studies have shown that remaining synapses compensate by increasing in size. Ruppin and colleagues use attractor-type associative memory models to study the effect of synaptic depletion and compensation on the recall ability of such networks. They observe that local compensatory mechanisms can, under some circumstances, maintain memory functions despite significant losses in other connections. Their models raise the possibility that the loss or saturation of local compensatory mechanisms plays a major role in the development of cognitive deficits.

A complete understanding of how the pathology of AD leads to its symptoms depends on answering fundamental questions related to the mechanisms of normal cognitive function. Human clinicopathological studies have demonstrated that many different brain regions must be intact for successful acquisition and consolidation of episodic memories. These regions include entorhinal cortex, hippocampus, amygdala, nucleus basalis, dorsal medial nucleus of the thalamus, mamillary bodies, mid-dorsolateral frontal cortex, and ventromedial frontal cortex (Petrides, 1989, 1994).

Alvarez and Squire (1994) proposed a connectionist-level model directed towards the role of some of these brain structures. They assume that learning between the neocortex and hippocampus (and then between hippocampus and neocortex) occurs quickly, but that forgetting occurs between these regions at a moderate rate. On the other hand, neocortical to neocortical learning occurs slowly, but forgetting is also very slow. In this model, the hippocampus slowly teaches the neocortex. An attractive feature of this model is that when lesioned it responds like patients with Alzheimer's disease. The model does well on associations it learned in early cycles, but less well on memories learned in later cycles.

The model of Alvarez and Squire makes assumptions and predictions that can be tested to some degree in physiologic or functional MRI studies. And it begins to address fundamental questions such as 1) how does hippocampal data get back to specific neocortical regions? and 2) how much data reduction is there between neocortex and hippocampus? In order to correctly answer these questions it is necessary to construct models at a more detailed level. One can postulate a variety of mechanisms, and construct "black-box" analogies, but the details of how the system actually works may be incompatible with many such schemes. For example, much of the current experimental evidence on hippocampus suggests that patterns of neuronal activations, representing events, are generated and ultimately stored in cortex, but are associated in a context-dependent fashion in the hippocampus. The "fusion" of cortical and hippocampal representations may occur through temporal synchronization of activity patterns. Buzsaki and colleagues have shown that this synchronization is probably mediated by super-networks of inhibitory GABA-ergic cells, many of which establish widespread, long-distance connections (Buzsaki and Chrobak, 1995). There are multiple classes of inhibitory cells, each with layer-specific patterns of connections, so that inputs to various regions of pyramidal cell dendrites (e.g., from perforant path, commissural path, etc.) can be specifically inhibited. Inhibition of a dendritic region may prevent calcium entry during back-propagating action potentials, preventing selected sets of synapses from becoming potentiated through LTP (Buzsaki and Chrobak, 1995). The point is that the details are critical, and can lead to models that are counter-intuitive. Synchronization by a network of inhibitory cells has very different properties as that achieved by excitatory-excitatory couplings. To appreciate the dynamics of such networks, a much more detailed understanding of cell properties is required. Once such detailed models have been studied, it may be possible to abstract the essence of the model in a computationally efficient manner. Thus, the scheme proposed by Buzsaki and Chrobak (1995) for how inhibitory supernetworks can synchronize pyramidal cells--based on extensive experimental investigation--actually turns out to be quite similar to the simple computational model proposed by Hopfield (1995) as a mechanism of representing spatial patterns in a temporal neural code (G. Buzsaki, personal communication). Without detailed modeling, however, there can be no assurance that the more abstract model represents the correct choice of mechanisms.

The studies of Hasselmo et al. (1992, 1993, 1994; Barkai et al, 1994a,b,c) represent an attempt to incorporate more detail into the modeling process. Both excitatory and inhibitory neurons are modeled with interconnection densities corresponding to those in vivo. In recent models, biologically realistic neurons are studied which contain 6 intrinsic ion currents and 3 synaptic currents. Hasselmo proposes that the cholinergic system might function to toggle networks between learning and recall states. Acetylcholine is proposed to suppress synaptic transmission at intrinsic connections and also to decrease adaptation of afferent input. Hasselmo and his colleagues showed that these two combined effects could enhance efficiency of learning more than either effect alone.

One prediction of Hasselmo's model is that studies of the effects of cholinesterase inhibitors should match neuropsychological task to periods of high or low cholinergic state. Their model would suggest that learning would occur best with high cholinergic state, but that recall would occur best with low cholinergic state. A subject with AD could be taught a task while receiving intravenous cholinesterase inhibitors, and then tested on recall after the drug is no longer active.

One goal for future models is to integrate additional cellular and network mechanisms with behavioral properties such as memory consolidation and recall. These models may help unravel the principles of higher cognitive function and the relationship between hippocampus and neocortex.

3. Parkinson's Disease

Parkinson's disease is a degenerative neurological disease characterized by resting tremor, rigidity, bradykinesia (slowing of movements), akinesia (difficulty initiating movements), and poor balance (Adams and Victor, 1993). Cognitive impairment and/or depression occur in a substantial percentage of patients (Mayeux et al, 1988).

The pathological hallmark of Parkinson's disease (PD) is loss of the dopaminergic neurons in the substantia nigra that project to the putamen. (Most surviving neurons will have a characteristic cytoplasmic inclusion called a Lewy body.) Other brain regions are often affected, but pathology in the substantia nigra is the sine qua non of the disease.

About 500,000 Americans have PD; the vast majority have idiopathic PD, although some cases are drug-induced. A specific form of PD developed among many survivors of the encephalitis epidemic of 1918-1921. However, few of these patients are still alive. Idiopathic PD is primarily a disease of middle age and late life.

A significant breakthrough occurred in the early 1980s when it was discovered that young people abusing the "designer drug" MPTP (a derivative of the narcotic meperidine) soon thereafter developed severe Parkinson's disease (Langston et al, 1983; Ballard et al, 1985). This neurotoxin became invaluable as a tool for developing animal models of PD. MPTP itself is not toxic, within the brain it is oxidized to itself toxic form, MPP+. Several investigators suggested that a similar process might occur in patients with idiopathic PD, and started studies asking whether drugs that blocked this oxidative step might slow the rate of progression of PD. Although several studies have suggested that PD patients treated with oxidase inhibitors do progress more slowly (Parkinson study group, 1989, 1993; Tetrud et al, 1989), interpretation of these data remain controversial (Schulzer et al, 1992)

The discovery that dopamine was deficient in the substantia nigra led to efforts to treat PD with L-DOPA, a precursor of dopamine (dopamine itself does not cross the blood brain barrier). Over 80% of patients with PD obtain substantial benefit with L-DOPA therapy (Adams and Victor, 1993). However, its efficacy frequently wanes after several years, and disabling side effects including dyskinesias and hallucinations can develop. Before L-DOPA therapy, stereotactic surgery with ablative lesions in the thalamus or globus pallidus was commonly performed. In recent years, interest in stereotactic surgery has revived, with newer surgical methods yielding more control over the size and site of the lesions. Efforts have been made to treat PD with transplantation into the brain of fetal cells from the adrenal medulla or from the fetal nigra. Several groups have recently shown that neural growth factors may improve the efficacy of transplanted tissues.

In Parkinson's disease the timing of the firing of agonist and antagonist muscle groups is dysfunctional. As a result, movements are slow and/or tremulous. To date, the mechanism by which dopaminergic deficiency leads to this symptomatology is not clear. Most investigators believe that dopamine deficiency leads to an imbalance of the direct and indirect pathways from the putamen to the internal part of the globus pallidus, but more precise mechanistic details are lacking.

Towards this end, Borrett and colleagues (1993) have studied the dynamics of a 4 layer neural network where the output layer feeds back to the input layer. They propose that such a network might model the type of calculations made by cortico-basal ganglia-thalamic-cortical loop that is dysfunctional in Parkinson's disease. Three types of stable states are possible from such nonlinear dynamic systems - a fixed attractor, a periodic attractor, or a chaotic attractor. Borrett showed that as the parameters of such a nonlinear system were gradually changed, the system suddenly reached a bifurcation point where output changed from a fixed attractor to a periodic attractor.

In their model, they simulated the effect of dopamine in cortico-ganglionic loops as a decrease in the threshold of excitability for units in the pre-output layer. They were able to show that as the threshold was gradually increased (simulating a decrease in dopamine levels) the output of the network first became slower and then changed from a fixed attractor state to a periodic (i.e. tremulous) state.

Even though Borrett's model consists of abstract units whose output is defined by a sigmoidal function, the model makes several points that underscore the role of computational models in understanding neurological disease. First, behavior results from the dynamic interaction of multiple units from different modular systems. Second, the model suggests that some behaviors such as tremor will develop suddenly when a bifurcation threshold is reached. The decrease in dopamine in the susbtantia nigra of Parkinson's disease occurs gradually over several years. It is likely that there must be very significant decrease in dopamine levels (some have estimated as much as 90%) before patients become symptomatic.

We believe that computational models will play an increasingly important role in understanding the pathophysiology of movement disorders such as Parkinson's disease. And a number of groups are beginning to apply methodologies used in understanding central pattern generators and neuronal oscillations to the study of Parkinson's tremor. These studies may yield insights that will eventually lead to better treatments for these disorders.

4. Epilepsy

Over 1.5 million Americans suffer from epilepsy (Engel, 1989). Although over two-thirds of patients with epilepsy can be well controlled with medication, a sizable minority cannot, and medication side effects frequently limit patient's quality of life (Adams and Victor, 1993). Epileptic seizures are the clinical manifestations of excessive abnormal neuronal firings. Clinical phenomenology of seizures can range from brief lapse of consciousness without loss of posture to a generalized tonic-clonic (grand mal) seizure with loss of consciousness and prolonged post ictal state (Engel, 1989).

Many different pathological processes including trauma, infection, hypoxia, and stroke can lead to the development of a seizure disorder. Certain parts of the brain are more epileptogenic than others. For example, the hippocampus and certain neocortical regions are most epileptogenic. Seizures probably never originate in such structures as the cerebellum, basal ganglia, or brain stem (Engel, 1989).

Epilepsy results from the exaggeration of two normal neuronal processes - neuronal excitation and synchronization of groups of neurons (Engel, 1989). In patients with epilepsy, the EEG shows sharp waves, in contrast to normally occurring (8-13 Hz) alpha waves. The sharp wave represents the summation of the potentials of up to hundreds of pyramidal cells that are repetitively firing riding on a sudden depolarization wave (Engel, 1989).

Some anti-epileptic drugs such as carbamazepine (Tegretol) and phenytoin (Dilantin) act by modulating Na (and Ca) ion currents. Other drugs including phenobarbital, valproate (Depakote), and benzodiazepines act by modulating the GABA-ergic system.

Computer models of single pyramidal cells have been used to study the effects of specific ion currents on bursting behavior and on repetitive firing. Lytton and Sejnowski (1991) developed a computer model to study the effects of inhibitory input on synchronization of pyramidal cells. In particular, they wanted to determine whether pyramidal cells receiving random afferent input could convert that data into regular repetitive output. They developed simple and complex models of pyramidal cells. The complex models had 406 compartments, and 11 types of ion channels were modeled. The simple models had 3 channels and 9 compartments. They were able to show that

IPSPs could entrain pyramidal cells receiving random input to fire at regular intervals.

Traub and colleagues (1992) developed models of CA3 in the hippocampus that contained 1000 pyramidal cells, 100 cells that simulated $GABA_A$ inhibition, and 100 cells that simulated $GABA_B$ inhibition. They attempted to adjust the density of intercellular connections to approximate that which occurs in vivo. Their models demonstrated that 1) recurrent excitation (in the absence of inhibition) can induce synchrony of the pyramidal cells; 2) in the presence of $GABA_A$ blockers, the network could produce synchronized bursts of activity; 3) with partial blockade of $GABA_A$ inhibition, the network could produce "synchronized synaptic potentials".

The use of such models has explained the basic mechanisms by which synchronized activity emerges. In particular, Traub and colleagues have been able to generate activity patterns, in realistic networks, that closely mimic epileptic activity recorded in vitro, and the types of EEG activity seen in patients. These models have been particularly useful in uncovering the roles of various cell types and connections in epileptogenesis, and in explaining the effects of various pharmacological agents. Traub's work serves as perhaps the best example of how detailed modeling can integrate neurobiological data, and serve as a means of generating testable experimental predictions.

5. Stroke and Neurological Injury

One clinical area in which there is an informative history of attempts to develop computational models is the reorganization of topographic maps in the somatosensory system as a consequence of injury. Over the last 20 years, a number of physiological experiments have been carried out to investigate in a controlled fashion, the central effects of peripheral nerve injury. Merzenich and his colleagues (Jenkins and Merzenich, 1987) made detailed mappings of areas 3b and 1 in monkey somatosensory cortex after a number of perturbations including nerve transections, nerve crush, digit amputation, syndactyly, and skin island pedicle transfer. They also studied the effects of focal correlated stimulation to a skin region under conditions in which the animal attended to the stimulus, or did not. Most relevant to stroke and CNS injury, they studied changes in representation as a consequence of focal cortical lesions. The general results of their extensive studies (reviewed in Merzenich and Jenkins, 1993) are that within the limits allowed by the anatomy, the cortical map reflects spatial relationships in the stimulus domain. Regions that are co-stimulated tend to be represented together. In addition, after a cortical lesion, skin sites formerly represented in the damaged region can come to be represented outside of the damaged area. These studies suggest that cortical representations are plastic, and may be alterable through some combination of the pattern of stimulation, control of synaptic plasticity, and the general excitability of cortical cells.

Several neural simulations have been developed to test these ideas in a quantitative fashion. Kohonen (1982) developed the first algorithm to model how changes in input correlations can lead to reorganization of computational maps. Studies by Cowan, von der Malsberg, and others had earlier shown how topographic maps can arise in development. Kohonen's algorithm was not intended to model physiological experiments. Rather it was directed towards the problem of how relations in feature space (e.g., topographic adjacency) can be preserved through a series of neural mappings. For each stimulus applied to the network, the algorithm picks the most strongly activated unit in the network, and the synaptic weights of that unit (and its nearest neighbors) are adjusted so as to increase the response to the applied stimulus. Kohonen showed that this rule leads to formation of topographically organized maps and that such maps obey a magnification rule. As the frequency of stimulation of a particular input region is increased, the fraction of the map devoted to the stimulated region proportionately increases.

In 1987, Pearson, Finkel and Edelman proposed a slightly more complex network specifically directed at modeling cortical map reorganization. The network contained excitatory and inhibitory cells, with a topographically organized set of inputs from a sensory receptor sheet (corresponding to the hand). Only excitatory cells in the network received an input from the receptor sheet, and these connections as well as the excitatory-excitatory connections within the network were plastic according to a voltage-dependent synaptic mechanism. Repeated stimulation of the receptor sheet led to the formation of clusters of strongly interconnected cells, neuronal groups. Cells in these groups had highly overlapped receptive fields. Each excitatory cell received equal numbers of inputs from receptors on the "glabrous" and "dorsal" aspects of the "hand". Thus, initially, all cells had receptive fields on both front and back of the hand. However, after neuronal groups had formed, all the cells in each group exhibited a receptive field either on the front or the back of the hand--but half of the input connections were weakened to subthreshold strengths.

Pearson and colleagues were able to demonstrate a number of reorganizational properties in the network that corresponded to those observed physiologically. Increased stimulation, manifested as tapping of a small skin region, led to an expansion of the representation of affected skin surface in the network--at the expense of the representation of adjacent skin regions. Resumption of a more balanced stimulation, was followed by a contraction of the map back to a representation similar to that originally found. A converse experiment involved transection of inputs corresponding to cutting the median nerve (which mediates touch perception for digits 1-3 on the glabrous surface of the hand). After transection, a representation of dorsal aspects of digits 1-3 emerged in the network locations formerly devoted to the glabrous representation. There were also silent regions in the network which could not be activated. But with tactile stimulation of the receptor sheet, these silent regions gradually shrank away, leaving an intact, topographic map of the back of the hand--just as is described experimentally.

In 1990, Grajski and Merzenich described a similar network model, which incorporated an intermediate "thalamic" stage. They were able to account for an additional important experimental finding, namely, that as the size of a cortical representation increases, the receptive fields of the cortical cells decrease in size -- the so-called inverse magnification rule.

More recently, Reggia and colleagues (Sutton, et al, 1994; Armentrout, et al., 1994) have shown that a competitive activation rule can also account for these findings. In addition, they have been able to account for the changes in representation seen after cortical lesions.

Thus, one can account for many, if not all, of the types of cortical reorganization seen after stimulation, deafferentation, and other manipulations by changes in either synaptic connection strengths or competitive distributions of activity in networks of interconnected cells. However, several recent experimental observations suggest that additional processes to those considered in these models may be at work.

First, in 1991, Pons and colleagues reported on the cortical effects of de-afferentation in a set of monkeys who had survived over 10 years after deafferentation. Whereas the effects Merzenich and others had observed had been limited to cortical shifts on the order of hundreds of microns (up to 1 mm in the most extreme cases), Pons reported map shifts on the order of 10-14 mm. In these animals, the cortical areas formerly devoted to representing the hand and arm were now occupied by a representation of the face. It was as if the representation of the lower face, chin and cheeks had been stretched, as if on a rubber sheet, over the centimeter of cortex formerly devoted to the arm.

Ramachandran (1993) has recently demonstrated similar findings in humans. He examined a set of patients who had recently undergone arm amputation, and were experiencing "phantom" limb syndrome. Ramachandran found that all of these patients had topographic representations of the missing arm which could be elicited by stimulation of a site on the remaining stump. And in several of the patients, there was a second site of representation of the missing hand, located on the lower portion of the face. Thus, in their cortices, the representation of the face must have expanded into the region formerly devoted to the hand. When the face was stimulated, it activated two sets of cells; the original, intact representation of the face, and also cells in the cortical region formerly devoted to the hand. Higher centers, viewing this latter activation, may "interpret" it as arising from the hand.

Further documentation for this view comes from combined MEG-MRI studies of these patients (reviewed in Ramachandran, 1993). The normal representational spacing of the face-arm-hand is observed in the hemisphere contralateral to the intact arm. However, in the affected hemisphere, the representation of the face is seen to shift towards the site of representation of the missing arm and hand.

In perhaps the most striking finding, Ramachandran had amputee patients view a mirror image of their remaining hand from such an angle that it visually appeared to be the missing hand. Patients were instructed to move both "hands" symmetrically through a range of motions. Remarkably, patients reported the disappearance of painful phantom sensations, and eventually, the disappearance of the phantom limb perception itself.

Ramachandran has also studied patients with right parietal lobe strokes who experience varying degrees of left hemisthesia, hemiparalysis, and hemineglect. Some of these patients also undergo somatoparaphrenic delusions, a syndrome of confabulation in which they deny the existence of their condition. Following earlier studies by Rubens, Bisiach and others, Ramachandran found that application of cold water to the external ear canal of these patients resulted in amelioration of their condition. Several minutes after cessation of the cold water, the temperature returns to normal, and the neurological deficits (and delusional state) return.

Cooling of the external ear results in a unilateral decrease in vestibular activation, and thus a shift of the perceptual "midline". Behavioral experiments confirm that after left ear cold water stimulation, when normal subjects with eyes closed are asked to point straight ahead, they instead point off to the left. Frackowiak and colleagues (Bottini, et al., 1995) have used PET to identify sites at which vestibular and somatosensory inputs are colocalized in the brain. They report that co-activation is found in secondary somatosensory cortex, in the putamen, insula, premotor cortex, and supramarginal gyrus. A patient with right parietal stroke (whose lesion spared putamen and insula) was found to have maximum PET activation of these regions when touch and vestibular stimulation were combined.

These observations are provocative and fascinating, and they imply that additional mechanisms to those considered in the above models must be at work. The anatomy underlying the shifts seen in Merzenich's data is limited to branching thalamic arbors, which can extend over 1-2 mm^2 in cortex. There is no way in which these arbors can account for shifts over 15mm. Given Darian-Smith and Gilbert's (1994) results on plasticity in striate cortex it is likely that these long-term effects result from new anatomical connections which are made in cortex. The consideration of sprouting adds a new dimension to the parameter space of modeling, but more importantly, to the possibilities for rehabilitation after neural injury.

A second set of recent experimental observations also calls for re-evaluation of some of the modeling assumptions.

Working in the cortex of the Australian flying fox, Calford & Tweedale (1988) studied changes in the hand representation that immediately followed digit amputation or application of local anesthesia. They found that, in addition to shifts in the location of receptive fields, there was an large and immediate expansion of the receptive field size. These changes were reversible when the anesthetic wore off. These results are analogous to those observed in visual cortex by Gilbert and Wiesel (1992) following creation of a focal scotoma.

The magnitude of these receptive field changes are large compared to the anatomical scales of the thalamo-cortical connections in the early models. More importantly, the fact that the change occurs before any significant stimulation of the skin takes place, suggests a mechanism different from that mediating the chronic map changes due to altered patterns of stimulation. And the immediate nature of the expansion leads these investigators to suggest that the change may be due to an alteration in the balance of excitation and inhibition, rather than due to synaptic plasticity, per se. In their article, Calford and Tweedale point out that the Pearson, et al. model is limited by the assumption that only excitatory cells receive a direct thalamic input. Thus, deafferentation affects excitatory cells directly, but inhibitory cells only indirectly, through the loss of inputs from local excitatory cells.

Some insight into the mechanisms responsible for these immediate changes in receptive field size come from an experiment by Pettet and Gilbert (1992) involving the creation of an "artificial" scotoma. The artificial scotoma is formed by a dynamic textured stimulus that has a small, homogeneous grey region whose luminance equals the average luminance in the surround The stimulus is placed such that the homogeneous region covers (and extends somewhat beyond) the classical receptive field of the recorded cell. Ramachandran and Gregory (1991) had shown psychophysically that when such a stimulus is viewed for several minutes, the texture appears to "fill-in" the homogeneous region (color also fills in with a slightly faster time course). Pettet and Gilbert reported that in cat cortex, there was a 5-fold expansion of receptive fields located within the scotoma region. This expansion was immediately reversible when the scotoma region was stimulated.

More recently, Freeman and colleagues (DeAngelis, et al, 1995) used reverse-correlation techniques to precisely determine receptive field changes during conditioning with similar artificial scotoma. They reported that many cells show no change in receptive field properties, and those that do change appear to have undergone a change in response gain. The overall responsiveness of a cell might be expected to change through contrast gain-control mechanisms as a result of decreasing the local contrast versus that in the surround. If response gain is increased, then inputs which were formerly sub-threshold, can become supra-threshold, and thus weak distant inputs can now be included in the receptive field. DeWeerd and colleagues (1995) present data consistent with this interpretation. They recorded from cells during the conditioning phase of the artificial scotoma, and found that cells in the scotoma region gradually increase their firing rates.

The explanation offered for these results (DeAngelis, et al., 1995; DeWeerd et al, 1995; Chapman and Stone, 1996) is that the conditioning stimulus (the texture surrounding the homogeneous "hole") leads to an adaptation of the inhibition onto cells in the scotoma region. Reduced inhibition translates into increased gain response. Restimulation in the scotoma region itself activates local inhibition which reduces the gain. The long-distance inhibition could be mediated by horizontal cortico-cortical connections, or by basket cell networks, or by a combination of both. This is consistent with the model of Xing and Gerstein (1994) who found that adaptation of inhibition can account for the types of receptive field expansions observed.

It is in fact conceivable that these immediate changes are solely the result of the decreased stimulation to the receptive field center, in the context of surround stimulation. Contrast normalization or gain control mechanisms would then up-regulate cell responsiveness--independent of any changes in inhibitory adaptation. Changes in gain control may have interesting effects particularly when considered in the context of the differential time courses of excitation and inhibition following cortical stimulation. For example, in the model recently proposed by Douglas and Martin (1991; 1995), thalamic inputs comprise a small fraction (on the order of 5%) of the connections received by cortical pyramidal cells, whereas the vast majority (85%) of those connections are from other pyramidal cells. Douglas and Martin therefore propose that the thalamic input serves more as a "trigger", unleashing a cascade of recurrent excitation that amplifies and sharpens the thalamic signal. Inhibitory cells are activated earlier than excitatory cells due to a faster, highly myelinated set of inputs (Somers, et al.,

1995). The extent of cortical activation is therefore a race over whether excitation can reach threshold levels before inhibition "wipes the slate clean". Receptive fields will tend to be localized as a consequence of the limited spatial domain over which excitation spreads before inhibition prevails. However, under conditions of deafferentation, and resulting changes in cell responsiveness, the balance between excitation and inhibition is changed. Stimuli which excite distant cortical locations are now capable of exciting cells in the deafferented region, due to a net increase in the positive feedback within the local recurrent circuits. Thus, the effect of a distant input is not merely strengthened due to increased cell responsiveness, but also as a result of the local recurrent excitatory circuits.

A number of other mechanisms are also possible, including effects mediated through inhibitory networks. Regardless, these results illustrate how the assumptions of the original models constrain their possible responses to altered stimulation conditions. Furthermore, it illustrates how the failure to incorporate a particular detail of cell physiology--in this case, overall cell responsiveness or gain--can have important implications for the ultimate success of the model.

It is possible that immediate changes in cell responsiveness can be translated into longer-term changes in synaptic plasticity. Increasing postsynaptic cell responses will lead, through any Hebb-type mechanism, to increased synaptic strengths. And it is further possible that these synaptic facilitations play a role in the even longer-term axonal sprouting processes that underlie the system's response to altered input stimulation. Thus, there may be a continuum of changes, over different time scales, that allow the system to measure the permanence of the alteration in input characteristics.

This graduated response to deafferentation suggests new approaches in neurological rehabilitation. In cases where deafferentation is not permanent, i.e., where input will be reestablished after some time, it may be beneficial to try to prevent synaptic facilitations and cortical sprouting. In cases where the lesion is irreversible, we may want to encourage whatever plasticity is possible. In either case, modulation of cell responsiveness through pharmacological means may serve as either a boost or a suppresser to intrinsic gain control mechanisms. It is conceivable that stroke patients might be given neuromodulatory agents (including those affecting cholinergic, adrenergic, serotonergic and other systems) to increase cell responsiveness, as a means of encouraging plasticity. And given the effect of vestibular stimulation in parietal strokes (Ramachandran, 1993; Bottini, et al., 1995) it may be possible to modulate neuronal responsiveness through stimulation of alternate anatomical pathways. Of course, increasing metabolic demands during a period when cortical regions remain ischemic may be counter-productive. But models can track the time course of both neuronal activity and cellular metabolic state, and in such a way, possibly suggest windows for therapeutic intervention. The development of treatment strategies may then be addressed through detailed simulations in which the anatomical, physiological, and pharmacological properties of cortical networks are studied under conditions emulating neurological disease.

6. Conclusions

The success of applying computational methods to understanding neurological disease will depend upon a number of factors. Models should be sufficiently detailed to capture the effects of the major contributing anatomical, physiological and pharmacological processes. However, once an understanding of the system is gained, the model should be simple enough to allow interpretation of its results. Whereas most modeling efforts culminate with reproduction of some subset of the known data, it is more valuable to use the model to try out new experimental predictions.

One of the most difficult initial decisions in constructing a model is the choice of level of detail to be considered. In any simulation, there is a trade-off between memory and speed, and thus a compromise must always be made between the level of detail (number of channels, anatomical structure, temporal resolution) and the number of units simulated. Should the network contain 5 different cell types with multiple channels and compartments--or is an abstract, artificial network sufficient to test the ideas behind the model. In general, the advantage of incorporating more biological detail into a model is the level of detail at which predictions can be made. The major disadvantage is the increase in model complexity as it becomes more realistic.

The choice of level always depends upon the particular problem, however, for many problems, a safe choice may be to construct the model at the level of integrate-and-fire units. Such units sum their inputs and generate an individual spike of activity whenever the firing threshold is exceeded. A growing body of evidence suggests that the temporal dynamics of cell activity is critical to neural function.

However, a major problem with modeling at the single spike level is that one is confined to a millisecond time scale, and thus behavioral events may require thousands of iterations to simulate. To model events transpiring over seconds or minutes, or to make correlations with MRI or MEG data, one may wish to move to a higher-level model in which only mean-firing rates are simulated. Neural models built of rate-coded units use a (usually nonlinear) transfer function to convert the summation of their inputs into a mean-firing rate. Such models are capable of representing the spatial aspects of network processing, but are not realistic in terms of the temporal aspects of network dynamics because they do not represent the instantaneous firing properties of cells.

Detailed models which simulate the actual Hodgkin-Huxley type dynamics of cell firing have the advantage of accurately computing these temporal dynamics, but introduce such a degree of complexity, and require such specific assumptions about channel properties as to be of limited use except in those cases where sufficient experimental evidence exists. The integrate-and-fire level model represents a reasonable compromise between these extremes. In addition, effects such as after-depolarizations, or transition to bursting modes, can be incorporated by appropriate terms in the equations of state. Most importantly, effects of various transmitters, modulators, and drugs can be modeled by their effect on cell excitability or firing characteristics. Understanding the detailed behavior of such interactions may require a channel-level model, but once the effect is understood, it may be sufficient to represent its effects on firing characteristics.

Perhaps the greatest challenge to the computational approach is to begin to explain how functional behavior emerges from the operation of cellular-level processes. A model constructed at the level of Ca-channels and NMDA receptors, which was also capable of high-level behavior--perception, memory, or motor action--would provide an invaluable illustration of how the system as a whole might work. Lesions to such a model, particularly if they can be made to resemble in some detail the pathologic changes in actual disease processes, can occur at the cellular level, but be manifested functionally. This approach may reveal unsuspected common mechanisms operating in different disease processes (relations between Parkinsonism and schizophrenia, or related problems in synchronization in Alzheimer's disease, epilepsy, and dyslexia). The goal is to move from the current situation, in which the "standard model" for a disease process is a flow chart of interconnections between brain regions, to a conceptual model that integrates, through simulations, the wealth of information at the molecular, cellular, network, systems, and behavioral levels.

Acknowledgements
We gratefully acknowledge the support of The Whitaker Foundation, Office of Naval Research N00014-93-1-0861, and the McDonnell-Pew Program in Cognitive Neuroscience (to L.F.) , and of The Joel and Maria Finkle Fund (to H.C.)

References

Adams RA and Victor M. *Principles of Neurology.* NY; McGraw Hill, 1993.

Allard, T., S.A. Clark, W.M. Jenkins, and M.M. Merzenich, *J. Neurophsiol.* **66** (1991) 1048.

Armentrout, S.L., Reggia, J.A., and Weinrich, M., *Artificial Intelligence in Medicine* **6** (1994) 383.

Alvarez P and LR Squire, *Proc. Natl. Acad. Sci. USA* **91** (1994) 7041.

Ballard PA, Tetrud JW, Langston JW. *Neurology* **35** (1985) 949.

Barkai E and ME Hasselmo, *J Neurophysiology* **72** (1994) 644.

Barkai E, Bergman RE, Horwitz G, Hasselmo ME., *J Neurophysiology* **72** (1994) 659.

Bick KL. in*Alzheimer's Disease,* eds. Terry RD, R Katzman R, Bick KL (Raven, New York, 1994).

Blessed G, Tomlinson BE, Roth M., *British J Psychiatry* **114** (1968) 797.

Borrett DS, Yeap TH, Kwan HC, *Candian Journal of Neurological Sciences* **20** (1993) 107.

Bottini, G., Paulesu, E., Sterzl, R., Warburton, E., Wise, R.J.S., Vallar, G., Frackowiak, R.S.J., and Frith, C.D., *Nature* **376** (1995) 778.

Braak H, Braak E., *Acta Neuropathologica* **82** (1991) 239.

Buzsaki, G., and Chrobak, J.J., *Curr. Opinion Neurobiol.* **5** (1995) 504.

Calford, M.B. and R. Tweedale, *Nature* **332** (1988) 446.

Chapman, B. and Stone, L.S., *Neuron* **16** (1996) 9.

Clark, S.A., T. Allard, W.M. Jenkins, and M.M. Merzenich, *Nature* **332**: (1988) 444.

Corder EH, Saunders AM, Strittmatter et al., *Science* **261** (1993) 921.

Darian-Smith, C. and Gilbert, C.D., *Nature* **368** (1994) 737.

Davies P Maloney AJ., *Lancet* **2** (1976) 1403.

Davis KL, Thal LJ, Gamzu ER et al., *NEJM* **327** (1992) 1253.

DeAngelis, G.C., Anzai,A., Ohzawa, I., and Freeman, R.D., *Proc. Natl. Acad. Sci. USA* **92** (1995) 9682.

deWeerd, P., Gattass, R., Desimone, R. and Ungerlieder, L.G., *Nature* **377** (1995) 731.

Douglas, R.J. and Martin, K.A.C., *J. Physiol.* **40** (1991) 735.

Douglas, R.J., Koch, C., Mahowald, M. Martin, K.A., and Suarez, H.H., *Science* **269** (1995) 981.

Drachman DA, Leavitt J., *Arch Neurology* **30** (1974) 113.

Evans DA, Funkenstein HH, Albert MS et al., *JAMA* **262** (1991) 2551.

Engel JE, *Seizures and Epilepsy.* (Davis, Philadelphia, 1989).

Gilbert, C.D. and T.N. Wiesel, *Nature* **356** (1992) 150.

Grajski, K. and Merzenich, M.M., *Neural Comput..* **2** (1990) 7.

270

Hasselmo ME, Anderson BP, Bower JM., *J Neurophysiology* **67** (1992) 1230.

Hasselmo ME and Bower JM., *Trends Neuroscience* **16** (1993) 218.

Hasselmo ME and Schnell E., *J Neuroscience* **14** (1994) 3898.

Honer WG, Dickson DW, Gleeson J, Davies P., *Neurobiology Aging* **13** (1992) 375.

Hopfield, J.J., *Nature* **376** (1995) 33.

Horn, D. and Ruppin E., *Neural Computation* **5** (1993) 736.

Horn, D. and Ruppin E., *Neural Computation* **7** (1995) 182.

Jenkins, W.M. and M.M. Merzenich, *Prog. Br. Res.* **71** (1987) 249.

Katzman R. Alzheimer's disease. *NEJM* **314** (1986) 964.

Kohonen, T., *Biological Cybernetics* **43** (1982) 59.

Kosik KS, Joachim CL, Selkoe DJ., *Proc. Natl. Acad. Sci. USA* (1986) 4044.

Langston JW, Ballard PA, Tetrud JW et al., *Science* **219** (1983) 979.

Lytton WW and TJ Sejnowski. *J Neurophysiology* **66** (1991) 1059.

Mayeux R, Stern Y, Rosenstein R et al., *Arch Neurol*. **45** (1988) 260.

Merzenich, M.M. and W.M. Jenkins. *J. Hand Therapy* **6** (1993) 89.

The Parkinson study group. *NEJM* **321** (1989) 1364.

The Parkinson study group. *NEJM* **328** (1993) 176.

Pearson, J.C., L.H. Finkel, and G.M. Edelman, *J. Neurosci.* **7** (1987) 4209.

Perry EK, Tomlinson BE, Blessed G et al., *Br Med J* (1978) 1427.

Petrides, M. in*Handbook of Neuropsychology, Vol 3;* , eds. Boller F, Grafman J (Elsevier Science Publishers, Amsterdam, 1989) p. 75.

Petrides M, in*Handbook of Neuropsychology, Vol 39* , eds. Boller F, Grafman J (Elsevier Science Publishers, Amsterdam, 1994) p 59.

Pettet, M.W. and C.D. Gilbert, *Proc. Natl. Acad. Sci. USA* **89** (1992) 8366.

Pons, T.P., P.E. Garraghty, A.K. Ommaya, J.H. Kaas, E.Taub, and M. Mishkin *Science* (1991) 1857.

Ramachandran, V.S., *Proc. Natl. Acad. Sci USA* **90** (1993) 10413.

Ramachandran, V.S. and Gregory R.L. *Nature* **350** (1991) 699.

Recanzone, G.H., M.M Merzenich, W.M. Jenkins, K.A. Grajski, and H.R. Dinse, *J. Neurophysiol.* **67** (1992) 1031.

Ruppin, E. and Reggia, J. *Br. J. Psychiatry* **166** (1995) 19.

Saunders AM, Streittmatter WJ, Schmecchel D et al.,*Neurolgy* **43** (1993) 1551.

Scheibel AB and Tomiyasu U., *Experimental Neurology* **60** (1978) 1.

Schulzer M, Mak E, Calne DB., *Annals Neurology* **32** (1992) 795.

Selkoe DJ. *Ann .Rev .Neuroscience* **17** (1994) 489.

Somers, D.C., Nelson, S.B., and Sur, M., *J. Neurosci.* **15** (1995) 5448.

Summers WL, Majorski LV, Marsh GM et al., *NEJM* **315** (1991) 1241.

Sutton, G.G., Reggia, J.A., Armentrout, S.L., and D'Autrechy, C.L., *Neural Computattion* **6** (1994) 1.

Terry RD, Masliah E, Salmon DP et al., *Ann Neurol* **30** (1991) 572.

Tetrud JW and JW Langston, *Science* (1989) 519.

Traub RD, Miles R, Buzsaki G., *J Physiology* **451** (1992) 653.

Wichmann T and MR DeLong, *Advances Neurology* , Raven Press, New York, 1993, p. 11.

Wolozin BL, Pruchnicki A, Dickson DW, Davies P., *Science* **232** (1986) 648.

Xing, J. and Gerstein, G.L., *Vision Res.* **34** (1994) 1901.

PHANTOM LIMBS, SELF-ORGANIZING FEATURE MAPS, AND NOISE-DRIVEN NEUROPLASTICITY

MANFRED SPITZER

Department of Psychiatry, University of Heidelberg
Voss-Str.4, 69115 Heidelberg, Germany
E-mail: Manfred_Spitzer@krzmail.krz.uni-heidelberg.de

ABSTRACT

Phantom limbs are sensations of the presence of an extremity that has been lost. A number of clinical features and recent findings of cortical map plasticity after deafferentation suggest that phantom limbs are caused by large scale cortical reorganization processes. However, paraplegics, who likewise suffer from cortical deafferentation, rarely develop phantom sensations, and if they do, these are weak, lack detail, and occur after months. This has been taken to suggest a non-cortical genesis of phantom limbs. A biologically plausible minimal neural network model is proposed to solve this apparent puzzle. In trained self-organizing feature maps, deafferentation was simulated. Reorganization is shown to be driven by input noise. According to the model, the production of input noise by the deafferented primary sensory neuron drives cortical reorganization in amputees. No such noise is generated and/or conducted to the cortex in paraplegics.

1. Introduction

Phantom limbs, i.e., tingling and often painful sensations of the presence of an extremity that has been lost, occur in 80 % to 100 % of amputees (Jensen & Rasmussen 1989), but only rarely and only negligibly in paraplegics (i.e., patients with lesions of the spinal cord). Phantom limbs in amputees have a number of remarkable clinical features (cf. Buchanen & Mandel 1986, Carlen et al. 1978, Cronholm 1951, Jensen et al. 1984, Katz 1992, Poeck 1963, Spitzer 1988, Weiss & Fishman 1963): (1) The *more severe* the trauma, the *more likely* and/or the *more extensive* is the phantom limb. Elective amputations, for example, cause fewer and less pronounced phantoms than traumatic amputations. Likewise, local anesthesia before elective amputations diminish phantom sensations thereafter. (2) Phantoms change over time in that they become subjectively experienced as shorter (the phenomenon is called "telescoping") and smaller ("shrinking"). As a result, a phantom hand may end up being experienced within the stump, having the size of a postage stamp. (3) Stimulation of the stump produces not only the experience in the stump, but also referred sensation, i.e., topographically organized sensations of the same modality on the phantom (called "referred sensations"). Water running down the stump, for example, is experienced as water running down the stump *and* the arm or the leg. (4) Sensory acuity of the stump is increased, i.e., the threshold of two-point-discrimination is decreased. (5) Phantom pain is highly correlated to the degree of cortical reorganization (Elbert et al. 1994, Flohr et al. 1995). (6) Both the extent and the clarity of these sensations vary greatly from case to case. Phantoms may not develop in patients with low intelligence or with senile dementia. There is some anecdotal evidence that characterological variables may modulate the development of phantom limbs (Schilder 1923, Zuk 1956; cf. Spitzer 1988 and Katz 1992 for critical discussions).

These clinical observations are compatible with the view that the experience of phantom limbs is produced by a cortical mechanism. This view was put forward decades ago (cf. Cronholm 1951) on the basis of the established map-like structure of the primary sensory cortex (cf. Penfield & Rasmussen 1950). It received further support by electro-physiological evidence of cortical reorganization due to changes in the general patterns of input signals (Recanzone et al. 1992a,b,c; Merzenich and Sameshima 1993). Pons et al. (1991) found cortical somatosensory maps to be capable of a particularly large degree of reorganization over distances of up to 14 mm. In one of their animals, the cortical area corresponding to the lost limb actually became responsive to stimuli applied to a region of the face.

Peripheral lesion experiments conducted by Merzenich and coworkers (1983; cf. Merzenich & Sameshima 1993) demonstrated self-organization capabilities in the somatosensory cortex after restricted deafferentation and provided evidence of dramatic cortical plasticity in adult primates. The authors advanced the hypothesis that it is the spatio-temporal coherence of input patterns which leads to their representation on the cortical surface. In this view, *input signals compete for representational space on the cortical surface*. The more similar the input signals, the closer they will eventually be located together. The process of translocation of input representation is driven by competition between cortical neurons.

Cortical reorganization in humans has since been demonstrated by a number of authors: When people learn Braille, the cortical somatosensory area that represents the tip of the right index finger becomes larger (Pascual-Leone et al. 1993), and when people learn to play the guitar or violin, the somatosensory cortex coding the fingers of their left hand becomes enlarged (Elbert et al. 1995). Finally, cortical reorganization is supposed to play a causal role when language impaired children get better at understanding spoken language after weeks of training with digitally stretched speech (Merzenich et al. 1996, Tallal et al. 1996).

Ramachandran et al. (1992) reported a clinical observation which provides further strong evidence in favor of the cortical view of the genesis of phantom limbs (cf. Halligan et al. 1993). Stimulation of the face in a patient with an amputated arm evoked localized and topographically mapped sensations in the phantom hand. As the face is not adjacent to the arm, but the *cortical representation* of the face is adjacent to the *cortical representation* of the arm, this finding supports the view that cortical reorganization drives the development of phantom limbs, i.e., that "tactile and proprioceptive input from surrounding tissue 'takes over' the brain areas corresponding to the amputated limb" (Ramachandran et al. 1992, p. 1160). In particular, the authors speculated that "spontaneous discharges arising from neurons innervating these tissues would be misinterpreted as arising from the missing limb." The authors "expect sensory input from both these regions [face and arm] to 'invade' the cortical hand area and provide a basis for referred sensations". In line with this view, Elbert et al. (1994), used magnetic source imaging to demonstrate that the topographic representation in the somatosensory cortex of the face area in upper extremity amputees was shifted an average of 1.5 cm toward the area that would normally receive input from the now absent nerves supplying the hand and fingers.

The cortical mechanism of phantom limb causation may be summarized as follows: The cortex is a two-dimensional computational map-like surface, which changes according to the spatio-temporal characteristics of the input. If an area becomes deafferented (i.e., deprived of its input), reorganization takes place. Either during this process or as a result of this process, neurons representing input patterns that are no longer present due to deafferentation become activated. This activation causes the phantom limb phenomenon.

This view of phantom limb causation has been challenged by a number of authors who suggested a peripheral mechanism or a mechanism at the level of the spinal cord. According to this non-cortical view, free nerve endings, neuromas and axons proliferating into scar tissue are regarded as the cause of phantom pain which in turn is supposed to lead to phantom sensations (Poeck 1963). In a recent review Katz (1992) proposed that phantom limbs are related to the sympathetic-efferent outflow of cutaneous vasoconstrictior fibers in the stump and stump neuromas. According to this view, phantom limb sensations are caused by efferent sympathetic activity finding its way back to afferent sensory fibers. Cronholm suggested that hyperexcitability of the spinal cord is the mechanism of phantom limb causation.

This non-cortical view of the causation of phantom limbs—either at the level of the peripheral nerve or the spinal cord—is supported by one striking clinical finding: Patients with lesions of the spinal cord and the clinical condition of paraplegia either do not develop phantom sensations or develop phantoms which are clinically different from the phantoms of amputees. Phantomsensations in paraplegic patients are weak, they lack detail, and occur months after the onset of paraplegia. In short, even if both, amputees and paraplegics have phantoms, there remain striking clinical differences in the way they are experienced. These differences—they are crucial for the analysis of the phenomenon and the arguments made in the discussion section — are highlighted by two case reports of thoracic spinal cord lesions and additional arm amputation (Bors 1951) which allow the intraindividual comparison of the effects of amputation and spinal cord lesion. Both patients experienced a pronounced and clear phantom of the arm but only a weak and hardly describable phantom of the lower body. Hence, individual differences cannot account for the differences in the phantom experience in amputees and paraplegics. The inevitable conclusion appears to be that the presence or absence of phantom sensations in this two patient groups has to be accounted for by differences located in the spinal cord or the peripheral nerve. Finally, Carlen et al. (1978, p. 216) point out that the observed differences between amputees and paraplegics render the cortical view of phantom causation unlikely: "If phantoms were generated by the activity of brain cells rather than cord cells, the paraplegic should report an even more vivid phantom sensation since his brain has lost even more input than an amputee's."

The non-cortical mechanism of phantom limb causation may be summarized as follows: Amputation and paraplegia are two clinically different conditions which both imply cortical deafferentation. Hence, cortical deafferentation cannot explain the differences. Hence, specific, clear, tingling phantom limbs cannot be caused by a cortical mechanism; they must be caused by a mechanism that involves the peripheral nerve endings and/or the spinal cord.

In this paper, computer simulations are reported, which use self-organizing feature maps as a minimal model of cortical reorganization in order to propose a model which solves the apparent puzzle posed by the two incompatible models of phantom limb causation.

2. Methods

Self-organizing feature maps are two-layered networks, in which every input node is connected to every output node. In addition, the neurons of the output layer have excitatory connections to nearby neurons and inhibitory to neurons further away (Kohonen 1989). The net result of this is the implementation of a general functional feature of the cortex, i.e., focused local activation and lateral inhibition (Creutzfeld 1995, Thomson & Deuchars 1994), which is critical to the network's self-organizing property. It has been shown that networks of this type, similar to the cerebral cortex (Ritter et al. 1991, Ritter & Kohonen 1989), have the general capability of organizing any coherent input according to its most frequent and most salient features over a given two dimensional neuronal layer. It spontaneously generates receptive fields that are ordered according to features of the input.

In order to simulate the cortical effects of deafferentation caused by amputation, a self-organizing feature map was trained and then partly deafferented. After deafferentation, the distribution of neuronal representations of the input was recorded under conditions of various degress of input noise.

This input noise was implemented by adding random numbers to the input patterns, which under conditions of no noise consisted of patterns of the values 0 and 1. As all input signals were scaled in the range of 0.0 to 1.0, possible noise levels fell into this range. Moreover, the addition of noise to each input signal was thresholded such that all input values remained in the range of 0.0 to 1.0. To give an example: Under the condition of a noise level of 10 %, random values between -0.1 and 0.1 were added to each of the 35 numbers (originally 0 or 1) of the 5 x 7 input pattern (cf. Caudill & Butler 1992, p. 20). This manipulation effectively degraded the clarity of any given input pattern, and, with increasing noise, allowed it to "resemble" other input patterns.

3. Results

Activation of neurons in the deafferented part of the network was found to significantly depend upon input noise (see Figures 1 and 2).

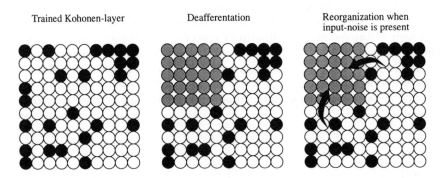

Trained Kohonen-layer   Deafferentation   Reorganization when
                                                  input-noise is present

Figure 1: Inexpensive and easy-to-use educational network modeling software (Caudill & Butler 1992) was used to implement a 100 neuron self-organizing feature map, which was trained to recognize the characters of the alphabet. After 400 training cycles, the characters of the alphabet were represented by neurons spread across the map in an orderly way, i.e., salient features of the characters determined the spatial distribution of the winning neurons (labeled black) within the network (left). Thereafter, deafferentation was simulated by removing those characters from the input file which had become represented in one quadrant (labeled grey) of the map (middle). Then the net was trained again with this restricted set of input patterns. Redistribution of the winning neurons over the entire network did not occur unless noise was added to the input: When the input patterns were degraded by random noise, the space on the map left empty by the removal of the respective input patterns was quickly "invaded" by representations of patterns of the restricted input (right).

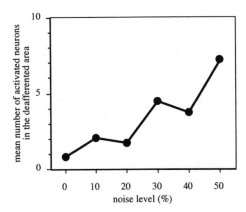

Figure 2: Number of invading winning neurons (mean and SEM) during 10 training cycles dependent upon noise level. Eight simulations were run, using each quadrant of two similarly trained networks, in which different random starting conditions had resulted in different distribution of input patterns. As the dependent variable, the frequency of winning neurons falling into the deafferented area was recorded. The increasing number of invading representations with increasing noise levels was significant (p < .02; data from Spitzer et al. 1995).

In order to examine the topographic changes of representations in detail, the representations in the non-deafferented parts of the network were grouped according to their distance to the deafferented part into five categories. In a 10x10 network with one quadrant lesioned, the remaining neurons are 1 to 5 steps (i.e., changes in the x and/or y coordinates) apart from the deafferented area. For each of the 8 quadrants of the two networks, the representations in the non-deafferented part of the network were grouped according to their distance to the deafferented part into five categories. As the number of invaders from each of these five categories depends upon the absolute number of neurons in that category, the percentage of invaders in each category was determined. Means and standard errors of the percentage scores of "invaders" clearly dependend upon the distance of the invading representation from the deafferented part of the network (see Figure 3).

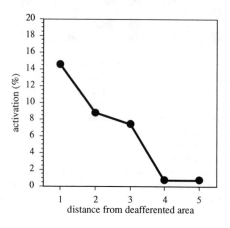

Figure 3: Means and standard errors of the percentage scores of "invaders" from each of five distance categories (distance of the invading representation from the deafferented part of the network). Representations "invade" from adjacent areas on the map.

4. Discussion

When limbs are amputated, the dorsal root ganglion cell as well as the pathways to the cortex remain intact. It is known that lesions of the primary afferent fibers lead to spontaneous activity of the dorsal root cell (Devor 1984, Welk et al. 1990), possibly generated at the site of the peripheral lesion. It is this production of input noise by the deafferented primary sensory neuron that degrades sensory input from adjacent areas of the body and thereby provides input to cortical neurons coding the lost limb in amputees. This gives rise to the subjective experience of the lost limb immediately after the amputation. It also triggers cortical reorganisation processes that sustain the sensations and are responsible for their changes over time. In paraplegics with lesions of the spinal cord, no such input-noise is carried to the cortex (see Figure 4).

This hypothesis suggests a parsimonious explanation for a number of otherwise unrelated and inexplicable features of phantom limbs.

(1) Phantom limbs are experienced immediately after amputation, because the very mechanism of amputation produces "sensory input noise" (i.e., random activity of the dorsal root ganglion sensory neurons). Because of such noisy input processing, new connections between previously unconnected or at least not functionally connected input fibers and cortical areas may be formed. These new connections may be the cause of chronification of the condition.

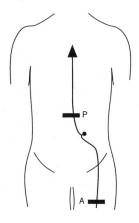

Figure 4: Schematic account of the model. In amutees (A), the lesion is distal from the first sensory neuron which generates noise that is propagated to the central nervous system. In contrast, no such noise is transmitted in paraplegics (P), where the lesion affects the spinal cord.

(2) Several lines of evidence suggest that severity of the trauma may be equivalent to the amount of noise generated in the course of it. It is not only known that (a) severity of the trauma correlates with severity of the phantom experience, and that (b) planned amputations with local anesthesia produce less pronounced phantoms than amputations after traumatic events. (c) Recent studies of cortical plasticity and phantom pain (Flohr et al. 1995) revealed a very high correlation of 0.93, which strongly suggests a common mechanism. As it is unlikely that, as one possible conclusion goes, cortical reorganization is itself painful, it appears likely that pain is either the source of cortical reorganization or, perhaps most likely, that pain and cortical reorganization are triggered by one and the same mechanism. This mechanism might consist of massive uncorrelated firing of sensory neurons. The clinical phenomena of telescoping and shrinking of the phantom over time are likely to correspond to the decrease of the size of the cortical area that codes for the amputated limb due to cortical reorganization. These processes occur on a larger time scale and must be accompanied by neurons of the deafferented area "unlearning" previous representations. It is likely that this process is facilitated by input noise.

(3) Stimulation of body surfaces represented by cortical areas adjacent to the deafferented area gives rise to "referred sensations", i.e., topographically organized sensory experiences in the phantom. This subjective phenomenon corresponds to the

finding that representations "invade" from map areas adjacent to the deafferented area. In any Kohonen-layer, similar patterns are coded by neurones that are close together on the map. Therefore, "invaders" move from areas adjacent to the deafferented area rather than "jump" in from distant areas. In short, the somatotopical organization of the referred sensations corresponds to the fact that the redistribution in feature maps is governed by the internal structure of the map.

(4) According to the model, amputation leads to an unused cortical area, which is taken over by adjacent areas. In other words, the deafferented cortical surface takes up computational functions of adjacent areas, which thereby increase their computational capacity. This increased capacity can be demonstrated: The receptive fields of sensory neurons in the stump become smaller, i.e., processing of sensory information from stump sensory neurons is improved as a result of the increased cortical computational surface.

(5) When the simulations were run with rather high noise levels, we observed that a given input pattern no longer activated the same neuron at every presentation. Instead, the added noise made the input activate neurons that used to code other input patterns. This led to the prediction that there should be clinical cases where similar "misplacements" of sensory input might occur, caused by processes that can be expected to lead to extra noise, as for example, in particularly severe and/or additional injuries. In such patients, touching an arm, for example, might result in the sensation of touch in the (non-amputated) leg. A search through the older (usually more descriptive) literature revealed that such cases exist (Cronholm 1951).

(6) The recent psychopathological literature suggests that neuromodulators such as dopamine and norepinephrine are involved in the regulation of the signal-to-noise ratio of cortical information processing (Servan-Schreiber et al. 1990, Cohen et al. 1992, Spitzer 1996). Though we do not have quantitative data on the effects of these neuromodulators on neuroplasticity, any modulation of noise, it appears, is likely to have an impact on neuroplasticity. Since we can assume genetic and possibly environmental influences on a person's "neuromodulatory setup" (which used to be called temperament) we may infer individual differences in the amount and speed of neuroplastic cortical changes. In short, the model provides a plausible account of how it might be possible that personality variables have an influence on the subjective experience of phantoms

The proposed model cannot account for reorganization processes after cortical damage (for such a model, cf. Sutton et al. 1994) and it does not explain the (though extremely rare) cases of phantoms in patients with birth defects. However, it belongs the small but growing number of instances where the presence of noise in nervous systems appears to be an important part of its function (cf. Collins et al. 1995, Douglas et al. 1993; Maddox 1994, Moss et al. 1994, Wiesenfeld & Moss 1995).

Finally, a general comment on the use of neural network simulations appears to be in order. Phantom sensations by definition consist of experiences which lack a corresponding reality, i.e., they are purely *subjective* phenomena and rely on a person experiencing them. The proposed model demonstrates therefore the wide scope of applications for neural network simulations. It shows—even if it turned out to be wrong—that neural network models can be applied to the study of even the most subjective and private experiences. The model therefore provides a counterexample for those who believe that neural network simulations, by their very nature, can only be applied to *objective* (i.e., intersubjectively accessible) facts, such as membrane potentials or neuronal assemblies. In short, there is no reason why neural network models cannot be applied to psychological and psychiatric phenomena of a purely subjective kind.

5. References

Bors, E. *Arch Neurol Psychiatr* **66** (1951) 610-631.
Buchanen, D.C. and Mandel, A.R., *Rehab. Psychol* **31/3** (1986) 183-188.
Carlen, P.L., P.D. Wall, P.D., Nadvorna, H. and Steinbach, T., *Neurology* **28,** (1978) 211-217.
Caudill, M. and Butler,C., *Understanding neural networks. vols 1 and 2.* (MIT Press, Cambridge, MA, 1992).
Collins, J.J., Chow, C.C. and Imhoff,T.T., *Nature* **376** (1995) 236-238.
Creutzfeld, O.D., *Cortex cerebri. Performance, structural and functional organization of the cortex* (Oxford University Press, Oxford, 1995).
Cronholm, B., *Phantom Limbs in Amputees* (Stockholm, 1951).
Devor, M., in: *Textbook of pain*, eds. P.D. Wall, M. Melzak (Churchill-Livingstone, Edinburgh, 1984), pp. 49-64.
Douglass, J.K., Wilkens, L., Pantazelou, E., and Moss, F., *Nature* **365** (1993) 337-340.
Elbert, T., Pantev, C., Wienbruch, C., Rockstroh, B. and Taub, E., *Science* **270** (1995) 305-307.
Elbert, T., Flor, H., Birbaumer, N., Knecht, S., Hampson, S., Larbig, W. and Taub, E., *Neuroreport* **5** (1994) 2593-2597.
Flor, H., Elbert, T., Knecht, S., Wienbruch, C., Pantev, C., Birbaumer, N., Larbig, W. and Taub, E., *Nature* **375** (1995) 482-484.
Halligan, P.W., Marshall, J.C., Wade, D.T., Davey, J. and Morrison, D., *Neuroreport* **4/3** (1993) 233-236.
Jensen, T.S., Krebs, B., Nielsen, J. and Rasmussen, P., *Acta Neurologica Scandinavica* **70/6** (1984) 407-414.
Jensen, T.S. and Rasmussen, P., in ed. P.D. Wall and R. Melzack, Textbook of Pain, 2nd ed. (Livingstone Churchill, Edinburgh, 1989).
Katz, J., *Canadian Journal of Psychiatry* **37** (1992) 282-298.
Kohonen, T., *Self-Organization and Associative Memory.* (Springer, Berlin, Heidelberg, New York, London, Paris, Tokyo, Hong Kong: 1989).
Maddox, J., *Nature* **369** (1994) 271.

Merzenich, M.M., Kaas, J.H., Wall, J., Nelson, R.J., Sur, M. and Felleman, D., *Neuroscience* **8** (1983) 33-55.

Merzenich, M.M.and Sameshima, K., *Current Opinion in Neurology* **3** (1993) 187-196.

Merzenich, M.M., Jenkins, W.M., Johnston, P., Schreiner, C., Miller, S.L. and Tallal, T., *Science* **271** (1996) 77-80.

Moss, F., Pierson, D. and O'Gorman, D., *International Journal of Bifurcation and Chaos* **4(6)** (1994) 1383-1397.

Pascual-Leone, A., and Torres, F., *Brain* **116** (1993) 39-52.

Penfield, W.and Rasmussen, T., *The Cerebral Cortex of Man: A Clinical Study of Localization and Function* (Macmillan, New York, 1950).

Poeck, K., *Nervenarzt* **34** (1963) 241-256.

Pons, T.P., Garraghty, P.E., Ommaya, A.K., Kaas, J.H., Taub, E. and Mishkin, M., *Science* **252** (1991) 1857-1860.

Ramachandran, V.S., Rogers-Ramachandran, D.and Steward, M., *Science* **258** (1992) 1159-1160.

Recanzone, G.H., Jenkins, W.M., Hradek, G.T. and Merzenich, M.M., *Journal of Neurophysiology* **67** (1992a) 1015-1030.

Recanzone, G.H., Merzenich, M.M., Jenkins, W.M., Grajski, K.A. and Dinse, H.R., *Journal of Neurophysiology* **67** (1992b) 1031-1056.

Recanzone, G.H., Merzenich, M.M. and Schreiner, C.E., *Journal of Neurophysiology* **67** (1992c) 1071-1091.

Ritter, H. and Kohonen, T., *Biological Cybernetics* **61** (1989) 241-254

Ritter, H., Martinetz, T. and Schulten, K., *Neuronale Netze. Eine Einführung in die Neuroinformatik selbstorganisierender Netzwerke.* (Addison-Wesley, Bonn, 1991).

Schilder, P., *Zeitschr f Neurol u Psychiat* **80** (1923) 424-431

Spitzer, M., *Halluzinationen.* (Springer, Berlin, Heidelberg, New York, London, Paris, Tokyo, 1988).

Spitzer, M., Böhler, P., Kischka, U. und Weisbrod, M. *Biological Cybernetics* **72** (1995) 197-206.

Spitzer, M., *Schizophrenia Bulletin* (in press).

Sutton, G., Reggia, J., Armentrout, S. and D'Autrechy, C., *Neural computation* **6** (1994) 1-13.

Tallal, P., Miller, S.L., Bedi, G., Byma, G., Wang, X., Nagarajan, S.S., Schreiner, C., Jenkins, W.M. and Merzenich, M.M., *Science* **271** (1996) 81-84.

Thomson, A.M., Deuchars, J., *TINS* **17:3** (1994) 119-126.

Weiss, S.A., Fishman, S., *J Abnorm Soc Psychol* **66** (1963) 489-497.

Welk, E., Leah, J.D. and Zimmermann, M., *J Neurophysiol* **63** (1990) 759-766.

Wiesenfeld, K. and Moss, F., *Nature* **373** (1995) 33-36.

Yang, T.T., Gallen, C., Schwartz, B., Bloom, F.E., Ramachandran, V.S. and Cobb, S., *Nature* **368** (1994) 592-593.

Zuk, G.H., *J Nerv Ment Dis* **124** (1956) 510-513.

Modeling Post-Stroke Cortical Map Reorganization

James Reggia, Sharon Goodall, Yinong Chen, Eytan Ruppin* and Carol Whitney

*Depts. of Computer Science and Neurology, Inst. Adv. Comp. Studies,
University of Maryland, College Park, MD 20742 USA*
E-mail: {reggia,goodall,cyn,cwhitney}@cs.umd.edu

** Dept. of Computer Science and Physiology, Schools of Mathematics and Medicine
Tel-Aviv University, Ramat-Aviv, 69978 Israel*
E-mail: ruppin@math.tau.ac.il

Abstract

We are using computational models to study how cortical maps reorganize following sudden, focal lesions. These models are explicitly intended to simulate small cortical ischemic strokes. Two prototypical models are described here. The first model has a topographic map of the hand region of primary somatosensory cortex. Following a sudden focal cortical lesion, portions of the hand originally represented in the lesioned area reappear in the perilesion cortex, as has been observed experimentally in animal studies. The second model, currently being studied, involves feature maps in proprioceptive and motor cortex regions that control a simulated arm moving in three-dimensional space. A sudden focal cortical lesion in this model can produce a very different result: a perilesion zone of decreased cortical activity. These two models make testable predictions, including that post-lesion map reorganization occurs in two phases, and that perilesion excitability is a critical factor in map reorganization. Current work is extending these studies to more realistic models incorporating biochemical and metabolic factors important in stroke.

1 Introduction

Efforts to understand the mechanisms of and recovery following a stroke have traditionally been based on either clinical studies or animal models. In this chapter we describe some first steps in developing an alternative approach: computational models of cerebral cortex and its reorganization following acute focal lesions. Ischemic stroke, where there is a loss of blood flow to a region of the brain, is a very complex, multifactorial process. Acute and post-stroke changes involve neural plasticity, metabolic and biochemical events, biophysical processes such as diffusion, mechanical displacement secondary to edema, altered autoregulation and metabolic regulation of blood flow, rheological changes, acute and chronic changes to blood vessels, collateral circulation, etc. [Caplan 1993]. These events and their interactions are only partially understood; their complexity has led some investigators to suggest that novel ways of thinking about stroke are needed [Hallenback and Frerichs 1993], such as the computational models described below. Computational models can be useful in furthering our understanding of these processes by supporting detailed examination of various hypotheses about stroke pathophysiology and recovery. In other words, the complexity of events in stroke suggests that computational models can be powerful tools for its investigation, much as they are in the analysis of other complex systems (global climate prediction, geological exploration, advanced engineering design, etc.).

Our focus here is on developing a computer model of the pathophysiological events occurring in ischemic stroke. Ultimately, one seeks a sufficiently powerful model that can be used to understand better the acute post-stroke changes in the ischemic penumbra, to determine which factors lead to worsening or recovery from stroke, and to suggest new pharmacologic interventions and rehabilitative actions that could improve stroke outcome. However, the complexity of stroke pathophysiology, and the limitations of current neural modeling technology and neuroscientific knowledge, make it impractical to begin with a detailed, large scale model of the brain and all of the effects of a major stroke. Here we consider the more limited objective of creating a computer model of circumscribed regions of cerebral cortex and of small, ischemic lesions. We further consider only the effects of acute lesions on cortical maps due to disruption of neural elements. MRI evidence suggests that small cortical and subcortical ischemic strokes are far more common and important than previously recognized [Hougaku et al. 1994], and they relate to the small cortical infarcts that can be produced with contemporary animal models of stroke. The reason for focusing on small lesions in restricted regions is the wealth of data on map organization in such regions and the fact that this size of model provides the best match with the current state of the art in neural modeling technology.

Two specific computational models are described here. The first model has a topographic map of the hand region of primary somatosensory cortex; the second model involves feature maps in primary sensorimotor cortex. The next section describes the first of these two models, and the subsequent section describes the second. This chapter concludes with a summary and overview of ongoing work that is examining more complex models involving metabolic and biochemical features relevant to stroke.

2 Acute Focal Lesions in Topographic Somatosensory Maps

Cortical maps can conveniently be classified as *topographic maps* [Udin and Fawcett 1988], which reflect the distribution and density of peripheral neurons over the body surface, or as *feature maps* ("computational maps") [Knudsen et al 1987] in which a computed feature varies across the cortical surface. For example, in primary visual cortex, line orientation and ocular dominance columns are organized into bands (a computational map) which are embedded within a topographic (retinotopic) map.

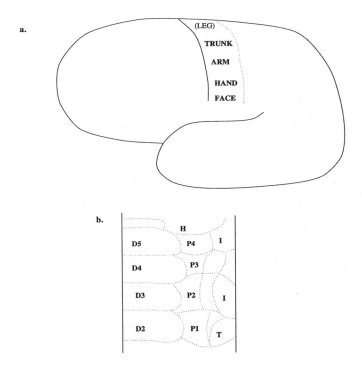

Figure 1: Primary somatosensory (SI) map. a) The contralateral body surface is represented in the post central gyrus in a systematic, order preserving fashion, forming a topographic map. b) Simplified, enlarged caricature of the hand region shown in a. Areas representing individual digits (D1 - D5; only four pictured here), palmar surfaces (P1-P4), thenar eminence (T), etc. are labeled. Unlabeled regions correspond to the back of the hand.

2.1   The Topographic Map in Primary Somatosensory Cortex (SI)

A familiar example of a topographic map, which we focus on in this section, occurs in primary somatosensory cortex, or SI cortex, as illustrated in Fig.1a. In this lateral view of the left hemisphere, the opposite side of the body is systematically projected onto the post-central gyrus. This representation is distorted in that parts of the body with the finest sensory discrimination (e.g., hand) have disproportionally large areas in the map. Electrophysiological studies in animals have carefully charted the details of this map. In the case of the hand, individual fingers and palmar areas can be identified (Fig. 1b) [Merzenich et al. 1983].

One of the most intriguing experimental observations in recent years is that maps in the sensory and motor cortex of adult animals are highly plastic (adaptable). For example, if a single finger of the hand is repeatedly stimulated over time, the area representing that finger in the SI cortical map increases substantially at the expense of areas of neighboring regions [Jenkins et al. 1990]. If a cortical finger region is deafferented, say by peripheral nerve sectioning, then that region of the cortical map becomes initially unresponsive to skin stimuli. Within a period of a few weeks, however, the representations of surrounding hand regions have expanded into the deafferented cortical region, which is once again responsive to peripheral stimuli [Kaas 1991, Merzenich et al. 1983].

Recent studies in humans following deafferentation indicate that map reorganization similar to that seen in animals occurs, sometimes very rapidly, and often associated with increased cortical excitability [Brasil-Neto et al. 1993, Cohen et al. 1991, Pascual-Leone and Torres 1993]. The extent to which such changes are due to neocortical plasticity, unmasking of normally silent subcortical pathways, or other mechanisms is unclear [Calford 1991, Killackey 1989]. Only limited animal data are available specifically about the effects of cortical lesions on map reorganization. These data indicate that following small focal lesions in primary somatosensory cortex, the body surface represented in the lesioned area eventually reappears in the perilesion region [Jenkins and Merzenich 1987]. Movements originally represented in a primary motor cortical area reappear outside that area when it is lesioned [Glees and Cole 1950], perhaps even in the somatosensory cortex [Sasaki and Gema 1984] or contralaterally [Chollet et al. 1991], although there is some conflicting evidence [Boyeson Jones and Harmon 1994, Nudo and Grenda 1992].

During the last few years there have been several efforts to develop computational models of cortical map self-organization and map refinement [Grajski and Merzenich 1990, Kohonen 1989, Obermayer Ritter and Schulten 1990, Pearson Finkel and Edelman 1987, Ritter Martinetz and Schulten 1989, von der Malsburg 1973]. These models typically take the form of a two-layer network, and use an unsupervised Hebbian learning method (often competitive learning). For example, such a computational model of the hand region of primary somatosensory cortex was able to demonstrate map refinement and map reorganization in response to localized repetitive stimulation and deafferentation [Pearson Finkel and Edelman 1987]. A similar study subsequently demonstrated that this type of model obeyed the inverse magnification rule [Grajski and Merzenich 1990].

These and related computational studies provide an impressive demonstration that fairly simple but plausible assumptions about network architecture and synaptic modifiability can qualitatively account for several fundamental facts about cortical map self-organization and reorganization. They have been less successful, however, in accounting for some map reorganization effects, particularly those of direct relevance here. For example, in the only previous computational model we know of that simulated a focal cortical lesion, map reorganization would not occur unless relatively implausible steps were taken (complete re-randomization of weights following a simulated focal lesion) [Grajski and Merzenich 1990]. Map reorganization following a cortical lesion is fundamentally different from that involving deafferentation or focal repetitive stimulation. In both of the latter situations there is a change in the probability distribution of input patterns seen by the intact cortex. Such a change has long been recognized to result in map alterations [Kohonen 1989]. In contrast, a focal cortical lesion does not affect the probability distribution of input patterns, so some other factors must be responsible for map reorganization.

2.2 A Model of Map Formation in SI

To examine these issues, we created and studied a computational model of the hand region of primary somatosensory cortex. In our model, cortex and thalamus are viewed as two-dimensional sheets of small volume elements (see Figure 2, left). Each cortical element represents a small patch of cortex containing on the order of 100 neurons, i.e., roughly a microcolumn. As indicated in Figure 2, each thalamic element x sends divergent excitatory connections to a set of cortical elements (circular region) centered on the corresponding cortical element x'. Each cortical element sends excitatory connections to nearby elements in cortex. In the simulations described here, each layer is a hexagonally tessellated grid of 32x32 nodes. Thalamic elements project into a radius four hexagonal region of cortex resulting in 61 connections per thalamic node. Accordingly, there are 62,464 thalamocortical connections and 6,144 corticocortical connections. To avoid possible edge effects, the top (right) and bottom (left) edges of each layer are connected, so that conceptually the two layers form nested tori. Competitive learning occurs along thalamocortical connections, but there is no intracortical learning. Inputs are presented directly to the thalamic layer which implicitly defines a skin surface with direct thalamic connections.

A Mexican Hat pattern of lateral interactions in cortex is brought about in two different ways in variations of our model. First, using *standard intracortical connectivity*, lateral/horizontal inhibitory connections are used as in past computational models of cortex. Second, peristimulus inhibition is produced by allowing cortical elements to *competitively distribute* their activity. We have presented arguments elsewhere that both forms of peristimulus inhibition are present in the cerebral cortex [Reggia et al. 1992]. The important point here is that from the viewpoint of cortical map formation and post-lesion reorganization, hundreds of simulations over the last few years have demonstrated that both mechanisms produce qualitatively similar results as long as an appropriate Mexican Hat pattern of lateral interactions is supported [Armentrout et al 1994, Cho and Reggia 1994, Goodall Reggia and Cho 1994, Reggia et al. 1992,

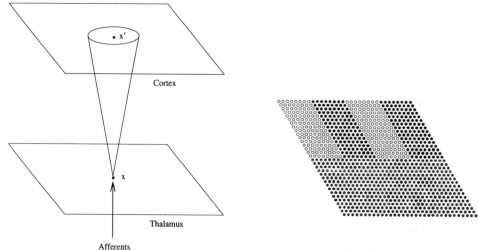

Figure 2: Left: network architecture; right: cortical map of hand surface after training.

Sutton et al. 1994]. An unsupervised, Hebbian synaptic weight change rule is used to simulate map formation in primary somatosensory cortex (area 3b). We refer to the resultant model here as the *SI model*. Starting with random thalamocortical weights, the SI model was trained by presenting stimuli to a simulated hand surface. Input patterns to the model consisted of hexagonal patches of fixed radius (a single thalamic node turned on is a hexagonal patch of radius zero, a thalamic node and its six immediate neighbors turned on is a patch of radius one, etc.). Patterns were presented in random order in a uniform distribution, and learning occurred only after cortical activations approximated equilibrium. The *Appendix* summarizes the dynamics of this model.

Summarizing the results of map formation in intact cortex, the coarse topographic map that existed before training due to the initially random weights and network structure was transformed by training into a finely tuned, uniform topographic map [Armentrout et al. 1994, Sutton et al. 1994]. Receptive fields decreased in size and changed from irregular to circular in shape (incoming weight vectors for cortical elements became roughly bell-shaped). These results were relatively insensitive to variations in input stimuli and the learning rule, i.e., the model was robust. Figure 2 (right) shows receptive fields of cortical elements plotted across the cortical surface after training with random, uniformly distributed sensory stimuli. Each ellipse in this figure provides a rough measure of receptive field size. The general location of the receptive fields is shown by shading to indicate four finger regions (upper half) and palm (lower half) of the cortical map representing the hand surface. A number of effects seen in animal studies were observed in the SI model. For example, if the relative frequency of input stimuli was increased to the second finger from the left, its cortical representation increased dramatically, similar to what occurs in animal experiments [Jenkins et al. 1990]. Conversely, if the same cortical finger region was deafferented, some of the cortical elements originally in that finger region developed new receptive fields in adjacent fingers, also as observed in animals [Kaas 1991].

2.3 Lesioning the Model

As noted above, the only previous cortical map model that has been subjected to simulation of a sudden, focal cortical lesion failed to reorganize spontaneously [Grajski and Merzenich 1990]. We originally hypothesized that a version of our model based on competitive distribution of activation would demonstrate spontaneous map reorganization following a cortical lesion. To test this hypothesis, a contiguous portion of the trained cortical layer (elements representing the second finger from the left in Figure 2) was deactivated after training. After this lesioning, the topographic map showed a two-phase reorganization process [Armentrout et al. 1994, Sutton et al. 1994]. Immediately after lesioning and before any retraining, the receptive fields of cortical elements adjoining the lesioned area spontaneously shifted towards the second finger and increased in size. As shown in Figure 3, left (contrast with Figure 2, right), parts of the finger region originally represented in the now-lesioned cortical area (solid black ovals) have shifted substantially into the surrounding intact cortex. This immediate shift was due to the competitive redistribution of thalamic output from lesioned to unlesioned cortical elements, which resulted in increased perilesion excitability. The second phase of map reorganization occurred more slowly with continued training and was due to synaptic weight changes. It resulted in further reappearance of the second finger in perilesion cortex, as shown in Figure 3, right. Receptive fields in perilesion cortex increased in size, consistent with an inverse magnification rule. This spontaneous map reorganization is consistent with that seen experimentally following small cortical lesions [Jenkins and Merzenich 1987]. It makes a testable prediction that can be examined experimentally: if competitive distribution of activity is present involving connections between thalamus and cortex, then significant shifts of sensory representation out of a lesioned cortical area should be observed immediately after a cortical lesion. It is not currently known whether this occurs.

Having demonstrated for the first time that spontaneous map reorganization can occur in a computational model of focal cortical damage, we examined how a number of factors influence the extent and nature of the reorganization process [Armentrout et al. 1994]. First, it was determined that with either thalamocortical competitive distribution alone or intracortical competitive distribution alone, as opposed to both as in the initial model, post-lesion map reorganization still occurred but was significantly reduced. Second, it was found that as circular lesion size increased from a radius of 1

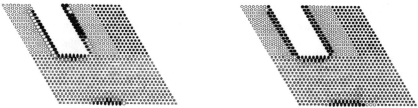

Figure 3: Hand tactile map immediately post-lesion (left) and after further training (right).

to 10 cortical elements, the mean distance that perilesion map representations moved increased at first but then leveled off; mean shift of receptive field location was always highest close to the lesion and diminished with increasing distance. Third, it was found that allowing learning on intracortical connections in addition to thalamocortical connections produced no qualitative differences in map reorganization. Fourth, only minor improvements in map reorganization occurred when increased plasticity was present on connections to cortex from thalamic elements originally represented in the lesioned area.

Variation of the post-lesion training stimuli also influenced map reorganization. As the input stimulus size was increased from radius 1 to 4, the speed of reorganization increased. Further, if the frequency of training stimuli to the region of sensory surface originally represented in the lesioned cortex was increased relative to other locations, there was a dramatic increase in the extent to which the lost sensory surface reappeared in the post-lesion cortical maps. Moreover, the receptive fields obtained were smaller [Weinrich et al. 1994]. Such results represent testable predictions that could be used to guide controlled clinical trials in stroke rehabilitation (the relative efficacy of current techniques for improving tactile feature detection in patients with sensory deficits is not well understood [Pediette and Zolten 1990]).

Finally, we simulated analogous lesions to a version of the SI model based on the use of lateral inhibitory connections rather than competitive distribution of activity. We found that map reorganization was in general more difficult to elicit and less marked than with the competitive SI model. However, with a suitable choice of parameters derived through a trial-and-error process, we were able to create a version of the standard SI model that demonstrated substantial, if irregular, reorganization. Like the competitive SI model, this reorganization could be enhanced by increased frequency of stimuli to the sensory surface in the region previously represented in the area of the cortical lesion.

Analysis of the factors that influence map reorganization in both types of models, and of why past efforts to demonstrate spontaneous map reorganization were unsuccessful, showed that increased perilesion excitability is a critical factor in map reorganization [Armentrout et al 1994]. Our results thus indicate that the increased perilesion excitability observed in some animal models of stroke, in addition to contributing to neurological impairment as some have suggested [Domann et al. 1993], may actually be an important aspect of brain recovery from focal injury.

2.4 Comments

In summary, the competitive SI model exhibits topographic map formation, and reorganization following both deafferentation and repetitive stimulation that is qualitatively similar to experimental findings reported in the literature [Jenkins and Merzenich 1987, Kaas 1991, Sutton et al. 1994]. More importantly, our model exhibited dramatic map reorganization in response to a focal cortical lesion. No special procedure such as post-lesion weight re-randomization was required for map reorganization: sensory regions originally represented in the lesioned cortex spontaneously reappeared in cortex outside the lesion area as long as synaptic plasticity was continued after the lesion. This spontaneous map reorganization seen when competitive distribution of activity is present is consistent with that seen experimentally in adult primates following small cortical lesions [Jenkins and Merzenich 1987]. Further, receptive fields increased in size in perilesion cortex as has also been described experimentally (inverse magnification rule) [Jenkins and Merzenich 1987].

Most intriguing is how and why map reorganization occurred following a cortical lesion to our model. Map reorganization involved a two-phase process where each phase, rapid and slow, was due to a different mechanism. Immediately after a cortical lesion there was a dramatic change in map organization associated with increased excitability in the perilesion cortex: some finger regions originally represented by the lesioned area of cortex 'shifted outward' and now appeared in adjacent regions of intact cortex. This first or rapid phase of map reorganization was due to the competitive distribution of thalamic activity to cortex. Individual thalamic elements that send connections to both lesioned and intact cortical elements redirected their output away from the lesioned cortex to intact adjacent cortex. Biologically, this redirected thalamic output would occur due to the loss of retrograde corticothalamic connections from the lesioned cortex (see [Reggia et al. 1992] for further explanation). This result provides a specific testable prediction: significant shifts of sensory representation out of a lesioned cortical area should be observed right after a cortical lesion. To the authors' knowledge there is no definitive experimental data yet available on this issue.

This first, rapid phase of map reorganization due to the competitive dynamics is followed by a second, slower phase due to synaptic plasticity. More of the hand region initially represented by the lesioned cortex appeared in the surrounding cortex. This second phase due to synaptic changes, like the first phase, occurred in spite of the fact that there was no change in the input stimuli. Increased perilesion excitability during the first phase of map reorganization appeared to be essential for jump-starting the second phase. The first phase provided the necessary receptive field changes to allow the second phase to take place. Synaptic modifications, however, ultimately accounted for most of the observed reorganization.

The extent of reorganization in the SI model following a cortical lesion increased dramatically using focal repetitive stimulation. Repeatedly stimulating the input region whose cortical representation was lesioned caused the number of cortical nodes which assumed that representation to increase sharply. Extrapolating this result into the clinical rehabilitation setting indicates some potential practical implications of this research and represents another testable prediction of the model. The efficacy of current rehabilitation techniques in promoting reorganization of the somatosensory cortex has been difficult to evaluate in the context of spontaneous recovery from stroke. Modeling the effects of different types of stimuli employed in treatment of cortical sensory deficits on simulated lesions may be a useful adjunct to controlled clinical trials, and predictions from them may serve to guide such trials. The current data suggest that stimulation of the anesthetic area and its immediate surround may be more beneficial in promoting reorganization than stimulation of larger areas.

3   Acute Focal Lesions in Sensorimotor Feature Maps

While both topographic maps [Grajski and Merzenich 1990, Pearson Finkel and Edelman 1987] and feature maps [Cho and Reggia 1994, Miller Keller and Stryker 1989, Ritter Martinetz and Schulten 1992, Kohonen 1989] have been modeled computationally in the past, only model SI topographic maps have been subjected to simulated focal lesions [Sutton et al. 1994, Armentrout Reggia and Weinrich 1994, Grajski and Merzenich, 1990]. As we saw above, whenever a focal lesion was introduced into the topographic map of that model, it reorganized such that the sensory surface originally represented by the lesioned area spontaneously reappeared in adjacent cortical areas, as has been seen experimentally in animal studies [Jenkins and Merzenich 1987]. Two key hypotheses emerged from that modeling work. First, post-lesion map reorganization is a two-phase process, consisting of a rapid phase due to the dynamics of neural activity and a longer-term phase due to synaptic plasticity. Second, increased perilesion excitability is necessary for useful map reorganization to occur. These results and others [Ruppin and Reggia 1995], indicate the important role of intracortical interactions in post-lesion brain reorganization. Following a *structural lesion* that simulates a region of damage and neuronal death, a secondary *functional lesion* can arise in surrounding cortex due to loss of synaptic connections from the damaged area to surrounding intact cortex. In the following we use the term "functional lesion" in this limited sense and not to indicate the ischemic penumbra.

We are now in the process of examining the generality of these two map reorganization hypotheses through simulations with a different cortical model. In doing this we are using a recently developed computational model of primary sensorimotor cortex that controls the positioning of a simulated arm in three-dimensional space [Chen and Reggia 1996]. This model involves both proprioceptive input as well as motor output in a "closed-loop" network. Maps initially form in the two cortical regions represented in the model: proprioceptive sensory cortex and primary motor cortex (MI). Unlike the SI model of the previous section, the maps involved here are feature maps rather than topographic maps, and involve motor output as well as sensory input information. This work is currently in progress; detailed results will be presented in [Goodall et al 1996].

3.1 Model Description

The computational model used in this study consists of two parts: a simulated arm that moves in three dimensional space, and a closed-loop of neural elements that controls and senses arm positions. Each neural element in the model again represents a population of real neurons, not a single neuron. The structure of the model is illustrated in Fig. 4.

The transformation of activity in lower motor neurons to proprioceptive sensory neural activity is generated using a simulated arm (bottom of Fig. 4). This model arm is a significant simplification of biological reality, and is described in more detail elsewhere [Cho and Reggia 1994, Chen and Reggia 1996]. It consists of upper and lower arm segments, connected at the elbow. It has six generic muscle groups, each of which corresponds to multiple muscles in a real arm. There are four muscle groups that control the upper arm and two that control the lower arm. Abductor and adductor muscles move the upper arm up and down through 180°, respectively, while flexor and extensor muscles move it forward and backward through 180°, respectively. The lower arm flexes and extends as much as 180°, controlled by lower arm flexor and extensor muscles. Activation of the lower motor neuron elements place the model arm into a specific spatial position. The simulated arm then generates input signals to the cortex via the proprioceptive neuron elements that indicate the length and stretch of each individual muscle group (see Fig. 4). The biologically-oriented proprioceptive input in this model, based on muscle stretch and tension, distinguishes it from previous robotically-oriented neural models of arm control where input is typically derived from a camera (e.g., [Ritter Martinetz and Schulten 1992]).

Activation flows in a closed loop through the four sets of neural elements: primary motor cortex (MI), lower motor neurons, proprioceptive neurons, proprioceptive cor-

294

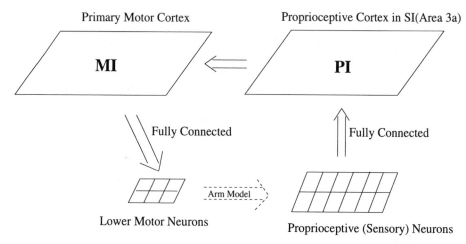

Figure 4: Structure of the motor control model: twelve proprioceptive receptor elements (lower right) form the proprioceptive input layer and are fully connected to the proprioceptive cortex layer (labeled PI). The PI layer and primary motor cortex layer (MI) are two dimensional arrays of neural elements with lateral (horizontal) intracortical connections. The projection from PI to MI is partial, with a coarse topographic ordering. Each MI element is connected to the six lower motor neuron elements. The transformation of activity in lower motor neurons to proprioceptive input is done by a simulated arm.

tex, and back to MI (Fig. 4). Activity in lower motor neurons sets the arm position, which in turn determines the length and tension of six simulated muscle groups. We use the non-standard abbreviation PI to designate the region of primary somatosensory cortex receiving proprioceptive input from the upper extremity; this roughly corresponds to Brodmann area 3a. The twelve receptor elements in the proprioceptive input layer are fully connected to PI; they provide six muscle length and six muscle tension measures. A length element becomes active when the corresponding muscle is stretched, while a tension element activates when the corresponding muscle is under increased tension. Similar to the SI model, the PI and MI layers are both two dimensional, hexagonally tessellated arrays of elements with lateral (horizontal) intracortical connections. Each element of these layers represents a cortical column, and is connected to its immediate neighboring elements up to a radius r. To remove edge effects, elements on the edges of the cortical sheet are connected with their corresponding neighbor elements on the opposite edges, forming a torus. Each element of PI sends synaptic connections to its corresponding element in MI and to the surrounding elements in MI within a radius 4, providing a coarse topographic ordering for the connections from PI to MI. Each MI element is fully connected to the lower motor neuron layer.

Each neural element i in the model has an associated activation level $a_i(t)$, representing the mean firing rate of neurons in that element at time t. The activation rule is similar to that used in the SI model of the preceding section; a full description of the activation dynamics is given in [Chen and Reggia 1996]. During simulations, inter-layer connection weights are modified using an unsupervised learning rule similar to that used in the SI model and elsewhere [Grajski and Merzenich 1990, Cho and Reggia 1994, Ritter Martinetz and Schulten 1992, Kohonen 1989, Sutton et al. 1994, von der Malsburg 1973]. This learning rule is quite typical of those used in neural models of cortical map formation and fully described in [Chen and Reggia 1996]. Intralayer connection weights remain constant.

3.2 Map Formation In the Intact Model

The model is initialized with small, random weights so that well-formed feature maps are not present in the cortical regions initially. The model is then trained as follows. A patch of external input is repeatedly provided at randomly selected positions in MI. This stimulus is applied as external *input* to the MI elements, i.e., none of the activation levels are clamped to a fixed value. Two thousand random stimuli to MI, covering the cortical space, are applied to the network during training, after which further training does not produce qualitative changes in the trained weights or the cortical feature maps that appear.

To examine the resultant *proprioceptive maps* in the cortical layer, these two layers are analyzed to determine to which muscle length and tension input each cortical element of a layer responds most strongly. Twelve input test patterns are presented, each having only one muscle length or tension element of the proprioceptive input layer activated. Since the proprioceptive input layer elements represent the length and tension of the six muscle groups of the model arm, each test pattern corresponds to the unphysiological situation of having the length or tension of only one muscle group activated (this situation was *never* present with the training patterns). A cortical element is taken to be "maximally tuned" to an arm input element if the cortical element's activation corresponding to the input element is largest and above a certain threshold. The pre-lesion maps are described in detail in [Cho and Reggia 1994, Chen and Reggia 1996] and are summarized briefly here.

Fig. 5 shows which PI and MI cortical elements are maximally responsive to stretch of specific muscles after training. For example, the third element to the right from the upper left corner of Fig. 5a is maximally responsive to stretch of the lower arm extensor (O). The input map in Fig. 5a is for all six muscle groups for the PI cortical layer; the map in Fig. 5c below it is the corresponding input map for MI. Prior to training, elements maximally responsive to the same muscle group's stretch or tension are irregularly scattered across the map.

a.

```
- - 0 0 - - - 0 0 - F - 0 0 - - B 0 0 -
D E - - D E E - - D E - - - D - - - - D
E C - - D E C C D D E C - D D E C F F D
C C B - - - C B - - C F B - E C C F - -
F B B 0 F F B B 0 - F B B 0 - - B B 0 -
F - 0 0 F - - 0 0 - - - 0 0 - - - 0 0 F
- E - - D - E - - D - - - F D E E - - D
E E C D D E E C D D E - F F D E C C D D
- C C - - - C C - E - C B - - - C B - -
F B - 0 - B F F 0 - - B - 0 F F B - 0 -
F - 0 0 - - F 0 0 - - - 0 0 F - - 0 0 -
- - - - D - - - - D - E - - D - E - - D
E - C D D E - C D D E E C D D E E C D D
E C F - E E C F F - - B F - - - C C - E
B B F 0 - - B F 0 - - B F 0 - B B F 0 -
B - 0 0 - - - 0 0 - - 0 0 - - F F 0 0 -
- - - - D E E - - D E E - - D - - - - D
E E C F D E - C D D E - C D D E - C D D
E C F F - - C B - - - C B - E E C F - E
- B B 0 - F F B 0 - F B B 0 - - B F 0 -
```

b.

```
- - 0 0 - - - 0 0 - - - 0 0 - - - 0 0 -
- - - - - - - - - - - - - - - - - - - -
- C - - - - C C - - - C - - - - C - - -
C C - - - - C - - - C - - - - C C - - -
- - - 0 - - - - 0 - - - - 0 - - - - 0 -
- - 0 0 - - - 0 0 - - - 0 0 - - - 0 0 -
- - - - - - - - - - - - - - - - - - - -
- - C - - - - C - - - - - - - - - C C - -
- C - - - - C C - - - C - - - C - - - -
- - - 0 - - - - 0 - - - - 0 - - - - 0 -
- - 0 0 - - - 0 0 - - - 0 0 - - - 0 0 -
- - - - - - - - - - - - - - - - - - - -
- - C - - - - C - - - - C - - - - C - -
- C - - - - C - - - - - - - - - - C C - -
- - - 0 - - - - 0 - - - - 0 - - - - 0 -
- - 0 0 - - - 0 0 - - - 0 0 - - - 0 0 -
- - - - - - - - - - - - - - - - - - - -
- - C - - - - C - - - - C - - - - C - -
- C - - - - C - - - - C - - - - C - - -
- - - 0 - - - - 0 - - - - 0 - - - - 0 -
```

c.

```
B F B B C - - - - C C D F F C - 0 0 - B
B B B F F F - 0 0 C - F F E - 0 0 0 - C
0 0 F F F B 0 0 0 B B F E E B - 0 0 C C
0 0 D F B B 0 0 - B B E E B B F - E C 0
0 D D C B - E C C B F D D B C C E E - 0
E D C C - E E C C F F D D C C D D - B -
E C C F - E - - F F - - E E E D F B B E
E 0 F F D D - 0 0 0 - E E E - F F B - E
0 0 - D D D - 0 0 0 0 - - C B B F - C C
0 0 D D E - - - - 0 0 - C C B F F C C -
C C - E E C D D D 0 0 F C B - F F F B B
C C E E C C D D E 0 F D 0 - 0 - F F B B
0 0 - B B B F E E - F D D 0 0 - D D B F
0 0 E B B F F - B F F E E 0 0 D D D F F
0 E E C F F - B B C - E E 0 0 E E - F F
E E C C - 0 0 - D C C - - 0 0 E E - F -
D D D - 0 0 - D - C B B 0 0 - C C F F D
D D D - 0 - E D D F B B 0 - C C B B - D
F D E E E E D D D D D - - C C B - - F
F - E C C E - D D D D D D F C C 0 0 - F
```

d.

```
- - - - C - - - - C C - - - C - 0 0 - -
- - - - - - - 0 0 C - - - - - 0 0 0 - C
0 0 - - - - 0 0 0 - - - - - - - 0 0 C C
0 0 - - - - 0 0 - - - - - - - - - - C 0
0 - - C - - - C C - - - - - C C - - - 0
- - C C - - - C C - - - - C C - - - - -
- C C - - - - - - - - - - - - - - - - -
- 0 - - - - - 0 0 0 - - - - - - - - - -
0 0 - - - - - 0 0 0 0 - - - C - - - - C
0 0 - - - - - - 0 0 - - C C - - - C C -
C C - - - C - - - 0 0 - C - - - - - - -
C C - - C C - - - 0 - - 0 - - - - - - -
0 0 - - - - - - - - 0 0 - - - - - - -
0 0 - - - - - - - - - - - - 0 0 - - - -
0 - - - - - - - - - - - - 0 - C C - - -
- - C C - 0 0 - - C C - - 0 0 - - - - -
- - - - 0 0 - - - C - - 0 0 - C C - - -
- - - - 0 - - - - - - - - 0 - C C - - -
- - - - - - - - - - - - - - - - C C - - -
- - - C C - - - - - - - - - C C 0 0 - -
```

Figure 5: Maps of intact proprioceptive cortex layer (a and b) and motor cortex layer (c and d) showing which cortical elements respond most strongly to stretch of specific muscle after training. Each cortical element is labeled by a letter indicating the muscle whose stretch (increased length) maximally activates that element. The labels are: E for upper arm extensor, F for upper arm flexor, B for upper arm abductor, D for upper arm adductor, O for lower arm extensor ("opener") and C for lower arm flexor ("closer"). Cortex elements marked "-" were found not to be responsive to stretching of any muscle above an activation threshold of 0.4. Maps (a) and (c) indicate cortical elements in PI and MI responding most strongly to stretch of all six muscle groups. Maps (b) and (d) show the same information but only for forearm extensor (O) and flexor (C) muscle groups, illustrating the clustering of cortical elements responsive to stretch for just these two antagonist muscles.

Although difficult to see in Fig. 5a and 5c, the maps form clusters of adjacent elements that respond to the same input. This map characteristic can be better seen in the maps of Fig. 5b and 5d, which show only those elements that are maximally activated for the stretch of the lower arm extensor (O) and lower arm flexor (C), in PI and MI respectively. Fig. 5b illustrates the regular size and arrangement of the clusters across the PI layer. Another characteristic of the input maps formed in PI and MI is that clusters responsive to antagonist muscle pairs tend to be separated, reflecting the constraint that simultaneous shortening of antagonist muscle pairs is not physically possible. For example, after training, the clusters of "O"s and "C"s are generally pushed apart (Figs. 5b and 5d). PI and MI maps of responsiveness to muscle tension inputs also exhibit uniformity in size and spacing of clusters responsive to the same muscle group. When the length map for PI is compared with the tension map for the layer, it is found that the length map of a particular muscle matches well with the tension map of its antagonist muscle [Chen and Reggia 1996]. The maps thus capture the correlated features of input patterns, reflecting the mechanical constraints imposed by the model arm.

For the MI *motor output map*, each MI element is examined to see which muscle group(s) it activates most strongly. With training, clusters of elements activating the same muscle group appear in this map as well. Further study reveals that the MI input map of a particular muscle's length matches very well with the MI output map of its antagonist muscle, while the MI input map of a particular muscle's tension matches well with the MI output map of its corresponding muscle [Chen and Reggia 1996]. The motor output map in MI (not pictured here) thus resembles the proprioceptive input map in Figure 5d very closely, except the C's and O's are reversed. The model's maps thus capture the proprioceptive feedback of an activated muscle from the increased stretch of its antagonist muscles and the increased tension of itself.

3.3 Lesioning the Model

To examine the effects of sudden, focal lesions to the cortex, systematic simulations are being done in which an area of focal damage is suddenly imposed upon a previously trained network. The results of these simulations will be presented in [Goodall et al, 1996]. We give only a single example here to illustrate how lesioning this model can produce quite different results than with the topographic map models described above.

For this example, we consider the effects of a structural lesion in PI. As with the SI model, changes to the feature maps in PI were observable immediately after a structural lesion occurs in this layer, as the first phase of a two-phase reorganization process. Following the primary structural lesion in P1, the activity of surrounding

```
a.                                    b.

- - O O F F E O O - F B O O - - B O O -    F F O O D F - E - - - - - O - - - O O -
D E - F D E E - - D D - - - - - - - - D    D E E - D D E E O - - - - - - - - - - D
E C C - D E C C - D E C F D D E C - - D    C E B - - C C O O D E C F D D E C - D D
C C B - - C C B O E C C F O E C C F - -    C B B - - C B F D E C B F D E C B - - -
F B B O - F F - O - - B - O - - B B O -    - F F O - - F F - - - - O - - B F O - -
F - O O - - - - - - - - - - - - O O F    D F O O - - - - - - - - - - - F O - -
D E - - D E * * * * * * * * - D E E - D    D - E E D - * * * * * * * * - D D E - D
E E C D E E * * * * * * * * - D E C - D    - - E D - - * * * * * * * * - D E C - -
- C C F E - * * * * * * * * - C C B - -    - C C F - - * * * * * * * * - - C B - -
- B B O - - * * * * * * * * - F B O O -    - B B O - - * * * * * * * * - - F O O -
- B O O - - * * * * * * * * - - O O F F    - - O O - - * * * * * * * * - - O O D -
- - - - D - * * * * * * * * - D E - F D    - - E D - - * * * * * * * * - - E D D -
E - C D E - * * * * * * * * D E E C D D    - E C C - - * * * * * * * * - - C C - -
E F F E E - * * * * * * * * - - C C - E    - - F B - - * * * * * * * * - C C F - -
- B B O - B B - - - - - - B O - F B - O -  - - B O O - - - - - - - - - - - B B O O
- B O O - B - O O F - B B O - F F O O -    - - - O E F - - - F - - E E - - - - O -
- - - F D E E O F D E E - - D - - - - D    - C - D D C B E E D C B E D D - C - D D
E - C F D E - C C D E - C D D E - C D D    C C - - - C B O D C C B F D D E C - D -
E - B - - - B B - - - C C - E E C F F E    E B - - - - - - - - C B F F - E E B F - E
- B B O - - B - O - F B B O - - B F O -    B F - O - F F - - - - - - O O B F - O O
```

Figure 6: Muscle length map of proprioceptive cortex layer PI (above threshold 0.4) for an 8x8 focal lesion of PI, (a) immediately post-lesion, and (b) following 2000 further random input stimuli in motor cortex layer MI. Same labeling conventions as in Fig. 5. Asterisks indicate the imposed structural lesion.

elements was decreased, forming a secondary *functional lesion*. For example, Fig. 6a shows the muscle length map of PI immediately after an 8x8 focal lesion in the center of this layer. The structural lesion site is marked by "*"s. A perilesion zone of relatively inactive cortical elements (marked by "-"s) can be seen immediately following the lesion; these elements do not respond to the stretch of any of the muscles above the threshold of 0.4. This perilesion zone represents a secondary functional lesion. The second phase of reorganization occurred more slowly with continued synaptic changes during the post lesion period. With time, as the map reorganized in the context of continued proprioceptive input and synaptic changes, the functional lesion gradually enlarged (Fig 6b).

4 Discussion

It is currently not well understood how the cerebral cortex adjusts to the sudden structural damage occuring with an ischemic stroke. In the work described here, we induced acute focal lesions in computational models of primary sensory and sensorimotor cortex to examine the resultant map reorganization in surrounding cortex. While our models involve substantial simplifications of reality, they are based on generally accepted concepts of cortical structure, activity dynamics and synaptic plasticity. Post-lesion effects in these models concerning cortical map reorganization represent testable predictions of the models.

Our initial simulations with topographic maps indicated that focal lesions resulted in a two-phase map reorganization process in the intact perilesion cortical region [Armentrout et al., 1994; Sutton et al, 1994]. The first, very rapid phase was due to changes in activation dynamics, while the second, slow phase was due to synaptic plasticity. Thus, the models make the prediction that perilesion map changes will be demonstratable within a few minutes of a cortical lesion, and then will increase gradually with time (presumably over days to weeks). To our knowledge only a single experimental study of post-lesion cortical map reorganization in an animal model has been done [Jenkins and Merzenich 1987]. This small experimental study showed long-term map reorganization, consistent with the predictions of our model, but did not examine map reorganization occurring immediately post-lesion. Recent experimental studies in animals have repeatedly shown map reorganization within minutes following focal deafferentation of cortex; our models predict that they will occur following cortical lesions as well. Thus, a critical issue in assessing the validity of our models is the experimental measurement of cortical map reorganization immediately after a cortical lesion.

The second prediction of our topographic models is that increased perilesion excitability is necessary for effective map reorganization in cortex surrounding an acute focal lesion. When increased perilesion excitability was present during the first phase of map reorganization the surrounding cortex consistently participated in the map reorganization process, even achieving a higher density feature map than in the prelesion cortex. Presumably such effective utilization of surrounding intact cortex following a lesion could contribute to behavioral recovery following an ischemic stroke. On the other hand, work now in progress indicates that when there is decreased excitation in perilesion cortex, this intact cortex consistently does *not* participate in map reorganization, and the perilesion cortex that "drops out" of the map can actually expand with time due to the normal modifications of synaptic strengths. Our computational models thus suggest that increased excitability may play an important and largely unrecognized role in recovery from stroke.

At the present time we are extending our models to encompass some biochemical and metabolic alterations occurring in the ischemic penumbra. In particular, we are interested in transient chemical and metabolic disturbances reminiscent of cortical spreading depression in the ischemic penumbra, a region of viable but non-functioning tissue that surrounds an infarction. This region is generally thought to be due to decreased blood flow that compromises neuronal functionality but does not immediately kill penumbra tissue [Caplan 1993, Heiss et al. 1993]. The secondary biochemical changes and depolarizations seen with cortical ischemia are remarkably similar to those of cortical spreading depression [do Carmo 1992, Lauritzen 1994].

We have already undertaken a series of computer simulations using an enhanced model of normal cortex that incorporates a few biochemical factors. The key result of these simulations is that a localized area of elevated potassium evokes a traveling wave of markedly elevated potassium that slowly propagates in an expanding annular region [Reggia and Montgomery 1994]. This model can exhibit several key features of cortical spreading depression. We have recently discovered that the patterns of cortical activity at the leading edge of spreading depression in the model, when projected onto the visual fields, resemble the visual hallucinations reported by patients with classic migraine [Reggia and Montgomery 1995].

Other state variables, such as metabolic supply and structural state, are fundamental to modeling the viability of cortex as biological tissue, and are currently being introduced into our cortex models. Once the enhanced model cortex is implemented, lesions will be simulated by producing a circumscribed zone of inadequate or absent metabolic supply. The perilesion cortex will not only lose input neuronal activity from the lesioned cortex, but it will also undergo marked biochemical and metabolic changes due to diffusion and adjustments in metabolic supply. We will use the enhanced model to examine the relative importance of different factors in causing the ischemic penumbra. Ultimately, we hope to use these models to suggest novel experimental investigations and new approaches to therapeutic intervention.

Acknowledgment: Supported by NINDS awards NS 29414 and NS 16332.

5 References

S. Armentrout, J. Reggia, M. Weinrich, *Artif Intel Med* **6** (1994) 383-400.

M. Boyeson, J. Jones and R. Harmon, *Arch. Neurol.* **51** (1994) 405-414.

J. Brasil-Neto, J. Valls-Sole et al., *Brain* **116** (1993) 511-525.

M. Calford, *Nature* **352** (1991) 759-760.

L. Caplan, *Stroke* (Butterworth-Heinemann, 1993).

R. do Carmo, ed. *Spreading Depression*, (Springer-Verlag, 1992).

Y. Chen and J. Reggia, *Neural Computation* **8** (1996), in press.

S. Cho and J. Reggia, *Internat. J. of Neural Systems* **5** (1994) 87-101.

F. Chollet et al., *Ann. Neurol.* **29** (1991) 63-71.

L. Cohen et al., *Brain* **114** (1991) 615-627.

R. Domann, G. Hagermann et al., *Neurosci. Lets.* **155** (1993) 69-72.

P. Glees and J. Cole, *J. Neurophys.* **13** (1950) 137-148.

S. Goodall, J. Reggia, S. Cho, *Proc 18th Symp Comp Applic in Med Care* (1994) 860-864.

S. Goodall, J. Reggia, Chen Y, et al, submitted, 1996.

K. Grajski and M. Merzenich , *Neural Computation* **2** (1990) 71-84.

J. Hallenback and K. Frerichs, *Arch. Neurol.* **50** (1993) 768-770.

W. Heiss, G. Fink, M. Huber and K. Herholz, *Stroke* **24** (1993) I50 - I53.

H. Hougaku, M. Matsumoto, N. Handa et al., *Stroke* **25** (1994) 566-570.

W. Jenkins and M. Merzenich, in *Progress in Brain Res.*, ed. Seil F et al., **71** (Elsevier, 1987), 249-266.

W. Jenkins et al., *J. Neurophys.* **63** (1990) 82-104.

J. Kaas, *Ann. Rev. Neurosci.* **14** (1991) 137.

H. Killackey, *Journal of Cognitive Neuroscience* **1** (1989) 3-11.

E. Knudsen, S. du Lac and S. Esterly, *Ann. Rev. of Neurosci.* **10** (1987) 41-65.

T. Kohonen, *Self-Organization and Associative Memory* (Springer-Verlag, 1989).

M. Lauritzen, *Brain* **117** (1994) 199-210.

C. von der Malsburg, *Kybernetik* **14** (1973) 85-100.

M. Merzenich, J. Kaas, J. Wall et al., *Neurosci.* **8** (1983) 33-55.

K. Miller, J. Keller and M. Stryker, *Science* **245** (1989) 605-615.

R. Nudo and R. Grenda, *Soc. Neurosci. Abs.* **18** (1992) 216.

K. Obermayer, H. Ritter, K. Schulten, *Proc Internat Joint Conf Neural Networks* **2** (1990) 423-429.

A. Pascual-Leone and F. Torres, *Brain* **116** (1993) 39-52.

J. Pearson, L. Finkel and G. Edelman, *J. Neurosci.* **7** (1987) 4209-4223.

W. Pediette and B. Zolten, *Occupational Therapy Practice Skills for Physical Dysfunction* (Mosby, 1990).

J. Reggia, C. D'Autrechy, G. Sutton and M. Weinrich, *Neural Computation* **4** (1992) 287-317.

J. Reggia and D. Montgomery, *Proc 18th Symp Comp Applic Med Care* (1994) 873-877.

J. Reggia and D. Montgomery, *Computers in Biology and Medicine* (1995), in press.

H. Ritter, T. Martinetz . and K. Schulten, *Neural Networks* **2** (1989) 159-168.

H. Ritter, T. Martinetz and K. Schulten, *Neural Computation and Self-Organizing Maps* (Addison-Wesley, 1992).

E. Ruppin and J. Reggia, *Neural Computation* **7** (1995) 1105-1127.

K. Sasaki and H. Gema, *Exp. Brain Res.* **55** (1984) 60-68.

G. Sutton, J. Reggia, S. Armentrout et al, *Neural Computation* **6** (1994) 1-13.

M. Weinrich, G. Sutton, J. Reggia et al, *J Artif Neural Networks* **1** (1994) 51-60.

S. Udin and J. Fawcett, *Ann. Rev. Neurosci.* **11** (1988) 289-327.

Appendix

We briefly summarize the dynamics of our models here; further details can be found in the references. Activation $a_j(t)$ of a cortical node j changes according to

$$\frac{d}{dt}a_j(t) = c_s a_j(t) + (M - a_j(t))in_j(t) \tag{1}$$

where $in_j(t)$ is the sum of the incoming thalamic and neighboring cortical outputs weighted by their respective connection strengths, M is the maximal activation of a cortical node, and c_s is a negative constant. The output dispersal rule is

$$out_{ji}(t) = c_p \left(\frac{w_{ji}(t)(a_j^p(t) + q)}{\sum_k w_{ki}(t)(a_k^p(t) + q)} \right) a_i(t) \tag{2}$$

when competitive distribution is used, where c_p is a network wide excitatory gain, w_{ji} is the weight from a node i to cortical node j, q is a small positive constant which varies the competitiveness of the output rule and prevents division by zero, and k varies over the cortical elements connected to i. The unsupervised learning rule used involves a change to the weight w_{ji} from a node i to cortical element j given by

$$\Delta w_{ji}(t + \delta) = \epsilon[a_i(t + \delta) - w_{ji}(t)]a_j(t + \delta) \tag{3}$$

where $0 < \epsilon \ll 1$ is the learning rate.

FUNCTIONAL VERSUS STRUCTURAL DAMAGE IN MULTI-INFARCT DEMENTIA: A COMPUTATIONAL STUDY

EYTAN RUPPIN
Departments of Computer Science & Physiology
Tel-Aviv University, Tel Aviv 69978, Israel
ruppin@math.tau.ac.il
and
JAMES A. REGGIA
Departments of Computer Science & Neurology
A.V. Williams Bldg.
University of Maryland
College Park, MD 20742
reggia@cs.umd.edu

ABSTRACT

Understanding the effects of damage on neural networks could lead to important insights concerning neurological and psychiatric disorders. We present a simple analytical framework for estimating the functional damage resulting from focal structural lesions to a neural network model. The effects of focal lesions of varying area, shape and number on the retrieval capacities of a spatially-organized associative memory are quantified, leading to specific scaling laws that may be further examined experimentally. It is predicted that multiple focal lesions will impair performance more than a single lesion of the same size, that slit like lesions are more damaging than rounder lesions, and that the same fraction of damage (relative to the total network size) will result in significantly less performance decrease in larger networks. Our study is clinically motivated by the observation that in multi-infarct dementia, the size of metabolically impaired tissue correlates with the level of cognitive impairment more than the size of structural damage. Our results account for the detrimental effect of the number of infarcts rather than their overall size of structural damage, and for the 'multiplicative' interaction between Alzheimer's disease and multi-infarct dementia.

1. Introduction

Understanding the response of neural nets to structural/functional damage is important for assessing the performance of neural network hardware, and in gaining understanding of the mechanisms underlying neurological and psychiatric disorders. Recently, there has been a growing interest in constructing neural models to study how specific pathological neuroanatomical and neurophysiological changes can result in various clinical manifestations, and to investigate the functional organization of the symptoms that result from specific brain pathologies (reviewed in (Reggia et. al. 1994, Ruppin 1995)). In the area of associative memory models specifically, early computational studies found an increase in memory impairment with increasing lesion severity (Wood 1978) (in accordance with Lashley's classical 'mass action' principle), and showed that slowly developing lesions can have less pronounced effects than equivalent acute lesions (Anderson 1983). More recently, it was shown that the gradual pattern of clinical deterioration manifested in the majority of Alzheimer's patients can be explained, and that different synaptic compensation rates can account for the observed variation in the severity and progression rate of this disease (Horn et. al. 1993, Horn et. al. 1995, Ruppin & Reggia 1995).

Previous work, however, is limited in that model elements have no spatial relationships to one another (all elements are conceptually equidistant). Thus, as there is no way to represent focal (localized) damage in such networks, it has not been possible to study the functional effects of focal lesions on memory and to compare them with those caused by diffuse lesions. This chapter presents the first computational study of the effect of focal lesions on memory performance with spatially-organized neural networks. It is motivated by the observation that in neural network models, a focal *structural lesion* (that is, the permanent and complete inactivation of some group of adjacent elements) is accompanied by a surrounding *functional lesion* composed of structurally intact but functionally impaired elements. This region of functional impairment occurs due to the loss of innervation from the structurally damaged region. It is the combined effect of both regions that determines the actual extent of performance decrease in the network. From a modeling perspective, this paper presents a simple but general approach to analyzing the functional effects of focal lesions. This approach is used to derive scaling laws that quantify the effects of spatial characterlstics of focal lesions such as their number and shape on the performance of network models of associative memory.

Beyond its computational interest, the study of the effects of focal damage on the performance of neural network models can lead to a better understanding of functional impairments accompanying focal brain lesions. In particular, we are interested in *multi-infarct dementia*, a frequent cause of dementia (chronic deterioration of cognitive and memory capacities) characterized by a series of multiple, aggregating focal lesions. The distinction made in the model network considered here between structural and functional lesions has a clinical parallel: 'structural' lesions represent regions of infarcted (dead) tissue, as measured by structural imaging methods such as computerized tomography, and 'functional' lesions represent regions of metabolically impaired tissue surrounding the infarcted tissue, as measured by functional imaging techniques such as positron emission tomography. Interestingly, in multi-infarct dementia the correlation between the volume of the primary infarct region and the severity of the resulting cognitive deficit is unclear and controversial (Meyer et. al. 1988, Del Ser et. al. 1990, Liu et. al. 1990, Tatemichi et. al. 1990, Gorelick et. al. 1992). In contrast, there is a strong relationship between the total volume of metabolically impaired tissue measured in the chronic phase and the severity of multi-infarct dementia (Mieke et. al. 1992, Heiss et. al. 1993a, Heiss et. al. 1993b). This highlights the importance of studying functional impairment after focal lesions.

The reader familiar with the clinical stroke literature should note that the functional lesions modeled in this paper are *not* the 'penumbra' perilesion areas of comprised blood supply and acute metabolic changes that surround focal infarcts during the acute post-infarct period. Rather, they are regions of reduced metabolic activity that are observed in chronic multi-infarct dementia patients months after the last infarct episode. The reduced metabolic activity in these areas is probably a result of both residual post-infarct neuropathological damage and the loss of innervation from the primary infarct region (Mies et. al. 1983, Heiss et. al. 1993a). Intuitively, it is clear that in large enough lesions the functional damage resulting from loss of innervation should scale proportionally to the lesion circumference. This entails, in turn, that the functional damage should depend on the spatial characteristics of the structural lesion, such as its shape and the number of spatially distinct sub-lesions composing it. This work is devoted to a formal and quantitative study of these dependencies, and to a discussion of their possible clinical implications.

In Section 2, we derive a theoretical framework that characterizes the effects of focal lesions on an associative network's performance. This framework, which is formulated in very general terms, is then examined via simulations with a specific associative memory network in Section 3. These simulations show a fair quantitative fit with the theoretical predictions, and are compared with simulations examining performance with diffuse damage. The effects of various parameters characterizing the network's architecture on post-lesion performance are further investigated in Section 4. Finally, our results are discussed in Section 5 and are evaluated in light of some relevant clinical data.

2. Analytical scaling rules

The model network we study consists of a 2-dimensional array of units whose edges are connected, forming a torus to eliminate edge effects. Each unit is connected primarily to its nearby neighbors, as in the cortex (Thomson & Deuchars

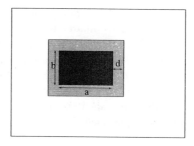

Figure 1: A sketch of a structural (dark shading) and surrounding functional (light shading) rectangular lesion. The a and b values denote the lengths of the rectangle's sides, and d is the functional impairment span.

1994). where the probability of a connection existing between two units is a Gaussian density function of the distance between them in the array. The unit of distance here is the distance between two neighboring elements in the array.

Our analysis pertains to the case where, in the pre-damaged network, all units have similar average activation and performance levels [1]. A focal *structural lesion* (anatomical lesion), denoting an area of damage and neuronal death, is modeled by permanently clamping the activity of the lesioned units to zero at the onset of the lesion. As a result of this primary structural lesion, the activity of surrounding units may be decreased, resulting in a secondary *functional lesion*, as illustrated in Figure 1.

We are primarily interested in large focal lesions, where the area s of the lesion is significantly greater than the local neighborhood region from which each unit receives its inputs. Throughout our analysis we shall hold the working assumption that, traversing from the border of the lesion outwards, the activity of units, and with it, the network performance level, gradually rises from zero until it reaches its normal, predamaged levels, at some distance d from the lesion's border (see Figure 1). We denote d as the *functional impairment span*. This assumption reflects the notion that units which are closer to the lesion border lose more viable inputs than units that are farther away from the lesion. Since s is large relative to each element's connectivity neighborhood, d is determined primarily by the effect of the inactive regions at the periphery of

---

[1]The analysis presented in this section is general in the sense that it does not rely on any specific connectivity or activation values. Note however that the above statement is true in general for associative memory networks, when the activity of each unit is averaged over a time span sufficiently long for the cueing and retrieval of a few stored patterns.

the lesion. We may therefore assume that the value of d is independent of the lesion size, and depends specifically on the parameters defining the network's connectivity and dynamics. In Section 4 we will use computer simulations to verify that d is invariant over lesion size, and examine its dependence on the network parameters.

Let the intact baseline performance level of the network be denoted as $P(0)$, and let the network area be A. The network's performance, is quantified by some measure P ranging from 0 to 1. For example, if the network is an associative memory (as we study numerically in the next section), P denotes how accurately the network retrieves the correct memorized patterns given a set of input cues (defined formally in Eq. (17) of the Appendix). In the pre-damaged network all units have an approximately similar level of activity and performance. Then, a structural lesion of area s (dark shading in Figure 1), causing an additional functional lesion of area Δ_s (light shading in Figure 1), results in a performance level of approximately

$$P(s) = \frac{P(0)\,[A - (s + \Delta_s)] + P_\Delta \Delta_s}{A - s} = P(0) - (\Delta P \Delta_s)/(A - s)\,, \qquad (1)$$

where P_Δ denotes the average level of performance over Δ_s and $\Delta P = P(0) - P_\Delta$. $P(s)$ hence reflects the performance level over the remaining viable parts of the network, discarding the structurally damaged region [2]. Bearing these definitions in mind, the effect of focal lesions on the network's performance level can by characterized by the following rules.

2.1 A single lesion

Consider a symmetric, circular structural lesion of size $s = \pi r^2$. The area of functional damage following such a lesion is $\Delta_s = \pi[(r + d)^2 - r^2] = \pi d^2 + \sqrt{4\pi}d\sqrt{s}$. In networks which operate well below the limit of their capacity and hence have significant functional reserves, the second term dominates since s is assumed to be large relative to d, and therefore

Rule 1:

$$\Delta_s \cong \sqrt{4\pi}d\sqrt{s}\,. \qquad (2)$$

The area of functional damage surrounding a single focal structural lesion is proportional to the square root of the structural lesion's area, as one would

---

[2] Alternatively, it is possible to measure the performance over the entire network. This would not affect our findings as long as the same measure is used in both the analysis and simulations, as the mapping between the two performance measures is order preserving.

308

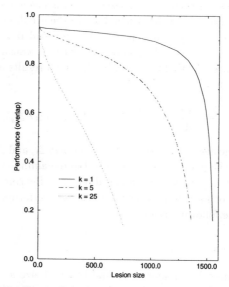

Figure 2: Theoretically predicted network performance as a function of a single focal structural lesion's size (area): analytic curves obtained for different k values; $A = 1600$.

expect. Substituting the expression for Δ_s in Eq. (1), we get

$$P(s) \cong P(0) - \frac{k\sqrt{s}}{A-s} \, , \tag{3}$$

for some constant $k = \sqrt{4\pi}d\Delta P$. Some analytic performance/lesioning curves for various k values are illustrated in Figure 2. Note the different qualitative shape of these curves as a function of k. As is evident, the shape of these curves reflects two conflicting tendencies; they are initially concave (in light of rule 1) and then turn convex (as s increases and the remaining viable area is decreased). Letting $x = s/A$ be the *fraction of structural damage*, we have

Corollary 1:

$$P(x) \cong P(0) - \frac{k\sqrt{x}}{1-x}\frac{1}{\sqrt{A}} \, , \tag{4}$$

that is, the same *fraction* x of damage results in less performance decrease in larger networks! This surprising result testifies to the possible protective value of having functional 'modular' cortical networks of large size. It arises from the fact that the functional damage does not scale up linearly with the structural lesion size, but only as the square root of the latter.

2.2 Varying shape and number

Expressions Eq. 3 and Eq. 4 are valid also when the structural lesion has a square shape. The resulting functional lesion of an s-size square structural lesion is $\Delta_s = 4d^2 + 4d\sqrt{s}$. To study the effect of the structural lesion's shape, we consider the area $\Delta_{s[n]}$ of a functional lesion resulting from a rectangular focal lesion of size $s = a \cdot b$ (see Figure 1), where, without loss of generality, $n = a/b \geq 1$. Then, for large n, (i.e., elongated lesions), the area of functional damage is

$$\Delta_{s[n]} = 2d(a+b)+4d^2 = (n+1)2d\sqrt{\frac{s}{n}}+4d^2 \cong 2d\sqrt{n}\sqrt{s}+4d^2 \cong \sqrt{n/4}\Delta_s \, , \tag{5}$$

where in the last step we neglect the contribution of the size-invariant term $4d^2$. The functional damage of a rectangular structural lesion of fixed size increases as its shape is more elongated. More quantitatively we have

Rule 2:

$$\Delta_{s[n]} \cong \sqrt{n/4}\Delta_s \, , \tag{6}$$

and

$$P(s) \cong P(0) - \frac{k\sqrt{ns}}{2(A-s)} \, . \tag{7}$$

Next, to study the effect of the number of lesions, consider the area $\Delta_s{}^m$ of a functional lesion composed of m focal rectangular structural lesions (with sides $a = n \cdot b$), each of area s/m. Using Eq. (5), we have

$$\Delta_s{}^m = m\left[2d(2d + \sqrt{n}\sqrt{s/m})\right] = \sqrt{m}\left[2d(2d\sqrt{m} + \sqrt{n}\sqrt{s})\right] \geq \sqrt{m}\Delta_{s[n]} . \quad (8)$$

The functional damage hence increases as the number of the focal lesions m increases (total structural lesion area held constant), in accordance with

Rule 3:

$$\Delta_s{}^m \geq \sqrt{m}\Delta_{s[n]} , \quad (9)$$

which is always valid, irrespective of the value of d, and

$$P(s) \cong P(0) - \frac{k\sqrt{mns}}{2(A - s)} . \quad (10)$$

At first glance, the second and third rules seem to indicate that the functional damage caused by varying the shape or by varying the number of focal lesions behaves according to scaling laws of similar order. However, while rule 3 presents a lower bound on the functional damage which may actually be significantly larger, and involves no approximations, rule 2 presents an upper bound on the actual functional damage. As we shall show in the next section, the number of lesions actually affects the network performance significantly more than its precise shape (maintaining the total structural area fixed).

Let $\Delta[x]$ denote the functional damage caused by a single focal square lesion of area x (so $\Delta[s]$ is Δ_s). Since $\sqrt{l}\Delta_s \cong \Delta[s \cdot l]$ (by rule 1), then following rules 2 and 3 we obtain the following corollaries:

Corollary 2:

$$\Delta_{s[n]} \cong \Delta[n/4 \cdot s] \quad (11)$$

That is, the functional damage area following a rectangular structural lesion of area s and sides-ratio n is approximately equal to the functional damage area following a larger single square structural lesion of area $n/4 \cdot s$ (for large n) .

Corollary 3:

$$\Delta_s{}^m \geq \Delta[m \cdot s] \quad (12)$$

In other words, the functional damage following multiple lesions composed of m rectangular focal structural lesions having a combined total area s is greater than the functional damage following a single square lesion of the much larger area $m \cdot s$.

As is evident, the analysis presented in this section is based on several simplifying approximations. As such, it cannot be expected to yield an exact match with numerical results from computer simulations. However, as demonstrated in the next section, the scaling rules developed have the same shape as the numerical data, matching quite well at times.

3. Numerical results

We now turn to examine the effect of lesions on the performance of an associative memory network via simulations. The goal of these simulations is twofold. First, to examine how accurately the general but approximate theoretical results presented above describe the actual performance degradation in a specific associative network. Second, to compare the effects of focal lesions to those of diffuse ones, as the effect of diffuse damage cannot be described as a limiting case within the framework of our analysis. Our simulations were performed using a standard Tsodyks-Feigelman attractor neural network (Tsodyks & Feigel'man 1988). This is a Hopfield-like network which has several features that make it more biologically plausible (Horn et. al. 1933), such as low activity and non-zero thresholds. Spatially-organized attractor networks can function reasonably well as associative memory devices (Karlholm 1993), and a biologically-inspired realization of attractor networks using cortical columns as its elements has also been proposed (Lansner & Fransen 1994). The recent findings of delayed, post-stimulus, sustained activity in memory-related tasks, both in the temporal (Miyashita & Chang 1988) and frontal (Wilson et. al. 1993) cortices, provides support to the plausibility of such attractor networks as a model of associative cortical areas.

A detailed formulation of the network used and simulation parameters is given in the Appendix. Each unit's connectivity is parameterized by σ, where smaller σ values denote a shorter (and more spatially-organized) connectivity range. The network's performance level is quantified by an *overlap* measure m ranging in the interval $[-1, +1]$. It measures the similarity between the network's end state and the cued memory pattern (which is the desired response), averaged over many trials with different input cues. We now describe the results of simulations examining the scaling rules derived in the previous section.

3.1 Performance decrease with a single lesion

Figure 3 plots the network's performance as a function of the area of a single square-shaped *focal* lesion. As is evident, the spatially-organized connectivity enables the network to maintain its memory retrieval capacities in the face of focal lesions of considerable size. As the connectivity dispersion σ increases, focal lesions become more damaging. Also plotted in Figure 3 is the analytical

312

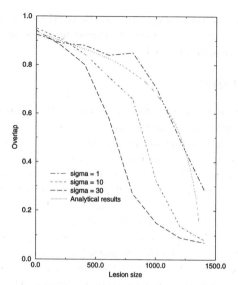

Figure 3: Network performance as a function of focal lesion size. Simulation results obtained in three different networks, each characterized by a distinct distribution of spatially-organized connectivity, and analytic results calculated with $k = 5$ using equation 2.

curve calculated via rule 1 and Eq. (3) with $k = 5$, which matches well with the actual performance of the spatially-connected network parameterized by $\sigma = 1$. Concentrating on the study of focal lesions in a spatially-connected network, we shall adhere to the values $\sigma = 1$ and $k = 5$ hereafter, and compare the analytical and numerical results.

The performance of the network as a function of the *fraction* of the network lesioned, for different network areas A, is displayed in Figure 4. The analytical curves, plotted using Eq. (4) (with $k = 5$) are qualitatively similar to the numerical results (with $\sigma = 1$). The sparing effect of large networks is marked.

3.2 The effects of shape and number

To examine rule 2, a rectangular structural lesion of area $s = 300$ was induced in the network. As shown in Figure 5a, as the ratio n between the sides is increased while holding the area constant, the network's performance further decreases, but this effect is relatively mild (note values on vertical axis). There

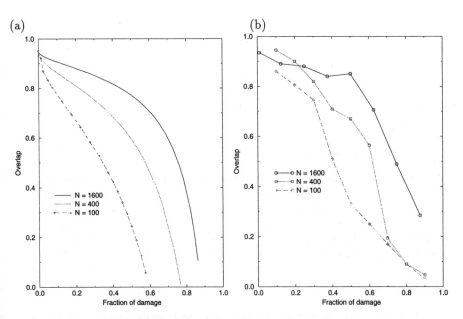

Figure 4: Network performance as a function of the fraction of focal damage, in networks of different sizes. Both analytical (a) and numerical (b) results are displayed.

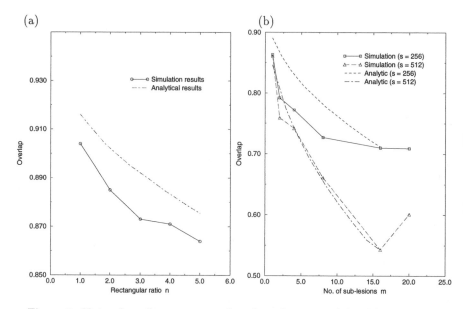

Figure 5: Network performance as a function of structural focal lesion shape (a) and number (b), while keeping total structural lesion area constant. Both numerical and analytical results are displayed. The simulations were performed in a network whose connectivity was generated with $\sigma = 1$. The analytical results are for the corresponding $k = 5$. In Figure 5b, the x-ordinate denotes the number of separate sub-lesions (1,2,4,8,16), and, for comparison, the performance achieved with a diffuse lesion of similar size is plotted arbitrarily on the 20'th x-ordinate.

is a fair quantitative agreement with the theoretical predictions obtained using Eq. (7), and these are also plotted in Figure 5. The effect of varying the lesion number while keeping the overall lesion area fixed stated in rule 3 is demonstrated in Figure 5b. This Figure shows the effect of multiple lesions composed of 2, 4, 8 and 16 separate focal lesions. This effect is much stronger than seen with lesion shape (note values on vertical axis). As is also evident, the analytical results computed using Eq. (10) correspond quite closely with the numerical ones. However, in both figures, the analytically calculated performance is consistently higher than that actually achieved in simulations, as the d^2 term is omitted in the analytic approximation. Note also (Figure 5b) that as the lesion size is increased the analytic results correspond better to the simulation results, as d becomes smaller in relation to $\sqrt{s}$.

To compare the effects of focal and diffuse lesions, the performance achieved with a diffuse lesion of similar size is arbitrarily plotted on the $20'th$ x-ordinate. It is interesting to note that a large multiple focal lesion ($s = 512$) can cause a larger performance decrease than a diffuse lesion of similar size. That is, at some point, when the size of each individual focal lesion becomes small in relation to the width of each unit's connectivity, our analysis loses its validity, and rule 3 does not hold any more. Hence, the effect of a diffuse lesion on the network's performance cannot be calculated by viewing it as a 'limiting case' of multiple focal lesions.

3.3 Diffuse lesions in spatially-organized networks

Figure 6 displays how the performance of the network degrades when *diffuse* structural lesions of increasing size are inflicted upon it by randomly selecting units on the lattice and clamping their activity to zero. While the performance of non-spatially connected networks manifests the classical sharp decline (denoted as 'catastrophic breakdown' (Amit 1989) at some critical lesion size (Figure 6, $\sigma = 30$), the performance of spatially-connected networks (Figure 6, $\sigma = 1$) degrades in a more gradual manner as the size of the diffuse lesion increases. It is of interest to note that this 'graceful' degradation parallels the gradual clinical and cognitive decline observed in the majority of Alzheimer patients (Katzman 1986, Katzman et. al. 1988). A comparison of Figures 3 and 6 demonstrates that diffuse lesions are generally more detrimental than a *single* focal lesion of identical area.

4. The functional impairment span d

The correspondence obtained between the theoretical and simulation results presented in the previous section testifies to the validity of the lesion-invariant impairment span that has been central to our analysis. This assumption is further supported directly by extensive simulations demonstrating that the span d remains practically invariant when the lesion size is varied (for large lesions). We now turn to study the influence of several factors such as the spatial connectivity distribution σ and the noise level T (defined in the Appendix) on the the functional impairment span. The simulation results described below are compared with analytical results obtained by iterating an overlap system of equations, derived in (Ruppin and Reggia 1995a). They describe the dependence of an overlap vector whose components are 'local' overlaps measured at consecutive distances from the border of the lesion (and hence termed *distance-overlaps*), on various parameters of the network.

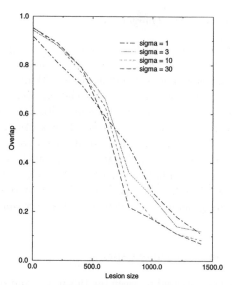

Figure 6: Network performance as a function of diffuse lesion size. Simulation results obtained in four different networks, each characterized by a distinct distribution of spatially-organized connectivity.

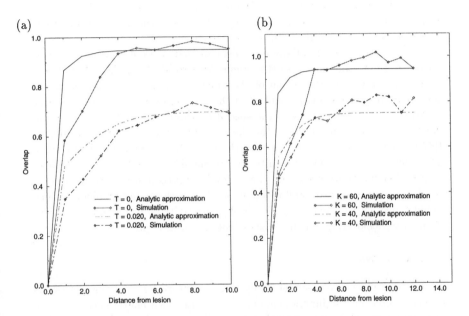

Figure 7: Performance levels as a function of distance from the lesion border. With different (a) Noise levels and (b) connectivity. Both analytical and simulation results are displayed; $s = 200$.

Figure 7a displays the distance-overlap span obtained with an almost noise-less ($T = 0.001$) network and with a network with noisy dynamics ($T = 0.020$). As is evident from the analytical results, as the noise level is increased the span d is markedly increased (e.g., from roughly $d = 3$ to $d = 6$ in Figure 7a). In other words, the functional damage is significantly larger for increased noise levels. As one would expect, increasing the noise levels also results in decreased performance levels. As shown in Figure 7b, after decreasing the synaptic connectivity by randomly eliminating some fraction of the synapses of each unit (leaving each unit with 40 instead of 60 incoming synapses), the network's performance decreases in a similar manner to the noisy dynamics case, but there is only a slight increase in d. In our simplified network the effects of random synaptic deletion are essentially equivalent to that of random neural damage (inactivation of some units), so that Figure 7b also illustrates how diffuse neuronal degeneration in the region of the functional lesion (as observed in the perilesion area after stroke) would effect the severity of multi-infarct dementia.

Studying the dependency of the span d on the connectivity dispersion parameter σ (or its equivalent r in the theoretical expressions (Ruppin & Reggia 1995a)) requires larger networks than those which we could practically simulate. Hence, only analytical results are presented in Figure 8. As is evident, increased connectivity dispersion (i.e., r levels) results in a marked increase in the distance-overlap span, and in a more gradual performance gradient. As one would expect, at sufficiently high levels of connectivity radii the typical gradient of the distance-overlaps' span vanishes (not shown in Figure 8).

5. Discussion

We have presented a simple analytical framework for studying the effects of focal lesions on the functioning of spatially organized neural networks. The analysis presented is quite general and a similar approach could be adopted to investigate the effect of focal lesions in other neural models, such as models of random neural networks (Minai & Levy 1993) or cortical map organization (Sutton et. al. 1994).

Using this analysis, specific scaling rules have been formulated describing the functional effects of structural focal lesions on memory retrieval performance in associative attractor networks. The functional lesion scales as the square root of the size of a single structural lesion, and the form of the resulting performance curve depends on the impairment span d. Surprisingly, the same fraction of damage results in significantly less performance decrease in larger networks, pointing to their relative robustness. As to the effects of shape and number,

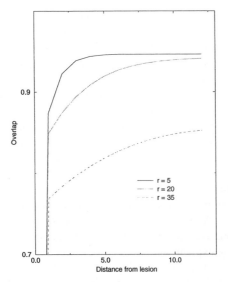

Figure 8: Performance levels as a function of distance from the lesion border, with different r values. Analytical results.

elongated structural lesions cause more damage than more symmetrical ones. However, the number of sub-lesions is the most critical factor determining the functional damage and performance decrease in the model. Numerical studies show that in some conditions multiple lesions can damage performance more than diffuse damage, even though the amount of lost innervation is always less in a multiple focal lesion than with diffuse damage.

The main parameter determining the relation between structural and functional damage is the length of the impairment span d. This span has been found to increase with noise level and connectivity dispersion. It should be noted that when d gets large (in relation to the network dimensions) multiple lesions are likely to 'interact' (i.e., their resulting functional lesions are likely to intersect) and increase the overall performance deterioration.

In the introduction we described the parallel between the structural/functional distinction that underlies this study and a similar distinction made with regard to infarcted tissue versus metabolically impaired regions in multi-infarct dementia. What are the clinical implications of this study with respect to the latter disease? Our results indicate a significant role for the number of infarcts in determining the extent of functional damage and dementia in multi-infarct disease. In our model, multiple focal lesions cause a much larger deficit than their simple 'sum', i.e., a single lesion of equivalent total size. This is consistent with clinical studies that have suggested the main factors related to the prevalence of dementia after stroke to be the infarct number and site, and not the overall infarct size, which is related to the prevalence of dementia in a significantly weaker manner (Del Ser et. al. 1990, Tatemichi et. al. 1990, Tatemichi 1990). As noted by (Hachinski 1983), "In general, the effect of additional lesions of the brain increases with the number of lesions already present, so that the deficits in the brain do not add up, they multiply".

We have found that decreasing the connectivity of each unit, and decreasing the fidelity of network dynamics by increasing the noise level, may not only lead to a decrease in the overall level of performance, but also to an increase in the length of the distance-overlap span in the perilesion area. The degenerative synaptic changes occurring as Alzheimer's disease progresses are known to lead to a reduction in the number of synapses in a unit volume of the cortex (e.g., (Dekosky & Scheff 1990)), and the accompanying synaptic compensatory changes increase the level of noise in the system (Horn et. al. 1993). This offers a plausible explanation for the 'multiplicative' interaction occurring between co-existing Alzheimer's and multi-infarct dementia (Tatemichi 1990), where cortical atrophy contributes as an independent variable to the severity of stroke symptomatology (Levine et. al. 1986) and increases the severity of stroke symptomatology in Alzheimer patients.

The loss of innervation from a focal stroke region to its immediate surroundings such as that studied in this paper may be viewed as sort of 'local diaschisis'. In contrast, global, interhemispheric diaschisis denotes the 'disconnection' of neural structures which are far apart in the brain, and may lead to structurally normal regions with reduced metabolism as observed in several neurological disorders (Feeney & Baron 1986). Such a metabolic depression of apparently intact structures involving Papez's circuit and basal anterior regions has been recently observed in human patients suffering from 'pure' amnesia (Fazio et. al. 1992). Given more information concerning the patterns of connectivity between these structures, it may be possible in the future to study the functional consequences of interhemispheric diaschisis. Future studies of diaschisis may also address the effects of subcortical infarcts, which frequently accompany cortical lesions in multi-infarct dementia. Interestingly, just very recently it has been shown that, as with cortical infarction, with subcortical infarction the number of infarcts but not the volume of infarction (as measured in computerized tomography scans) are significantly associated with cognitive impairment in stroke patients (Corbett et. al. 1994).

Acknowledgements: This research has been supported in part by a Rothschild Fellowship to Dr. Ruppin and in part by Awards NS29414 and NS16332 from NINDS. It has first been presented in *Neural Computation* 7(5), 1995.

References

D.J. Amit (1989). *Modeling brain function: the world of attractor neural networks*. Cambridge University Press.

J.A. Anderson (1983). Cognitive and psychological computation with neural models. *IEEE Trans. on Systems,Man, and Cybernetics*, 13 (5):799–815.

A. Corbett, H. Bennett, and S. Kos (1994). Cognitive dysfunction following subcortical infarction. *Arch. Neurol.*, 51:999–1007.

S. T. DeKosky and S.W. Scheff (1990). Synapse loss in frontal cortex biopsies in alzheimer's disease: Correlation with cognitive severity. *Ann. Neurology*, 27(5):457–464.

T. Del Ser, F. Bermejo, A. Portera, J.M. Arredondo, C. Bouras, and J. Constantinidis (1990). Vascular dementia: a clinicopathological study. *Journal of Neurological Sciences*, 96:1–17.

F. Fazio, D. Perani, M.C. Gilardi, F. Colombo, S.F. Cappa, G. Vallar, V. Bettinardi, E. Paulesu, M. Alberoni, S. Bressi, M. Franceschi, and G.L. Lenzi (1992). Metabolic impairment in human amnesia: A PET study of memory networks. *Journal of cerebral blood flow and metaboism*, 12(3):353–358.

D.M. Feeney and J.C. Baron (1986). Diaschisis. *Stroke*, 17:817–830.

P.B. Gorelick, A. Chatterjee, D. Patel, G. Flowerdew, W. Dollear, J. Taber, and Y. Harris (1992). Cranial computed tomographic observations in Multi-Infarct Dementia. *Stroke*, 23:804–811.

V. Hachinski (1983). Multi-infarct dementia. *Neurol. Clin.*, 1:27–36.

W.D. Heiss, H.G. Emunds, and K. Herholz (1993a). Cerebral glucose metabolism as a predictor of rehabilitation after ischemic stroke. *Stroke*, 24:1784–1788.

W.D. Heiss, J. Kessler, H. Karbe, G.R. Fink, and G. Pawlik (1993b). Cerebral glucose metabolism as a predictor of recovery from aphasia in ischemic stroke. *Archives of Neurology*, 50:958–964.

D. Horn, E. Ruppin, M. Usher, and M. Herrmann (1993). Neural network modeling of memory deterioration in alzheimer's disease. *Neural Computation*, 5:736–749.

D. Horn, N. Levy, and E. Ruppin (1995). Locally-driven synaptic compensation in alzheimer's disease: A computational study. In *Fourth Annual Computation and Neural Systems Meeting*.

D. Horn and E. Ruppin (1995). Compensatory mechanisms in an attractor neural network model of schizophrenia. *Neural Computation*, 7(1):182–205.

J.M. Karlholm (1993). Associative memories with short-range higher order couplings. *Neural Networks*, 6:409–421.

R. Katzman (1986). Alzheimer's disease. *New England Journal of Medicine*, 314(15):964–973.

R. Katzman and et. al. (1988). Comparison of rate of annual change of mental status score in four independent studies of patients with alzheimer's disease. *Ann. Neurology*, 24(3):384–389.

A. Lansner and E. Fransen (1994). Improving the realism of attractor models by using cortical columns as functional units. In *Third Annual Computation and Neural Systems Meeting*.

D.N. Levine, J.D. Walrach, L. Benowitz, and R. Calvino (1986). Left spatial neglect: effects of lesion size on severity and recovery follwoing right cerebral infarction. *Neurology*, 36:362–366.

C.K. Liu, B.L. Miller, J.L. Cummings, C.M. Mehringer, M.A. Goldberg, S.L. Howng, and D.F. Benson (1990). A quantitative MRI study of vascular dementia. *Neurology*, 42:138–143.

J.S. Meyer, K.L. McClintic, R.L. Rogers, P. Sims, and K.F. Mortel (1988). Aetiological considerations and risk factors for multi-infarct dementia. *J. Neurol. Neurosurg. Psychiatry*, 51:1489–1497.

R. Mieke, K. Herholz, M. Grond, J. Kessler, and W.D. Heiss (1992). Severity of vascular dementia is related to volume of metabolically impaired tissue. *Archives of Neurology*, 49:909–913.

G. Mies, L.M. Auer, H. Ebhardt, H. Traupe, and W.D. Heiss (1983). Flow and neuronal density in tissue surrounding chronic infarction. *Stroke*, 14(1):22–27.

A.A. Minai and W.B. Levy (1993). Setting the activity level in sparse random networks. *Neural Computation*, 6:85–99.

Y. Miyashita and H.S. Chang (1988). Neuronal correlate of pictorial short-term memory in the primate temporal cortex. *Nature*, 331:68–71.

J. Reggia, R. Berndt, and L. D'Autrechy (1994). Connectionist models in neuropsychology. In *Handbook of Neuropsychology*, volume (9), pages 297–333. Elsevier Science, Amsterdam.

E. Ruppin (1995). Neural modeling of psychiatric disorders. *Network*, 6:1–22.

E. Ruppin and J. Reggia (1995). A neural model of memory impairment in diffuse cerebral atrophy. *Br. Jour. of Psychiatry*, 166(1):19–28.

E. Ruppin and J. Reggia (1995a). Patterns of functional damage in associative memory models. *Neural Computation*, 7(5):1105–1127.

G. Sutton, J. Reggia, S. Armentrout, and C. D'Autrechy (1994). Map reorganization as a competitive process. *Neural Computation*, 6:1–13.

T. K. Tatemichi (1990). How acute brain failure becomes chronic: a view of the mechanisms of dementia related to stroke. *Neurology*, 40:1652–1659.

T.K. Tatemichi, M.A. Foulkes, J.P. Mohr, J.R. Hewitt, D. B. Hier, T.R. Price, and P.A. Wolf (1990). Dementia in stroke survivors in the stroke data bank cohort. *Stroke*, 21:858–866.

A. M. Thomson and J. Deuchars (1994). Temporal and spatial properties of local circuits in the neocortex. *Trends in neuroscience*, 17(3):119–126.

M.V. Tsodyks and M.V. Feigel'man (1988). The enhanced storage capacity in neural networks with low activity level. *Europhys. Lett.*, 6:101 – 105.

F.A.W. Wilson, S.P.O Scalaidhe, and P.S. Goldman-Rakic (1993). Dissociation of object and spatial processing domains in primate prefrontal cortex. *Science*, 260:1955–1958.

C.C. Wood (1978). Variations on a theme by Lashley: lesion experiments on the neural model of Anderson, Silverstien, Ritz and Jones. *Psychological Review*, 85(6):582–591.

Appendix: The Associative Network Used In The Simulations

The attractor network used in this study is composed of N units, where each unit i is described by a binary variable $S_i = \{1, 0\}$ denoting an active (firing) or passive (quiescent) state, respectively. M distributed memory patterns ξ^μ, where superscript μ indicates a pattern index, are stored in the network. The elements of each memory pattern are randomly chosen to be 1 or 0 with probability p or $1 - p$, respectively, with $p \ll 1$.

With each set of parameters characterizing a given network, the behavior of the network is monitored over many trials. In each trial, the initial state of the network $S(0)$ is random, with average activity level $q < p$, reflecting the notion that the network's baseline level of activity is lower than its activity in persistent memory states. Each unit's state is updated stochastically, in accordance with its input. The input (post-synaptic potential) h_i of element i at time t is the sum of internal contributions from other units in the network and external contribution F_i^e, given by

$$h_i(t) = \sum_j w_{ij} S_j(t - 1) + F_i^e \tag{13}$$

where $S_j(t)$ is the state of unit j at time t and w_{ij} is the weight on the directed connection to unit i from unit j. The updating rule for unit i at time t is given by

$$S_i(t) = \begin{cases} 1, & \text{with probability } G(h_i(t) - \theta) \\ 0, & \text{otherwise} \end{cases}, \tag{14}$$

where G is the sigmoid function $G(x) = 1/(1 + \exp(-x/T))$, T denotes the noise level, and θ is a uniform threshold which is optimally tuned to guarantee perfect retrieval in the network's premorbid state (Horn and Ruppin 1995).

The weights of the internal synaptic connections are assigned based on the stored memory patterns ξ^μ using

$$w_{ij} = \frac{1}{N} \sum_{\mu=1}^{M} (\xi^\mu{}_i - p)(\xi^\mu{}_j - p), \tag{15}$$

and in each trial the external input component F_i^e is used to present a stored memory pattern (say ξ^1) as an input cue to the network, such that

$$F_i^e = e \cdot \xi^1{}_i \tag{16}$$

where $0 < e < 1$ is a network-wide constant. Following the dynamics defined in Eq. (13) and Eq. (14), the network state evolves until it converges to the vicinity of an attractor stable state.

The network's performance level is measured by the similarity between the network's end state S and the cued memory pattern ξ^μ (which is the desired response), conventionally denoted as the *overlap* m^μ (Tsodyks & Feigel'man 1988), and defined by

$$m^\mu = \frac{1}{p(1-p)N} \sum_{i=1}^N (\xi_i^\mu - p)S_i \ . \tag{17}$$

where the sum is taken only over the viable, non-lesioned units. This overlap measure, ranging in the interval $[-1, +1]$, keeps track of the neurons which should correctly fire and also counts with lower negative weighting the erroneously firing ones. In all simulations we report the average overlap achieved over 100 trials.

In all simulations, $M = 20$ sparse random memory patterns (with a fraction $p = 0.1$ of 1's) were stored in a network of $N = 1600$ units, placed on a 2-dimensional lattice. The external input magnitude is $e = 0.035$ and the noise level is $T = 0.005$. Unlike in the original Tsodyks-Feigelman model which is fully-connected, the network in our model has spatially organized connectivity, where each unit has $K = 60$ incoming connections determined randomly with a Gaussian probability $\phi(z) = \sqrt{1/2\pi} \exp(-z^2/2\sigma^2)$, where z is the distance between two units in the array, and σ determines the extent to which each unit's connectivity is concentrated in its surrounding neighborhood. A structural lesion of the network is realized by clamping the activity state of the lesioned units to zero.

Minimal biophysical models of oscillations and waves in thalamus and hippocampus

David Golomb

*Zlotowski Center for Neuroscience and Dept. of Physiology, Faculty of
Health Sciences, Ben-Gurion University of the Negev, Beer-Sheva, Israel*
E-mail: golomb@bgumail.bgu.ac.il

and

John Rinzel

Mathematical Research Branch, NIDDK, National Institute of Health
9190 Wisconsin Ave., Suite 350, Bethesda, MD 20814, U.S.A.
E-mail: rinzel@helix.nih.gov

ABSTRACT

The value of using minimal biophysical computational models is addressed and illustrated. We describe with such models the dynamical
behavior of seizure-like rhythms in thalamic and hippocampal slices.
The Hodgkin-Huxley-like models include the essential description of the
intrinsic ionic channels, synapses and network architecture but they neglect unessential complexity. In the thalamus, we model the propagation of spindle waves in a network of excitatory thalamocortical and
inhibitory reticular cells. As the wave advances, cells are recruited into
the population rhythm, with reticular cells bursting almost every cycle
at 7–10 Hz while thalamocortical cells burst only every few cycles. When
$GABA_A$ receptors are blocked all cells burst on nearly every cycle at 3-
4 Hz, reminiscent of absence seizure-like activity. For the hippocampal
slice we use a 2-compartment model for a CA3 neuron, a reduction of
Traub's 19-compartment model. Currents for generating fast sodium
spikes are located in the soma-like compartment; slower calcium and
calcium-mediated currents are located in the dendrite-like compartment.
Bursting occurs only for an intermediate range of the electrical coupling
conductance between the compartments. A network of hippocampal
CA3 neuron models coupled by fast AMPA and slow NMDA synapses
produces multiple synchronized population bursts. We distinguish between the discontinuous, "lurching" nature of the thalamic waves and
the continuous nature of the hippocampal waves. The rhythms in both
cases are collective phenomena, since isolated cells are quiescent.

1. Introduction

1.1. Minimal biophysical models

Despite the enormous development of experimental techniques in recent years, it has become clear that to understand the brain's complexity demands the usage of computational and theoretical tools for research. The development of faster computers makes the simulations of biophysical models of neuronal networks plausible. These models take into account the various intrinsic and synaptic ionic channels. The channel dynamics and parameters are determined according to voltage-clamp and current clamp experiments. Evolution of a single-cell's membrane potential in time is determined by the nonlinear combination of all the ionic channels involved. In most of the dynamical network models that have been developed and systematically analyzed, the neuronal unit is assumed to be equipotential; in some cases a few compartments are assumed. A network model incorporates, in addition to the single cell behavior, information about the synaptic dynamics and about the architecture, *i.e.*, the network connectivity scheme.

The enormous complexity of neurons and networks poses a difficult questions for the modeler: which details should be ignored? Taking all the known biological details into account yields a model with many parameters, and only a few that are constrained by experiments. On the other hand, over-simplified models may ignore important biological factors. Useful modeling involves the art of neglecting the right things. Indeed, some of the most successful applications of theory in understanding neuronal systems and predicting new nontrivial results have relied on using *minimal* biophysical models. Such models have been used to describe and explain the behavior of *in vitro* slice preparations, whereas the complexity of *in vivo* experiments often precludes them. In particular, they are useful for analyzing healthy and pathological population rhythms such as sleep oscillations (spindle and delta) and epileptic activity, such as petit mal and hippocampal epileptiform (see the experimental work of Coulter *et al.* 1989, 1990, Huguenard and Prince 1994a,b; and the modeling work of Lytton and Sejnowski 1992). The properties of the intrinsic and synaptic currents are treated as parameters in the model, and changing them mimics the effects of neuromodulators and anti-seizure drugs.

In this Chapter we illustrate the use of reduced models by presenting computational models of two different brain slice preparations that exhibit spatiotemporal rhythmic behavior. One model describes spindle oscillations in thalamic slices, and the second one describes epileptic bursting in CA3 hippocampal slices. Both preparations have been investigated extensively in experimental laboratories, and are considered model systems for studying epileptic activity and sleep, as well as information processing and memory.

1.2. Spindle and petit mal oscillations in the thalamus

The thalamus is a gateway interposed between the peripheral sensory areas and the neocortex. It plays a major role in the generation of various sleep oscillations and in the transition between sleep to awareness. The 7-14 Hz spindle oscillations during early stages of sleep originate from the thalamus (Morison and Bassett 1945, Steriade *et al.* 1985, 1990, Steriade and Deschênes 1984). It is also involved in the onset and synchronization of the 0.5-5 Hz delta rhythm during later stages of quiet sleep (Leresche *et al.* 1991, McCormick and Pape 1990).

Cellular properties. Thalamic cells can fire in two different modes. When depolarized, they fire tonically depending on their synaptic input. At membrane potentials more negative than rest they show a rebound burst response when released from hyperpolarization. The biophysical origin of the post-inhibitory rebound was elucidated with the discovery of the T-type, low threshold calcium current in thalamic cells (Deschênes *et al.* 1984, Jahnsen and Llinás 1984a,b). This inactivating inward current requires a long-lasting hyperpolarization to be de-inactivated. Two ensembles of thalamic neurons contribute to rhythmogenesis. Thalamocortical (TC) cells are excitatory, but do not excite each other; they excite cortical cells and cells in the reticular thalamic (RE) nucleus, a thin neuronal sheet embracing partially the dorsal thalamus. Inhibitory RE cells inhibit each other and the TC cells.

Network properties. It was found that spindles in thalamic nuclei could be abolished by depriving them from RE inputs (Steriade *et al.* 1985, 1987). Therefore, the RE is crucial for spindle generation. A major breakthrough in the search for the origin of spindles emerged when McCormick and coworkers (Bal *et al.* 1995a,b, Kim *et al.* 1994, 1995, Lee and McCormick 1995, Lee *et al.* 1994, McCormick and Bal 1994, von Krosigk *et al.* 1993) discovered spontaneous spindle waves in ferret thalamic slices. When the excitation from TC to RE cells was blocked, either pharmacologically or by a knife cut, the oscillation disappeared. In addition, several other important phenomena were observed: 1. In intact slices (with no pharmacological manipulation of synaptic transmission), RE cells fire bursts almost at every cycle in coherence with the local population rhythm. TC cells fire bursts only at every two, three, or more cycles, again in phase with the local population rhythm (2:1 bursting mode). 2. The bursting pattern is hardly changed when the slow inhibitory

GABA$_B$ synapses are blocked. 3. When the fast inhibitory GABA$_A$ synapses are blocked, the activity pattern slows and changes form: the population frequency drops by about half, and both RE and TC cells fire prolonged bursts at almost every cycle (1:1 bursting mode). These oscillations are said to have absence seizure-like character (Adams and Victor 1981, von Krosigk *et al.* 1993). 4. When both GABA$_A$ and GABA$_B$ receptors are blocked, the network is quiescent. 5. Spindle episodes propagate with a slow velocity (around 1 mm/s).

Here we present a model of the RE-TC thalamic network (Golomb *et al.* 1995, 1996, Wang *et al.* 1995), that is consistent with the experimental results of McCormick and colleagues. The effects of both local and sparse connectivities are considered, and predictions are made regarding synaptic and circuitry properties.

1.3. Synchronized epileptic bursting in hippocampal area CA3

The hippocampus is a cortical structure, part of the limbic system, which is involved in memory formation and spatial learning. Neuronal activity in the hippocampus is highly synchronized during certain behavioral states and during epileptiform activity. Such synchronous activity includes rhythmical EEG waves, sharp waves and other EEG transients (both normal and pathological) and seizure discharges. As in the thalamus, the synchronous activity depends on the cell's intrinsic biophysical properties, the synaptic properties, and the network architecture (Getting 1989). Most isolated hippocampal cells are regular spiking cells, and the remaining are endogenous bursters (McCormick *et al.* 1985). We concentrate here on area CA3 of the hippocampus.

Cellular Properties. The functional role of intrinsic neuronal properties was demonstrated by Traub, Wong and coworkers (Traub *et al.* 1991, Traub and Miles 1991, Traub and Wong 1982). They developed a multi-compartmental model for the behavior of CA3 pyramidal neurons. As observed experimentally (Traub and Miles 1991, Traub and Wong 1982) the model exhibits low-frequency bursts endogenously or when small depolarizing current is injected; it fires tonically at high rate when the depolarizing current is strong.

Network properties. In partial epilepsy (interictal spike discharge in the EEG), thousands of neurons exhibit synchronized bursting. Similar network bursts can be created in hippocampus and cortex *in vitro* by blocking GABA$_A$ inhibition (Schwartzkroin and Prince 1978). Network models of

CA3 pyramidal cells were studied with all-to-all (or sparse, but geometry-independent) synaptic coupling (Traub *et al.* 1993, Traub and Miles 1991). In the simulations, as well as in the *in vitro* experiments, brief stimulation of a single cell in a resting network produces multiple synchronized population bursts. The fast excitatory AMPA synapses provide the dominant synchronizing mechanism in the model, while the slow excitatory NMDA synapses contribute to prolonging the bursting episode; for strong enough NMDA levels synchronized bursting repeats indefinitely. Propagation of waves in networks with one dimensional architecture and a synaptic coupling which decays exponentially with distance were studied by Traub and colleagues (Miles *et al.* 1988, Traub *et al.* 1993). With inhibition blocked, synchronous burst firing spreads throughout the neuron array. The velocity increases with the spatial extent of the excitatory connectivity.

The Traub model is rather complex and difficult to analyze. We review a first step towards a mathematical treatment for understanding CA3 pyramidal cells (Pinsky and Rinzel 1994). The Traub model is reduced from 19 to 2 compartments. The dynamical properties of the Pinsky–Rinzel (PR) model and the Traub model are found to be similar. Here we also study the wave-like behavior of the PR model with localized synaptic connectivity.

2. The models

2.1. Thalamic cells

Single cell models. The single cell models have only one compartment and are represented by coupled differential equations according to the Hodgkin-Huxley-type scheme. Sodium spike-generating currents are not included for simplicity. The equations and parameters of the model neurons are given in (Golomb *et al.* 1996).

RE CELL

$$C\frac{dV}{dt} = -I_{Ca-T} - I_{AHP} - I_{KL} - I_{NL} - I_{GABA-A}^{RR} - I_{AMPA} \,, \qquad (1)$$

where I_{Ca-T} is the low-threshold T-type calcium current, I_{AHP} is a calcium-activated potassium current and I_{KL} and I_{NL} are the potassium and non-specific leak currents respectively. I_{GABA-A}^{RR} is the GABA$_\mathbf{A}$ synaptic current an RE cell receives from other RE cells, and I_{AMPA} is the AMPA excitation an RE cell receives from TC cells.

TC CELL

$$C\frac{dV}{dt} = -I_{Ca-T} - I_h - I_{KL} - I_{NL} - I_{GABA-A} - I_{GABA-B} , \qquad (2)$$

where I_h is the slow "sag" current and the other currents are of the same types as in the RE cell, but with different gating kinetics, conductance strengths and reversal potentials. I_{GABA-A} and I_{GABA-B} are the GABA$_\mathbf{A}$ and GABA$_\mathbf{B}$ synaptic currents a TC cell receives from RE cells.

Synaptic models. The gating variables s for AMPA and GABA$_\mathbf{A}$ synapses, representing the fractions of open channels, are assumed to increase fast during a pre-synaptic burst and decay after it with a time constant of $\sim$ 10 ms. The dynamics of GABA$_\mathbf{B}$ synapses are different. GABA$_\mathbf{B}$ receptors are modeled as strongly nonlinear, and capable of eliciting a significantly stronger response to a prolonged burst than to a single spike or a short burst (Destexhe and Sejnowski 1995). The decay time of GABA$_\mathbf{B}$ inhibition following a burst is $\sim$ 100 ms.

Network architecture. The slice is treated as a one-dimensional array of cells. We assume that the synaptic coupling between two cells decays either exponentially or as a step function with the distance between them, with a characteristic length scale λ denoted as "synaptic footprint length". The footprint lengths λ_{RR}, λ_{RT} and λ_{TR} have subscripts denoting the type of the pre- and post-synaptic cells. In order to analyze the effects of sparseness we use also a second architecture in which each cell receives synaptic input from only a few other cells at random, independent of the cell's location.

Initial conditions. At time $t = 0$, all the neurons are at their rest state, except a few RE cells at the left end of the model slice that are depolarized to 0 mV. These neurons may recruit TC cells to burst and initiate a wave of activity.

2.2. Hippocampal cells

Single cell models. The single pyramidal cell model has two compartments. A soma-like compartment with potential V_s has fast currents for generating brief Na action potentials: sodium I_{Na} and delayed rectifier potassium I_{K-DR}. A dendrite-like compartment with potential V_d has slower currents: high-threshold (L-type) calcium current I_{Ca} and two types of calcium-dependent potassium currents, I_{K-C} and I_{K-AHP}. Both compartments have leak currents I_L, and the compartments are coupled electrically with strength

g_c; p is the proportion of the cell area taken up by the soma. The equations and parameters of the model neuron are given in (Pinsky and Rinzel *et al.* 1994).

$$C\frac{dV_s}{dt} = -I_L - I_{Na} - I_{K-DR} + \frac{g_c}{p}(V_d - V_s) , \qquad (3)$$

$$C\frac{dV_d}{dt} = -I_L - I_{Ca} - I_{K-C} - I_{K-AHP}$$

$$+\frac{1}{(1-p)}\left[g_c(V_s - V_d) - I_{AMPA} - I_{NMDA}\right] . \qquad (4)$$

The fast AMPA excitation and the slow NMDA excitation affect the dendritic compartment. There are no inhibitory synapses, since we are modeling the disinhibited slice preparation.

Synaptic models. One goal in building this hippocampal model is to confirm that results of Traub and colleagues can be duplicated with a significantly reduced model; one that can easily be implemented by other workers. Hence, we retain the synaptic model of Traub *et al.* (1992). AMPA and NMDA synaptic variables increase fast during a spike. The decay rates are 2 ms for AMPA and 150 ms for NMDA.

Network architecture. Pinsky and Rinzel (1994) examined networks of CA3 pyramidal cells in which the coupling does not depend on the distance between cells; each cell receives inputs from 20 out of 100 cells. Here we also study the case of local coupling. The synaptic conductance between two cells decays exponentially with the distance between them with a footprint length λ.

Initial conditions. All the cells are at rest at $t = 0$, except a few cells that initiate a wave.

3. Results

3.1. Thalamic cells

Single cell dynamics. The isolated RE and TC cells are conditional oscillators. With the reference parameter set they are at rest. However, depolarizing the RE cell or hyperpolarizing the TC cell may cause the cell to oscillate (McCormick 1992). Neuromodulators such as acetylcholine, norepinephrine and serotonin may affect the potassium leak conductance g_{KL} of RE and TC cells and change their dynamical states, as shown in Fig. 1. If the cell's rest potential is more depolarized than the (usually unstable) steady state in the oscillatory regime, the cell exhibits post-inhibitory rebound and bursts upon release from hyperpolarization (Jahnsen and Llinás 1984a,1984b); such is the case for our TC cells with the reference parameter set. If the rest potential is more hyperpolarized than the steady state in the oscillatory regime (as the RE cell with reference parameter set), the cell can be excited by synaptic excitation. The sodium action potentials that ride on the calcium burst are not included in our model.

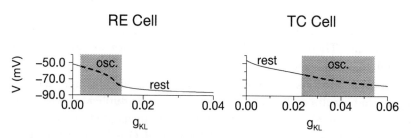

Figure 1: Dynamics of single RE and TC cell models. The resting membrane potential versus g_{KL} is represented by a solid line in the regimes where the rest state is stable and by a wide dashed line in the regime where it is unstable. The shaded areas represent the regime of endogenous oscillation. Bistability occurs in narrow regimes of overlap (on the right of the shaded area for the RE cell and on the left of the shaded area of the TC cell), where both the rest state and the periodic oscillations exist and are stable there. Adapted from Golomb *et al.* (1996).

Network dynamics. The coupled RE-TC network exhibits a traveling wave that recruits resting cells to participate in the spindle oscillation. In the tissue a spindle wanes after 2–4 seconds, but our model contains no waning mechanism. This wavefront propagates at a constant velocity and corresponds to a moving transition between spatial regions of two different activity levels: neurons ahead of the wavefront are at rest, and the others, behind it, are oscillating. The oscillations persist because TC cells rebound from inhibition and re-excite the RE cells. Then, the RE cells inhibit the TC cells again and de-inactivate the T-current, eliciting rebound bursts. Membrane potential traces of 8 RE and 8 TC neurons equally spaced along the slice are shown in Fig. 2. In the "intact" slice model, a 2:1 bursting mode is observed with population frequency of 10.1 Hz. RE cells tend to fire bursts simultaneously. TC cells burst every second cycle. The effect of blocking GABA$_A$ receptors is prominent. The population frequency drops to 4.15 Hz, and the bursting pattern changes to 1:1; both RE and TC cells now fire bursts at every cycle. If both $GABA_A$ and $GABA_B$ are blocked, or if the AMPA excitation is blocked, the neurons are quiescent and no wave propagation occurs (not shown). Thus our model is consistent with the six main experimental observations (Bal *et al.* 1995a,b, Kim *et al.* 1995).

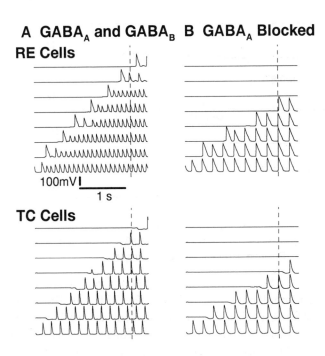

A $\mathbf{GABA_A}$ **and** $\mathbf{GABA_B}$ **B** $\mathbf{GABA_A}$ **Blocked**
RE Cells

100mV

1 s

TC Cells

Figure 2: Membrane potential time courses of 8 RE neurons and 8 TC neurons equally spaced along the slice. The vertical dashed lines help to show how TC and RE cells fire in a 2:1 bursting mode when both $GABA_A$ and $GABA_B$ are intact (A), and in a 1:1 bursting mode when $GABA_A$ is blocked (B). In (B), the phase shift between bursting neurons in this mode is close to zero for our reference parameter set. Adapted from Golomb *et al.* (1996).

As stated above, we may view the wavefront propagation as a recruitment process (Fig. 3). Here, we follow the recruitment process in the 1:1 state (with $GABA_A$ blocked), because in this mode the neuronal dynamics near the wavefront is relatively regular and repeats itself as the wave propagates. In

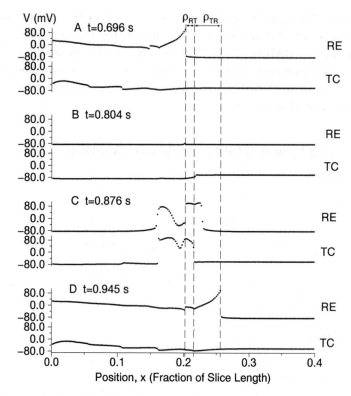

Figure 3: Analysis of the lurching wave. Snapshots of the spatial profile along the slice of cells' membrane potentials, taken at four different times within a recruitment cycle. The vertical dashed lines represent, from left to right, the wavefront position at subsequent steps of the recruitment cycle, corresponding to snapshots A, C and D respectively. A. RE cells fire a burst. B. RE cells are at rest, TC cells are hyperpolarized, including the cells within a distance ρ_{RT} ahead of the wavefront. C. TC cells within ρ_{RT} from the RE wavefront fire a rebound burst, and excite the RE cells. RE cells start to burst. D. RE cells at a distance of ρ_{TR} ahead of the TC wavefront fire a burst, and the cycle starts again. Adapted from Golomb *et al.* (1996).

each step of the cycle (RE bursting or TC bursting) we define the wavefront location as the position of the rightmost RE or TC cell (with the largest x) that bursts at this cycle. Suppose that at a certain time, RE cells behind the wavefront position have just fired a burst (Fig. 3A). These RE cells inhibit TC cells, including some within a distance (denoted by ρ_{RT}) in front of the wavefront position. The TC cells remain hyperpolarized for a certain time interval (Fig. 3B), until the T-current de-inactivates sufficiently and these TC cells fire a rebound burst (Fig. 3C). At that moment the wavefront position moves forward by ρ_{RT} in the TC cell population, hence ρ_{RT} is the RE-to-TC *recruitment length*. During the rebound burst the TC cells in turn excite RE cells within a distance ρ_{TR} of the rightmost TC cell that has just burst; ρ_{TR} is the TC-to-RE recruitment length (Fig. 3D). The wavefront position is moved by an additional distance ρ_{TR}, and the cycle starts again. Hence, the wavefront lurches forward instead of propagating continuously.

Numerical simulations have been performed in order to study the wavefront velocity's dependence on parameter values. Its dependence on the synaptic footprint length is presented in Fig. 4. The velocity is expressed as fraction of slice length per second. The velocity v_F changes only slightly with the AMPA

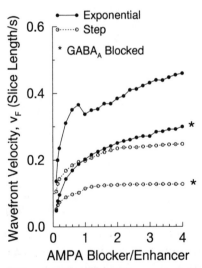

Figure 4: Dependence of the wavefront velocity v_F on the maximal synaptic conductances for AMPA, measured here as the ratio with respect to their respective reference values (unity corresponds to the standard parameter set); $\lambda_{RT} = \lambda_{TR} = 0.0156$. Filled circles: exponential footprint shape, Open circles: step footprint shape. Curves for the case with GABA$_A$ blocked are indicated by asterisks. In general, the wavefront propagation is accelerated by increasing the AMPA coupling strength, more significantly so for the exponential than for the step footprint shape. Adapted from Golomb *et al.* (1996).

synaptic coupling strength in the case of a step footprint shape, except for small g_{AMPA}. With an exponential footprint shape, the dependence of v_F on the coupling strength is more significant, and consistent with the estimated logarithmic relationship (Golomb *et al.* 1996). The steep drop in v_F for small g_{AMPA} is a result of the near-threshold behavior for the onset of network oscillations.

Introducing sparse connectivity into the network architecture causes both RE and TC cells to skip bursts (Wang *et al.* 1995). Still, synchrony is maintained even if the number of inputs each cell receives is not large (*i.e.*, between 5 and 10). We define the bursting ratio of a cell population to be the ratio between the population frequency and the average bursting rate. For example,

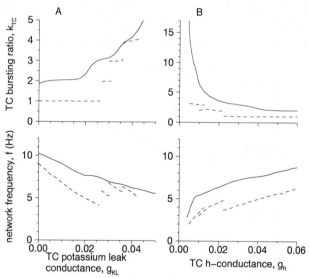

Figure 5: Dependence of the TC bursting ratio k_{TC} and the population frequency f on the potassium leak conductance g_{KL} (A) and g_h (B) in TC cells. Comparison for sparse coupling (each cell receives synaptic inputs from 10 cells of the other type at random, solid lines) and for all-to-all coupling (dashed line). The bursting ratio increases and the population frequency decreases with g_{KL} as the TC cells become more hyperpolarized. Distinct regimes are observed for all-to-all coupling, sparseness smoothes the transitions. With sparse coupling, the bursting ratio becomes large at small g_h values, as many neurons are quiescent and the remaining ones burst at low rates. Adapted from Wang *et al.* (1995).

in the 2:1 mode the bursting ratio of the TC population is 2 and that of the RE population is 1. While without sparseness the network usually bursts in a distinct mode (1:1, 2:1, 3:1 etc), the bursting ratios of the RE and TC populations in a sparse network do not have to be integers, and they vary continuously as the network parameters are changed. The dependence of the TC bursting mode and the population frequency on the TC potassium leak conductance g_{KL} and the TC sag conductance g_h is shown in Fig. 5. Increasing g_{KL} or decreasing g_h both cause bursting rate increase and frequency reduction. In a model without sparseness these magnitudes vary discontinuously.

3.2. Hippocampal cells

Single cell dynamics. The isolated hippocampal cell exhibits three prototypical repetitive behaviors in response to tonic somatic and dendritic input — periodic somatic spiking, very low frequency bursting and low frequency

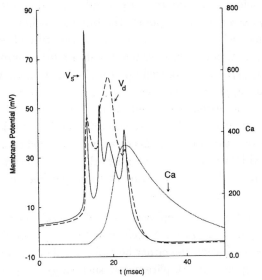

Figure 6: Time courses of somatic voltage, V_s, dendritic voltage, V_d, and dendritic calcium concentration Ca during a burst. Burst is initiated by somatic action potential which triggers a subthreshold dendritic Ca spike. This is followed by full Ca spike in the dendrite leading to somatic burst pattern. Dendritic spike, and hence burst, is terminated by I_{K-C} current which turns on when Ca reaches appreciable levels. Adapted from Pinsky and Rinzel (1994).

bursting. The soma and dendritic compartments, when uncoupled, can fire repetitively under constant stimulation, although the dendrite voltage spike is considerably longer in duration. When electrotonically coupled, these two spike generators give rise to complex spatiotemporal patterns and bursting. The burst is initiated by a sodium action potential in the soma which then triggers a dendritic calcium spike. The time courses of voltage and calcium variables during a burst are presented in Fig. 6. The electrotonic interaction between soma and dendrite involves significant coupling current that flows back and forth and results in a burst duration twice that of an isolated dendritic spike. The dendritic calcium spike, and hence the burst, is terminated by I_{K-C}.

Network dynamics We have investigated a network of hippocampal cells coupled by AMPA and NMDA synapses, first with *random sparse* coupling. The network exhibits a stable rest state. When it is stimulated by a brief current pulse, population oscillations may develop. The number of cycles that the network oscillates before returning to rest depends strongly on the level of NMDA conductance g_{NMDA}, which supports the bursting behavior, and the AHP conductance g_{AHP}, which tends to shut off the bursting (Fig. 7). For smaller g_{NMDA} the population response terminates after a finite number of cycles; for large enough g_{NMDA} synchronized bursting is maintained. While the bursting oscillations are approximately synchronized, they are not perfectly synchronized even for a homogeneous population. These simulation results are consistent with the analyses of Hansel *et al.* (1995) and of Pinsky (1995), showing that mutual excitation does not necessarily fully synchronize a neuronal network. After AMPA is blocked, the network rapidly desynchronizes; the primary mechanism for desynchronization at these parameter settings is that the NMDA-saturated orbit is chaotic.

With *local* synaptic interaction, depolarization of several neurons at one edge can lead to a propagating pulse of excitation (Fig. 8). Similar to the random sparse case, the oscillation can either be maintained or terminate after a certain time, depending on network parameters such as g_{NMDA} and g_{AHP}. The wave propagates at a constant velocity far from the edges, and therefore the first bursts of neurons are synchronized (with a phase shift). Synchrony is maintained during the first few cycles, but it is destroyed after that (if oscillations are maintained) because the synchronized state is not stable. The local dynamics of neurons is then aperiodic, probably chaotic.

We follow the recruitment process of neurons by the wave by plotting snapshots of all the cells' voltages at four different times (Fig. 9). At each time, quiescent cells are continuously recruited by the wavefront due to the excitatory effect of their neighbors. Behind the wavefront, the firing pattern of cells looks very similar at different times, but shifted in space.

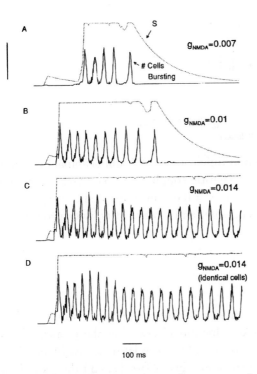

100 ms

Figure 7: Population burst patterns for a network of 100 cells with random sparse coupling for different values of NMDA conductance g_{NMDA}. The solid line represents the number of cells bursting, i.e., with $V_s > 20$ mV. The dotted line is the value of the synaptic variable $S(t)$ from a typical cell where $g_{NMDA}S(t)$ is the voltage independent part of I_{NMDA}. Vertical bar represents 50 cells (out of 100 in this simulation) or 50 S units. The number of population bursts increases with g_{NMDA}. Past a threshold g_{NMDA} level, bursting continues indefinitely. In panels A-C the heterogeneous network (10% variation in g_{Ca}) was used while in D the network is homogeneous, *i.e.*, identical cells. In each case the system was initially at rest when a single cell was stimulated with a brief excitatory input at $t = 0$. Adapted from Pinsky and Rinzel (1994).

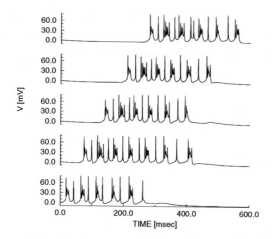

Figure 8: Membrane potential time courses of 5 hippocampal neurons equally spaced along the slice. The synaptic coupling between neurons decays exponentially with a space constant $\lambda = 0.06$ (in units of slice length). The slice is stimulated at the left hand side, and a wave of activity propagates to the right.

4. Discussion

In this Chapter we presented two biophysically-motivated, but minimal, models of neuronal networks. One model describes the propagation of spindle waves and so-called perverted absence seizure waves (Kim *et al.* 1995, von Krosigk *et al.* 1993) in thalamic slice networks, and the second describes paroxysmal (*"in vitro* epileptic"*) wave propagation in CA3 hippocampal slices. The wavefront velocity of thalamic waves is about 1 mm/sec, whereas the wavefront velocity of hippocampal waves is 100 times faster. In both models, the collective dynamical patterns were investigated mainly by numerical simulations. The thalamic model mimics successfully the main experimental observation from thalamic slices (Golomb *et al.* 1996), and the hippocampal model yields results similar to the Traub 19-compartment model (Traub and Miles 1991, Traub *et al.* 1991, 1992, 1993). These examples demonstrate the importance of such models in reproducing several experimental observations together, understanding the dynamical mechanisms behind these observations, and predicting the results of new experiments, as reported in Golomb *et al.*

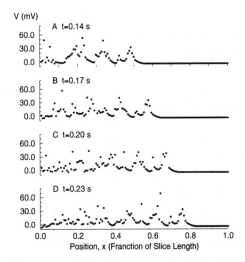

Figure 9: Analysis of the continuous wave. The parameters are the same as in Fig. 8. Snapshots of the spatial profile along the slice of cells' membrane potentials, taken at four different times. At each time step, new cells are recruited by the wave under the effect of the nearby, already bursting neurons. Except for a shift to the right, the network (spatial) profile of neuronal firing patterns is similar at subsequent times. The four snapshots are at arbitrary times, not chosen specially to be at the same phase of subsequent oscillation cycles.

(1996). Our models take into account the essential biophysics of neurons and synapses. Further reduced descriptions, such as firing rate models, are typically too incomplete to allow for understanding effects of synaptic kinetic time scales and phenomena such as post-inhibitory rebound.

Our thalamic model demonstrates the lurching, discontinuous characteristics of the recruitment process. Aspects of the wavefront propagation are affected by both intrinsic and network properties. The wavefront velocity is limited by the post-inhibitory rebound properties of TC cells (intrinsic), and by the spatially localized synaptic footprints (network) (Golomb *et al.* 1996). The wave speed increases linearly with the footprint lengths but only gradually with the synaptic coupling strengths, and it decreases gradually with enhanced hyperpolarization of the RE cell population.

The hippocampal model exhibits a continuous recruitment process. As in the thalamic slice, the wavefront velocity depends linearly on the synaptic footprint length. However, the dependence of the velocity on the synaptic strength is much stronger and close to being linear (data not shown).

The reason for this difference in propagation characteristics is that the velocity of thalamic waves is restricted because of the post-inhibitory rebound mechanism. The recruitment occurs in cycles. At each cycle, the recruitment length (or the number of cells that are recruited into the wave) is determined by the anatomic footprint length and shape. For a step footprint shape, the recruitment length must be smaller than the footprint length, and for an exponential footprint shape it depends only logarithmically on the synaptic strength (Golomb *et al.* 1996). In contrast, the notion of "recruitment cycle" is meaningless in the context of the hippocampal network, despite the fact that behind the wavefront the system oscillates, and the recruitment is done continuously. When the synaptic coupling is stronger, quiescent cells in front of the wave are affected by stronger excitation and therefore burst more rapidly. The excitatory recruitment mechanism still needs to be compared with experimental results about wave propagation in hippocampus and neocortex (Chervin *et al.* 1988, Wadman and Gutnick 1993). On the other hand, it should be mathematically analyzed using even simpler neuronal models, such as integrate-and-fire models (see Ermentrout and McLeod 1993, Idiart and Abbott 1993).

At this state, we have modeled *in vitro* preparations. Our results about the circuitry and dynamical mechanisms in thalamus and hippocampus illuminate the range of behaviors of brain tissues more generally and may play a role in the understanding of the more complicated *in vivo* preparations during information processing, sensory and motor tasks.

Acknowledgments

We are grateful to B. Ermentrout, M. Gutnick, D. Hansel, P. Pinsky and X.-J. Wang for helpful discussion.

References

Adams, R.D., and Victor, D. *Principles of Neurology*, 2nd edition, McGraw-Hill, New-York, 1981.

Bal., T., von Krosigk, M., and McCormick, D.A. *J. Physiol. (Lond.)* **483**, 641-663, 1995a.

Bal., T., von Krosigk, M., and McCormick, D.A. *J. Physiol. (Lond.)* **483**, 665-685, 1995b.

Chervin, R.D., Pierce, P.A., and Connors, B.W. *J. Neurophysiol.* **60**, 1695-1713, 1988.

Coulter, D.A., Huguenard, J.R., and Prince, D.A. *Neurosci. Lett.* **98**, 74-78, 1989.

Coulter, D.A., Huguenard, J.R., and Prince, D.A. *Br. J. Pharmacol.* **100**, 800-806, 1990.

Deschênes, M., Paradis, M., Roy, J. P., and Steriade, M. *J. Neurophysiol.* **51**, 1196-1219, 1984.

Destexhe, A., and Sejnowski, T.J. *Proc. Natl. Acad. Sci. (USA)*, in press, 1995.

Ermentrout, G.B., and McLeod, J.B. *Proc. Royal Society of Edinburgh* 123A: 461-478, 1993.

Getting, P.A. *Ann. Rev. Neurosci.* , **12**, 185-204, 1989.

Golomb, D., Wang, X.-J., and Rinzel, J. In *The Neurobiology of Computation*, Jim Bower Ed., Boston, MA: Kluwer, 215-220, 1995.

Golomb, D., Wang, X.-J., and Rinzel, J. *J. Neurophysiol.*, in press, 1996.

Hansel, D., Mato, G., and Meunier, C. *Neural Comp.* **7**, 307-337, 1995.

Huguenard, J.R., and Prince, D.A. *J. Neurophysiol.* **71**, 2576-2581, 1994a.

Huguenard, D.A., and Prince, D.A. *J. Neurosci.* **14**, 5485-5502, 1994b.

Idiart, M.A.P., and Abbott, L.F. *Network* 4:285-294, 1993.

Jahnsen, H., and Llinás, R. R. *J. Physiol. (Lond.)* **349**, 205-226, 1984a.

Jahnsen, H., and Llinás, R. R. *J. Physiol. (Lond.)* **349**, 227-247, 1984b.

Kim, U., Bal, T., and McCormick, D.A. *Neuroscience Abstr.* **20**, 133, 1994.

Kim, U., Bal, T., and McCormick, D.A. *J. Neurophysiol.* **74**, 1301-1323, 1995.

Lee, K., Bal, T., and McCormick, D.A. *Neuroscience Abstr.* **20**, 133, 1994.

Lee, K.H., and McCormick, D.A. *J. Neurophysiol.* **73**, 2123-2128, 1995.

Leresche, N., Lightowler, S., Soltesz, I., Jassik-Gerschenfeld, D. and Cruneli, V. *J. Physiol. (Lond.)*, **441**, 155-174, 1991.

Lytton, W.W., and Sejnowski, T.J. *Ann. Neurol.* **32**, 131-139, 1992.

McCormick, D.A. in neuromodulation of thalamocortical activity. *Progress in Neurobiology* **39**, 337-388, 1992.

McCormick, D.A., and Bal, T. *Current Opinion in Neurobiology* **4**, 550-556, 1994.

McCormick, D. A., and Pape, H.-C. *J. Physiol.* **431** 291-318, 1990.

McCormick, D.A., Connors, B.W., Lighthall, J.W., and Prince, D.A. *J. Neurophysiol.* **54**, 782-806, 1985.

Miles, R., Traub, R.D., and Wong, R.K.S. *J. Neurophysiol.* **60**, 1481-1496, 1988.

Morison, R.S., and Bassett, D.L. *J. Neurophysiol.* **8**, 309-314, 1945.

Pinsky, P.F. *SIAM J. on Applied Math.* **55**, 220-241, 1995.

Pinsky, P.F. and Rinzel, J. *J. Comp. Neurosci.* , **1**, 39-60, 1994.

Schwartzkroin, P.A., and Prince, D.A. *Brain Research* **147**, 117-130, 1978.

Steriade, M., and Deschênes, M. *Brain Res. Rev.* **8**, 1-63, 1984.

Steriade, M., Deschênes, M., Domich, L., and Mulle, C. *J. Neurophysiol.* **54**, 1473-1479, 1985.

Steriade, M., Domich, L., Oakson, G., and Deschênes, M. *J. Neurophysiol.* **57** 260-273, 1987.

Steriade, M., Jones, E.G., and Llinás, R.R. *Thalamic Oscillations and Signaling*, New York: John Wiley, 1990.

Traub, R.D., and Miles, R. *Neural Networks of the Hippocampus.* Cambridge University Press, Cambridge, 1991.

Traub, R.D., Miles, R., and Buzsaki, G. *J. Physiol. (Lond.)* **451**, 653-672, 1992.

Traub, R.D., Miles, R., and Jeffery, J.G.R. *J. Physiol. (Lond.)* **461**, 525-547, 1993.

Traub, R.D., and Wong, R.K.S. *Science* **216**, 745-747, 1982.

Traub, R.D., Wong, R.M., Miles, R., and Michelson, H. J. Neurophysiol. **66**, 635-650, 1991

von Krosigk, M., Bal, T., and McCormick, D.A. *Science* **261**, 361-364, 1993.

Wadman, W.J., and Gutnick, M.J. *Neuroscience* **52**, 255-262, 1993.

Wang, X.-J., Golomb, D., and Rinzel, J. *Proc. Natl. Acad. Sci. USA*, **92**, 5577-5581, 1995.

A NEURAL NETWORK MODEL FOR KINDLING OF FOCAL EPILEPSY

Mayank R. Mehta
ARL Division of NSMA, University of Arizona
Tucson AZ, 85724 5115
E-mail: Mayank@NSMA.Arizona.EDU

Chandan Dasgupta
Department of Physics and
Jawaharlal Nehru Center for Advanced Scientific Research
Indian Institute of Science, Bangalore 560012, India
E-mail: cdgupta@physics.iisc.ernet.in

Gautam R. Ullal
Department of Physiology
M. S. Ramaiah Medical College, Bangalore 560054, India

Abstract

Various aspects of kindling — the phenomenon of generating epileptic seizures by means of repeated electrical or chemical stimulations — are modeled using a simple neural network. The model incorporates a number of biologically relevant features such as synaptic specificity, low average activity, synaptic delays and synaptic refractoriness. We argue that kindling of epilepsy occurs due to the formation of a large number of excitatory synaptic connections through a Hebbian learning mechanism. Several experimentally observed phenomena, such as the initial rapid growth and eventual saturation of the amplitude and duration of the afterdischarge, the insensitivity of the rate of kindling to the amplitude of the stimulus, drop in afterdischarge threshold due to repeated stimulations, and frequency dependence of kindling rate, are qualitatively reproduced by simulations of the model and explained. We show that one of the reasons for the termination of epileptic afterdischarge is that the neuronal network gets trapped in 'normal', low activity attractors of the network dynamics. It is argued that the first subthreshold shock induced afterdischarge is caused by the linking of originally present low activity attractors via stimulus driven synapse formation. New experiments, which would test the validity of the proposed mechanism of kindling and shed some light on the nature of memory storage in the brain, are suggested.

1. Introduction

Neural networks (Amit 1989, Rumelhart and McClelland 1986) exhibit many functional properties of the brain, such as associative memory, learning, fault tolerant computing etc. This has made neural networks a popular model for understanding the functioning of the brain. To this end it is desirable to construct realistic neural network models and use these models to understand some of the experimentally observed neurobiological phenomena.

In this work we study kindling (Delgado and Sevillano 1961, Goddard *et al* 1969, Lothman *et al* 1991, McNamara 1989) using neural networks. Kindling is the phenomenon of generating epileptic seizures by repeated stimulations of some part of the brain. The stimuli can be electrical pulses or microinjections of chemicals. This phenomenon has been extensively studied for the last thirty years. It is believed that an understanding of kindling would lead to new insights into the nature and causes of epilepsy.

We first summarize some of the experimental observations which we later model. In the resting state, the brain has low activity and the cortical electroencephalograph (EEG) signal is often rhythmic. If a large electrical stimulus is applied to some region of the brain, say the hippocampus, the resulting EEG shows spikes which indicate increased and synchronous neuronal activity. Such a spiky EEG is called an afterdischarge (AD) (Lothman *et al* 1991). The smallest amplitude of the stimulus which yields an AD on the first application is called the AD threshold. Stimuli of larger amplitude are called suprathreshold. If the stimulus amplitude is small, it takes a large number of these so called subthreshold stimuli to elicit an AD. Once an AD is elicited, repeated applications of the (supra or subthreshold) stimuli lead to an initial rapid increase in the AD amplitude and duration. These parameters quickly reach saturation values and further stimulations produce only a slow increase in them. The poststimulus AD at this stage is also accompanied by epileptic seizures. This is the kindled state. The kindled state is permanent, i.e. a stimulation of the subject after a prolonged absence of stimuli immediately leads to a seizure (Goddard *et al* 1969). The rate of kindling depends on various parameters. It has been observed that the number of ADs needed to reach the kindled state is fairly insensitive to the amplitude of the stimulus (Lothman *et al* 1991, McNamara 1989, Racine 1972b). The AD threshold falls rapidly with repeated elicitation of ADs (Racine 1972a).

The kindling rate is sensitive to the frequency of the stimulus (Cain 1981, Cain and Corcoran 1981). If the amplitude and the number of pulses of the stimulating signal are kept constant, the number of ADs needed to reach the kindled state is larger for high frequencies than for low frequencies.

Kindling has also been produced by repeated topical administration of chemicals such as penicillin (Prince 1968) which suppress the action of inhibitory neurotransmitter such as γ-amino butyric acid (GABA). This phenomenon is known as chemical kindling. The phenomenology of chemical kindling is similar to that of electrical kindling described above.

A simple neural network model for kindling was set up and the stimulus amplitude dependence of the kindling rate was studied in Mehta *et al* (1993). In this work we present a detailed study of this neural network model and discuss the modeling of other kindling related phenomena mentioned above.

In Section 2 we discuss the biological motivations for setting up the basic neural network model and describe the way it functions. The results of computer simulations of various phenomena studied using this model are presented in the following Sections. Electrical kindling and its amplitude dependence is discussed in Section 3. Dependence of the AD threshold on the number of stimuli is presented in Section 4 and the frequency dependence of kindling in Section 5. Chemical kindling is described in Section 6. Section 7 contains a discussion of the main results and conclusions.

2. The Neural Network Model

The neural network model studied in this work is the one developed in Mehta *et al* (1993). We briefly describe the motivation and structure of the neural network model. The details may be found in Mehta *et al* (1993). The high or low firing rate of a neuron i is represented by a McCulloch-Pitts (McCulloch and Pitts 1943) variable S_i which takes corresponding values 1 or 0. The subscript i takes values from 1 to N, where N is the number of excitatory neurons. The network satisfies Dale's hypothesis (Eccles 1964) which states that the afferent synapses from a neuron are either all excitatory or all inhibitory. The network also incorporates time delays which are inherent in the signal transmission between different neurons (Kleinfeld and Sompolinsky 1988). All the inhibitory neurons are collectively modeled by a background inhibition which is proportional to the number of excitatory neurons firing at that time. A Hebbian learning rule (Hebb 1949) is also incorporated for the excitatory synapses.

The fast excitatory synapses are denoted by J_{ij} and the slow or delayed excitatory synapses are denoted by K_{ij}. The state of a neuron depends on the net postsynaptic potential, which is a sum of fast and slow excitatory and inhibitory inputs. This is called a local field h_i and is given by

$$h_i(t) = \sum_{j=1}^{N} [\{J_{ij}S_j(t) - wS_j(t)\} + \lambda\{K_{ij}S_j(t-\tau) - wS_j(t-\tau)\}]. \qquad (1)$$

Various terms in this equation are explained below. The transmission delays, which can be of various lengths, are modeled for simplicity by a delay of fixed length τ. The strength of delayed signals, relative to that of the fast signals, is given by λ. $S_i(t)$ is the state of the neuron i at a time t and $S_i(t-\tau)$ is the state of the same neuron at an earlier time $t-\tau$. Further, w ($0 < w < 1$) is the averaged strength of inhibition. The net inhibitory input is assumed to be proportional to the total number of excitatory neurons firing ($= \sum_{i=1}^{N} S_i(t)$ or $\sum_{i=1}^{N} S_i(t-\tau)$ for fast or slow inhibitory synapses respectively).

A number, q, of random low activity patterns $\xi_i^\mu (i = 1, \cdots, N; \mu = 1, \cdots, q;$ each $\xi_i^\mu = 0$ or 1) are initially stored in the fast and slow excitatory synapses of the network. Low values of average activity are guaranteed by choosing $u^\mu = \sum_{i=1}^{N} \xi_i^\mu$ to be small, of the order of $N/20$, for all μ. These patterns are encoded in the synapses as follows.

$$\begin{aligned} J_{ij} &= 1 \; if \; \sum_{\mu=1}^{q} \xi_i^\mu \xi_j^\mu > 0 \;\; (i \neq j) \\ J_{ij} &= 0 \; \text{otherwise.} \\ J_{ii} &= 0 \end{aligned} \qquad (2)$$

$$\begin{aligned} K_{ij} &= 1 \; if \; \sum_{\mu=1}^{q} \xi_i^{\mu+1} \xi_j^\mu > 0 \;\; (i \neq j) \\ K_{ij} &= 0 \; \text{otherwise} \\ K_{ii} &= 0 \end{aligned} \qquad (3)$$

with $\xi_i^{q+1} = \xi_i^1$.

As in the Willshaw (Willshaw *et al* 1969) model, the synaptic strengths take only two values, 1 or 0. This is clearly an idealization, meant to simplify analysis. In fact, even if one used the usual Hebbian prescription for encoding patterns, i.e. $J_{ij} = \sum_{\mu=1}^{q} \xi_i^\mu \xi_j^\mu$, for a small number of random low activity patterns, very few J_{ij}s will differ from 1 or 0 and hence eqns 2 and 3 are a good approximation. Further, the Willshaw model is particularly suited for storage and retrieval of low activity patterns (Golomb *et al* 1990).

Given various excitatory and inhibitory inputs to a neuron, it fires or does not fire depending on whether the total input is excitatory or inhibitory. This is modeled by the following update rule for the state of the neuron, $S_i(t+1)$ at a time $t+1$.

Rule 1 *If the local field $h_i(t) \geq 0$ make $S_i(t+1) = 1$, and if $h_i(t) < 0$ make $S_i(t+1) = 0$.*

Note that we have assumed that a neuron fires even if the net excitatory and inhibitory inputs cancel out. That is, we have taken the threshold for firing to have a small negative value, corresponding to small spontaneous activity exhibited by neurons *in vivo*. The updates are performed asynchronously, in a random sequence.

Whenever a neuron fires, all the afferent synapses release neurotransmitters, which lead to excitatory or inhibitory inputs in the postsynaptic neuron. If a neuron fires rapidly for a long time t_{max}, the neurotransmitters in the synapses get exhausted and the synapse becomes refractory for a period t_{ref} (Guyton 1986), during which these neurotransmitters are slowly replenished. Activation of the neuron during this period leads to the release of the accumulated small stock and its quick exhaustion. The synapse will then be refractory for a further period t_{ref}. Since we have modeled synaptic efficacies by 1 or 0, even if a neuron fires during t_{ref}, the small release of neurotransmitters is approximated by saying that the afferent synapse contributes nothing to the local field of the postsynaptic neuron. This sort of refractoriness of a synapse, say $A_{ij}(= J_{ij} or K_{ij})$, is modeled by the following rule.

Rule 2 *If a synapse A_{ij} is active for a period t_{max}, then it contributes nothing to the local field h_i for a following period t_{ref}. If the synapse is activated at any time during the period t_{ref}, it remains refractory for a further period t_{ref} from that instant.*

Thus we have some hysteresis in the synaptic refractoriness algorithm. Since we have modeled the inhibitory neurons by a background inhibition, we ignore refractoriness of any synapse related to the inhibitory neurons.

We also incorporate a Hebb like learning rule (Hebb 1949) in the excitatory synapses of our network. As we will see, the following learning rule plays a very important role in our model of kindling.

Rule 3 *If, over a certain period, $S_i = 1$ and $S_j = 1$ more often than some average value, make the synaptic strength $J_{ij} = 1$.*

Biologically, Hebbian learning may be manifested in formation of new synapses, activation of existing but inactive synapses and/or strengthening of existing active synapses (Sutula *et al* 1988, Gustafsson and Wigstrom 1988, Ben-Ari and Represea 1990, Geinisman, Morrell and Toledo-Morrell 1988). Since we have modeled synaptic efficacies by 1 or 0, these different processes are modeled in rule 3 by changing the value of a synapse from 0 to 1. A neuron can affect another neuron directly via a synaptic connection or indirectly via a long path involving other neurons. The direct connections are modeled here by the fast synapses and the indirect ones are the slow synapses of our model. A Hebbian learning mechanism, which is local, is therefore included in our model only for the fast synapses and not for the slow synapses.

In the absence of external stimulations, the above network models the resting brain. The stimulations (chemical or electrical) are modeled as follows. Chemical stimuli such as penicillin suppress inhibitory neurotransmitters for some time. This can be modeled by reducing the relative strength of inhibition w throughout the network to $(w - s)$ for some time, where $0 < s < w$ is the strength of the chemical stimulus, measured in the same units as w.

The electric shocks affect the network in two ways. The injection of positive current induces the neurons to fire whereas the injection of negative current tends to reduce neuronal activity. Thus neurons near one of the electrodes would be hyperexcitable and those near the other would be hypoexcitable. For a biphasic pulse, the effect during the second half of the pulse would be the reverse of the effect during the first half.

Thus electric pulses of amplitude $s(0 < s < w)$ are modeled by changing the weight of inhibition to $w - s(w + s)$ for the neurons near +ve (–ve) electrodes and leaving it unchanged, i.e. equal to w in the rest of the network. [1]

Let us now discuss the time evolution of such a network. Consider a network in the absence of stimulations. Various parameters (i.e. number of patterns q, average activity of the stored patterns u, weight of inhibition w, strength of the delayed signal λ and delay time τ) are chosen such that the network performs stable, smooth, low activity oscillations in the resting state. The state of a neuron S_i now evolves as follows. If the state of the neuron at a time $t - \tau$ coincides with the νth stored pattern, i.e. if $S_j(t - \tau) = \xi_j^\nu$ for all j, then due to the structure of the slow synapses K_{ij} (eqn 3), the terms enclosed by the second set of curly brackets in eqn 1 yield a net +ve (–ve) contribution to h_i if

---

[1] The effect of an electrical stimulus is therefore similar to that of a chemical stimulus, in that the relative strength of inhibition changes in both the cases. The difference lies in the fact that while most chemical stimuli either increase or decrease the strength of inhibition, the electrical stimuli do both. Also the shortest duration for which the electrical stimuli can be applied is much smaller than that for chemical stimuli. Finally, the effect of electrical stimuli can be localized in a much smaller region than that for chemical stimuli.

$\xi_i^{\nu+1} = 1$ (0), i.e. if i is (is not) one of the active neurons in the pattern $\xi_i^{\nu+1}$. If simultaneously $S_j(t) = \xi_j^{\nu+1}$ for all j, then the contribution of the fast synapses, i.e. of the terms in the first set of curly brackets in eqn 1 also yields a +ve (−ve) contribution for h_i if $\xi_i^{\nu+1} = 1(0)$. Thus $S_i(t+1) = \xi_i^{\nu+1}$ for all i, i.e. the system converges to the pattern $\xi_i^{\nu+1}$. After a period τ the delayed state becomes $\xi_i^{\nu+1}$ and the slow synapses will try to push the network state to $\xi_i^{\nu+2}$. However, the fast synapses will try to keep the network in the state $\xi_i^{\nu+1}$. If the relative strength λ of the delayed signals is greater than 1, the delayed contribution will be greater than the fast signal and the state of the network will quickly converge to $\xi_i^{\nu+2}$. Thus for $\lambda > 1$ and for $\tau >$ the time required to converge to the next pattern, the network goes through all the stored patterns sequentially, leading to stable periodic oscillations. If one monitors the total activity of the network, it oscillates smoothly with a period $q\tau$. The firing pattern of individual neurons also varies with a period $q\tau$. Evidently, if the stored patterns have similar activities, the total activity will vary with a smaller period, of the order of τ.

Rhythmic oscillations of the net activity can also be generated without the slow excitatory synapses K_{ij}, i.e. a model with only fast excitation and both fast and slow inhibition. In that case, the network would exhibit random (rather than sequential) transitions between the patterns stored in J_{ij}. However, in order to reproduce some of the observed phenomenology of kindling, the slow excitatory synapses appear to be essential.

Except for a small time, during which the network shifts from one stored pattern to the next one, the firing pattern of the network corresponds to one of the stored patterns. Hence the J_{ij} corresponding to $S_iS_j = 1$ are already equal to 1 (eqn. 2). Therefore almost no new synapses are formed during the resting state. Also, since the time the network spends in each memory state is assumed to be smaller than t_{max}, the synaptic refractoriness does not come into play.

Although the model described above is far too simple to be considered realistic for any region of the brain, it is interesting to note that the basic features incorporated in the model are believed to be present in the hippocampus. The hippocampus is known to be centrally involved in the acquisition and storage of memories (Squire et al 1989). The occurrence of Hebbian synaptic modifications in hippocampal slices has been demonstrated by long-term potentiation experiments (Kelso et al 1986). The sparse connectivity among the excitatory neurons assumed in our model is similar to the connectivity among the CA3 pyramidal cells of the hippocampus (Squire et al 1989). A neural network model proposed recently (Gibson and Robinson 1992) as a realization of Marr's ideas (Marr 1971) about memory storage in the hippocampus has several features (sparse connections among excitatory neurons, clipped Hebbian synapses, inhibition proportional to the net activity of the excitatory neurons) in common with our model. Storage of temporal sequences of patterns has recently been proposed (Reiss and Taylor 1991) as one of the many possible activities that may be performed by the hippocampus. The time delay mechanism assumed in this work for the storage of temporal sequences is similar to that incorporated in our model. Finally, the synaptic refractoriness incorporated in our model is similar to that assumed in earlier modeling (Knowles *et al* 1985) of the hippocampal slice.

The maximum number of patterns q that can be stored such that the network performs stable oscillations depends on the relative strength of inhibition w, the average activity u of the patterns and the relative strength λ of the delayed signal. This dependence has been worked out, using the techniques of statistical mechanics, for a simpler model where there are no delays (i.e. the terms in the second set of curly brackets in eqn. 1 are absent), no synaptic refractoriness and no dynamic learning (Golomb *et al* 1990). It is very difficult to do the same calculations for the present model, due to the presence of delays, synaptic refractoriness and learning. We have studied this dependence using computer simulations.

The network described above was simulated using a system of 200 neurons. The neurons were updated sequentially in a random fashion. The time needed for one pass (i.e. random sequential update of all the neurons) was chosen to be the unit of time. In the absence of shocks, it was found that about 40 patterns, each with only about 10 neurons firing, could be stored in a stable fashion. The optimum value of the weight w, for the above choice of parameters, was found to be around 0.6-0.7. We chose the number of patterns $q = 20$, $\lambda = 2$ and $w = 0.6$. The delay period τ was chosen to be equal to that needed for two passes. A synapse could continuously fire for a period $t_{max} = 10$ passes after which it was refractory for a period t_{ref}, which was chosen randomly between 6 and 12 passes. We used a learning rule in which two neurons have to fire at least three times in the last ten passes to form a new synapse between the two. External shocks were assumed to change the local fields of two distinct groups of 20 neurons near the two electrodes. Each electrical pulse lasted for two passes and the interpulse interval T was varied from 6 passes to 20 passes.

Figure 1 shows a typical time evolution of the network in the absence of any external stimulus. The network was started off in the memory state ξ_i^1 at $t = 0$. The bottom panel shows the time evolution of the overlaps of the network with the first five memory states, $m^\mu(t) = (\sum_{i=1}^N \xi_i^\mu S_i(t))/(S_{up}(t)), \mu = 1, 2, \cdots, 5, S_{up}(t) = \sum_{i=1}^N S_i(t)$. The sequence of transitions, $\mu = 1 \to 2 \to 3 \to 4 \to 5$, is clearly seen. The top panel shows the variation of the net activity,

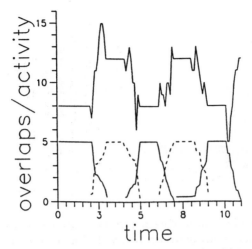

Figure 1: Overlap of the state of the network $(m^\mu(t), \mu = 1, 2, 3, 4, 5,$ multiplied by 5) with the first five stored patterns are shown in the bottom panel as a function of time or number of passes. The top panel shows the resulting small amplitude oscillations of the net activity $S_{up}(t)$. The network was started off in the state ξ_i^1 at a time t=0.

$S_{up}(t)$, of the network during the same period.

The pyramidal neurons in the superficial layers of the cortex and in the hippocampus are arranged parallel to each other, with their dendritic arborizations pointing in the same direction [2] The injection of synaptic currents would make the excitatory neurons act like electrical dipoles and the EEG would be preportional to the sum of synaptic currents flowing into these neurons.

In the neural network language, the sum of excitatory and inhibitory inputs to a given neuron is equal to the local field h_i (eqn. (1)). Thus the EEG is modeled by the sum of local fields $H = \sum_i h_i$, where the sum runs over all the neurons near the measuring electrode. Since only a small fraction of the neurons fire in the resting state, there is more net inhibition than excitation; hence H is always −ve. When a large number of neurons fire simultaneously, there is less inhibition and H is less −ve or even +ve. During an AD, when the activity drops to very low values (due to delayed inhibition, see next Section), H drops to large −ve values, much smaller than the resting value. Thus in the neural network language, the plot of H vs time corresponds to the (−ve of) unipolar

---

[2]The inhibitory neurons do not exhibit such orderly arrangement.

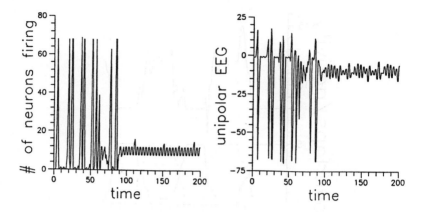

Figure 2: (a) The number of neurons firing ($S_{up}(t)$) is plotted as a function of time for an AD obtained from a kindled network. The AD lasts for 90 passes. The last part of the plot correspond to the resting state. (b) The sum of local fields near one electrode ($H_1 = \sum_i S_i$, with the sum running over the neurons near the electrode) is plotted as a function of time (for the same event as in Figure 2a). This corresponds to a unipolar EEG.

EEG.

Thus the EEG or H are clearly related to the number of neurons firing. This is illustrated in Figures 2a and 2b where we have shown the variation of both S_{up} and H over a short segment of the time evolution of a kindled network (see below). The similarity between the two graphs is evident. So, in our study, we have used S_{up} as a measure of the EEG signal. Note that S_{up} counts the number of active excitatory neurons. Since in our simplified description of the inhibitory neurons, the net activity of the inhibitory neurons is assumed to be proportional to S_{up}, inclusion of this would correspond to an overall scale factor which is unimportant.

If the stored patterns have slightly different activities, the total activity varies by small amounts as the network goes through the patterns in the resting state (see Figure 1). According to the arguments above, this leads to a low amplitude smooth and rhythmic EEG, similar to that observed experimentally in the absence of any external stimulation.

3. Electrical Kindling

In our study of electrical kindling, different subjects (modeled using networks with different realizations of initial patterns ξ^μ) were given shocks with different amplitude and frequency, depending on the phenomenon being studied. For all values of frequency and amplitude, the number of pulses given in one "session" was kept fixed at 35 and each biphasic pulse lasted for 2 passes. The network was then allowed to relax without any external stimulation for 160 passes. It was then reset to a resting state and this 'schedule' was repeated sixty times (each application of the shock will be referred to as one 'day' in the actual experiment). The following parameters were monitored as a function time: the EEG (which is represented by the net activity of the network $S_{up}(t)$), the total number of excitatory synaptic connections, J_{ij}, in the block of neurons which feel the shock (J_{shock}), in the block of neurons which do not feel the shock ($J_{noshock}$), and in the block connecting the above two blocks of neurons (J_{cross}). The total number of synapses is denoted by $J_{sum} = J_{shock} + J_{noshock} + J_{cross}$.

3.1 Suprathreshold Shocks

As discussed earlier, the effect of electric shocks is modeled by increasing (decreasing) the weight of inhibition near the -ve (+ve) electrode. If the amplitude of the shock is large, there will be a significant change in the weight of inhibition. This will lead to turning on (off) of a large number of neurons near the +ve (-ve) electrode. During the resting state, only a few neurons fire at any instant of time. The effect of the -ve electrode will be to turn off a fraction of these in its vicinity. This is a very small number. Thus the net effect of a large biphasic pulse is to turn on greater than average number of neurons, most of which are located near the electrodes.

When the first pulse is over, the weights of inhibition return to the resting value. However, after a period τ, the delayed state corresponds to the large activity state. Due to sparse coding, very few K_{ij} are nonzero. Hence, for a large activity state $S_i(t-\tau)$, the contribution from delayed excitation $\sum_j K_{ij} S_j(t-\tau)$ is much less than the delayed inhibition $(-w \sum_j S_j(t-\tau))$. The net result is an excess delayed inhibition, which tends to switch off most of the neurons. Thus, once the pulse is switched off, the total activity drops rapidly, from a large value to a very small value, after a period τ. After another period of time τ, the delayed state (as well as the present state) corresponds to one with very low activity. Hence the net inputs are mostly zero. Since we have assumed that neurons exhibit spontaneous firing, although there is no excitatory input on any neuron, some S_is become 1. The activity of the network now starts rising slowly. Since the delayed inputs are still mostly equal to zero, the network evolution is now largely governed by the fast synapses. At this stage two things can happen. First, if the state S_i of the network has a large overlap with one of the stored patterns, then due to the absence of the delayed inputs, the fast synapses immediately trap the network into the corresponding low activity state. After this, as described before, the network again starts performing smooth low activity oscillations. If on the other hand, the state of the network does not have a large overlap with one pattern, the activity keeps rising above the average value and the entire process discussed above repeats, till the network gets trapped into one of the attractors in J_{ij}.

During this process, a set of neurons which do not correspond to any stored pattern fire simultaneously. If this activity persists for some time, the learning rule has its effect and some fast excitatory synapses are formed near the electrodes. Thus the net excitability of the network increases. When the next pulse arrives, the above sequence of events is repeated. Due to the increased excitability of the network, a larger number of neurons fire simultaneously, leading to oscillations in net activity with larger amplitude and longer duration. Thus the rate of synapse formation and the oscillation amplitude increase rapidly with the first few pulses. When the first series of pulses is over, i.e. the shock is discontinued, the network continues the violent oscillations between very large and very small activity for a relatively long time before getting trapped in the originally stored sequence of low activity attractors. The post stimulation EEG therefore shows spikes i.e. an afterdischarge is elicited. A typical AD, which relaxes into smooth oscillations is shown in Figure 2a.

Notice that as discussed above and as can be seen from Figures 2a and 2b, the network gets trapped into a low activity attractor only when the activity of the network is rising form very low values. In fact we have seen in our simulations that this is always the case, and the network never gets trapped into the original attractors while evolving from a very high activity state. This is due to the following reason. When the network has been in the high activity state for a time τ, the state of the network at the next instant will be where both the delayed state and the present state have large activity. As discussed above, due to sparse coding of K_{ij} and because $\lambda > 1$, the strength of the delayed inhibition overrides the contribution of fast synapses and the network activity shows a sharp downward trend. During this process, even if the network state S_i has a large overlap with one of the stored patterns, the contribution from

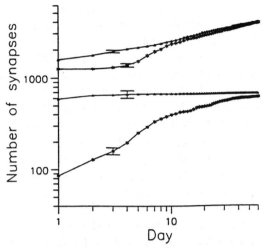

Figure 3 : The rate of synapse formation, averaged over 23 (43) subjects each for suprathreshold and subthreshold shocks, in different regions of the network. The plots from top to bottom are; $J_{noshock}$ for suprathreshold and subthreshold shocks, J_{shock} for suprathreshold and subthreshold shocks. Typical error bars are shown. The network parameters used are: shock amplitude $s = 0.40(0.56)$ for subthreshold (suprathreshold) shocks, interpulse interval $T = 7$ passes.

delayed inhibition overrides the contribution from the fast synapses, forcing the network to a very low activity state. However, as we have seen above, while the activity is rising from low values, *it is possible* for the network to get trapped into one of the low activity attractors coded in the fast synapses, thereby starting the smooth oscillations.

Thus whenever the unipolar EEG returns to smooth oscillations from large spikes, it should do so predominantly from the direction corresponding to low activity. Such an observation would confirm the attractor mechanism proposed here.

If the high activity state persists for a long time, i.e. some set of neurons fire at a high rate for a long time, the synaptic refractoriness, Rule 2, has its effect. These neurons are then unable to excite each other or the rest or the network. Thus the network remains in the very low activity state for a relatively long time — equal to the synaptic refractoriness period t_{ref}. When this period is over, the network activity starts rising and it is possible for the network to get trapped into the low activity attractors by the mechanism discussed above. Thus the synaptic refractoriness not only decreases the activity of the network but also increases the probability of the network relaxing to the resting state. If this does not happen, the entire process repeats. Thus the EEG acquires a typical "spike and wave" kind of pattern. According to our modeling, the synaptic refractoriness is responsible for the "wave" part of the EEG. The duration for which the bunch of spikes occurs corresponds to t_{max} and the smooth part of the EEG corresponds to the synaptic refractoriness period t_{ref}.

Further suprathreshold stimulations lead to a rapid increase in AD duration and amplitude. The number of synapses in the region near the electrodes, J_{shock} also increases rapidly during this period. The increased excitability of the network leads to a larger excitatory input to the neurons which are not in the vicinity of the electrodes, making them fire. Thus some synapses also start forming in the region of the network which does not get the shocks, i.e. $J_{noshock}$ starts increasing (Figure 3). Almost all the J_{ij} in the vicinity of each of the electrodes become 1 within a few suprathreshold stimulations. The AD amplitude (Mehta et al 1993) and the total number of synapses rise rapidly for about 10-12 suprathreshold stimuli, after which they increase very slowly. Such a dependence of the AD amplitude, or the severity of seizures, on the number of stimulations has also been observed experimentally (Lothman et al 1991, McNamara 1989, Racine 1972b). The first epileptic seizures occur when these parameters reach the saturation value and the network is then said to be kindled.

As the number of stimulations increases, the fraction of time that the network spends in the original low activity attractors in the absence of stimulations also reduces. The activity of a network which has been stimulated by 10 suprathreshold shocks (s=0.56) is plotted as a function of time in Figure 4a. The network is put into one of the original low activity attractors in the beginning and is not stimulated during this period. As can be seen, occasionally the network makes short excursions to the high activity states (even without stimulations) and is quickly trapped back in the original attractors. These spontaneous transitions to high activity states are called spontaneous ADs and are also observed in kindled laboratory animals (Pinel and Rovner 1978). A similar plot for a network which has been stimulated 30 times is shown in Figure 4b. The network has now learned a large number of high activity patterns. Therefore, unlike the earlier plot, Figure 4a, most of the time the network is in the high activity state and spends a very small amount of time in the original attractors. This is similar to "status epilepticus", i.e. a permanent epileptic state, observed in animals which receive a large number of stimulations. Such

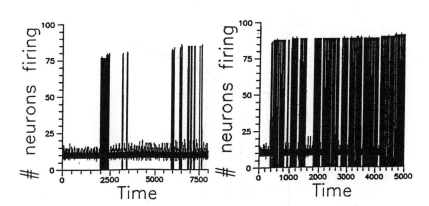

Figure 4 : (a) The activity of a network which has been given 10 suprathreshold stimulations ($s = 0.56, T = 7$ passes) is plotted as function of time. No stimuli are given immediately before or during this period. The network remains in the resting state most of the time. (b) A plot similar to Figure 4a for a network which has been given 30 suprathreshold stimuli ($s = 0.56, T = 7$ passes). The network spends a large amount of time in the high activity state.

a network will return to the resting state after a relatively long time, by mechanisms such as after-hyperpolarization (Hotson and Prince 1980) and neuronal fatigue which are not included in our model.

The attractor mechanism is also responsible for the fact that sometimes the suprathreshold stimulations do not lead to any ADs, or yield an AD with small amplitude and short duration, even though some large ADs have already been elicited. This is observed in simulations (Figure 5) and also in laboratory experiments (Lothman *et al* 1991). The reason for this phenomenon is that at any time there is a finite probability that the network gets trapped in the original low activity attractors. This can also happen as soon as the shock is discontinued, thereby leading to no AD.

As the number of stimulations increases, the excitability of the network is enhanced due to learning and the probability of finding the network in the low activity patterns reduces, i.e. the probability of seeing no AD decreases. Similarly, once an AD begins, depending on the order of update of neurons, there

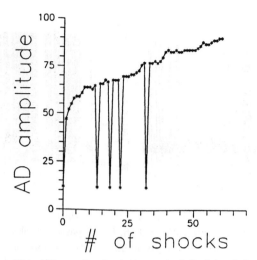

Figure 5 : The AD amplitude for a typical "subject" is plotted as a function of the number of suprathreshold stimuli of amplitude 0.56 and interpulse interval of 9 passes.

is a finite probability of the network getting trapped in the original low activity attractors, i.e. the AD terminates. Therefore, the AD duration fluctuates as a function of the number of stimuli and the average AD duration increases with the number of stimulations (Figure 6).

3.2 Subthreshold Shocks

If the amplitude of the stimulus is small, the dynamics of kindling reveals the structure of the underlying network in an interesting way. Consider first the unkindled network. Neurons which fire together in any of the originally stored pattern are connected to each other via excitatory synapses. Due to sparse connectivity and low activity of patterns stored in the network, neurons have a very low probability of being active in more than one pattern. Thus the (fast) synaptic matrix J_{ij} looks like clusters of tightly connected neurons, linked together by those few neurons which are common to more than one pattern.

Consider for simplicity a network with q distinct patterns such that only two of the patterns, μ and ν, have one common active neuron and all the other patterns have no overlap with each other. When any pattern except μ or ν is active, neurons which are a part of that pattern receive excitatory inputs,

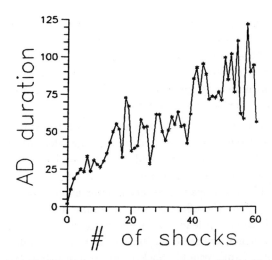

Figure 6 : The AD duration, averaged over 20 subjects, is plotted as a function of the number of stimulations for 60 suprathreshold stimulations of amplitude 0.56 and interpulse interval of 9 passes.

and all the other neurons receive an inhibitory input equal to $-wu$ where w is the weight of inhibition and u is the number of active neurons [3]. If pattern μ is active, all the neurons which do not belong to the patterns μ and ν receive the same background inhibition $-wu$. However, due to the one common neuron between patterns μ and ν, all the neurons which belong to ν but not to μ receive a net input of $1-wu$. Thus the neurons belonging to pattern ν are less inhibited than all the other neurons when pattern μ is active (similarly for neurons of μ when ν is active).

If the network is in any state except μ and ν, the minimum amplitude of a stimulus which can turn on a neuron which is not a part of that state is $s = w$. However, if the network is in either of the states μ and ν, the minimum stimulus amplitude is lower, given by $s = w - 1/u$.

It is easy to see that in an arbitrary network, with randomly chosen patterns, the lowest amplitude of the shock which will induce neurons outside an active pattern to fire is equal to $s = w - C/u$ where C is the highest number of common neurons between any two patterns.

---

[3]Here we ignore for simplicity the contributions of the delayed excitatory and inhibitory connections. These terms may be taken into account in a similar but more complicated analysis.

Thus the afterdischarge threshold is a decreasing function of the highest number of common neurons between any two patterns, which in turn depends on the structure of the memory storage. For example, in a network of randomly chosen patterns, the highest number of common neurons between any two patterns would be an increasing function of the fraction of neurons active in any pattern and the number of stored patterns.

When very low amplitude shocks are applied and the state of the network happens to be μ, those neurons in pattern ν which are close to the positive electrode will get a net excitatory input and fire, thereby leading to the strengthening of synapses between all the neurons in pattern μ and these additionally active neurons. This would lead to an even larger number of common neurons between μ and ν. Thus the effect is self sustaining and eventually a stage is reached when activation of μ leads to the activation of most of the neurons in ν, including the ones which are far from the stimulating electrodes. At this stage the application of a subthreshold shock leads to more than twice the normal number of neurons to be active simultaneously and this constitutes the first afterdischarge. Unlike the original low activity patterns the high activity "pattern" formed by the linking of two attractors is not stable. The main reason for this is that the slow synapses K_{ij}, which are unmodified, tend to pull such a mixed pattern in two different directions corresponding to the (distinct) patterns that are temporal successors of μ and ν. Due to increased excitability the network activity undergoes large amplitude oscillations, for reasons described in the previous subsection, leading to a typical AD. Thus the first afterdischarge produced by subthreshold stimulations arises due to the linking up of some of the low activity attractors.

The rate of synapse formation due to subthreshold stimulations evolves as follows. Initially, the number of synapses in the shocked region and the excitability of the network increase by small amounts with repeated subthreshold stimulations. However, the total excitability is still not large, i.e. the strength of the original low activity attractors is much larger than the strength of the newly learned (low activity) patterns. Hence there is no AD, and very few synapses are formed in the unshocked region. As the number of stimuli increases, the number of synapses J_{shock} in the region near the electrodes increases beyond a threshold value which leads to the activation of neurons outside the shocked region too. After this stage the number of synapses in the unshocked region $J_{noshock}$ increases rapidly (Figure 3). Soon the AD amplitude and $J_{noshock}$ reaches saturation values, comparable to the ones obtained after the same number of ADs elicited by suprathreshold stimulations. Thus the kindled state is reached by the same number of ADs, independent of the stimulus being suprathreshold or subthreshold. However, due to the smallness of the subthreshold stimulus, all neurons near the electrodes are not turned on and hence not all the possible synapses are formed near the electrodes. Thus, unlike the situation for suprathreshold stimuli, J_{shock} continues to rise slowly even after kindling.

The dynamics of kindling due to subthreshold and suprathreshold stimuli is therefore quite different until an AD is elicited. For suprathreshold shocks, most of the neurons near the electrodes are induced to fire irrespective of the nature of overlaps between the patterns, thereby establishing synaptic connections between them and all the other neurons. In contrast, synapse formation for subthreshold stimuli is more dependent on the structure of the patterns stored in the memory.

After a large number of stimuli (nearly 50), the average AD amplitude, J_{shock} and $J_{noshock}$ are all nearly the same for supra and subthreshold stimuli. This behavior is also observed in laboratory experiments (Racine 1972b).

Although the number of ADs needed to reach the kindled state is insensitive to the amplitude of the stimuli, the number of subthreshold stimuli needed to elicit the first AD depends strongly on the amplitude of stimulation. For example, suprathreshold stimulations of amplitude greater than 0.5 lead to an AD in one or two applications whereas subthreshold stimuli of amplitude less than 0.3 do not lead to any AD even after 100 applications (Mehta *et al* 1993). As argued above, if the amplitude of the shock is smaller than a certain minimum value determined by the highest number of common neurons between any two pattern, the subthreshold stimuli produce very small deviations in the firing pattern of the network and therefore, a very slow rate of learning. Hence the number of subthreshold stimulations needed to elicit the first AD depends strongly on the amplitude of the subthreshold stimulus.

4. AD Threshold as a Function of Number of Stimulations

The dependence of the network response on the amplitude of the shock depends crucially on whether some ADs have already been elicited or not. This fact can be better understood by studying the dependence of the AD threshold on the number of stimulations.

The following simulations were done to study the dependence of the AD threshold on the number of stimuli. The network was given 20 suprathreshold stimuli of amplitude 0.56. After every two stimulations, the AD threshold was measured by ramping the amplitude of the shock in small steps (of 0.02), starting from small values (0.04), till an AD was elicited. Each subthreshold shock was of

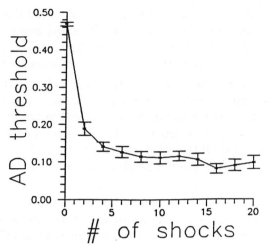

Figure 7 : The AD threshold, averaged over 20 subjects, is plotted as a function of number of suprathreshold ($s = 0.56, T = 7$ passes) stimulations.

the same frequency and duration as the daily suprathreshold stimulus. The AD threshold so measured, averaged over twenty subjects is plotted as a function of the number of suprathreshold stimulations in Figure 7. We see that the AD threshold sharply drops from the initial value of 0.46 to below 0.3 within a few suprathreshold stimulations. However, as discussed above and in Mehta *et al* (1993), before any ADs are elicited, a large number of stimulations of amplitude less than 0.3 failed to produce an AD. The (average) amplitude and duration of the ADs produced by suprathreshold stimulations and these (new low) subthreshold stimulations are the same.

These observations can be understood as follows. If no ADs have been elicited, the only attractors are the original low activity ones, and it needs one or two large stimulations to pull the network away from these attractors towards higher activity. Elicitation of a few ADs leads to a substantial increase (nearly 30 %) in the number of excitatory synapses (Figure 3). The network has an increased excitability due to learning of some high activity patterns. This has a twofold effect on the reduction of the AD threshold. First, the increased excitability enhances the excitatory effect of the shock, as discussed in subsection 3.1. Second, even if a subthreshold shock puts the network in a slightly higher activity state, a large overlap of this transient state with the newly formed high activity patterns can pull the network towards large activity, leading to an AD.

As long as the amplitude of the shock is large enough to shift the network by a small amount from the resting state, it leads to an AD by these two mechanisms. Therefore a suprathreshold shock has nearly the same effect as a subthreshold shock on the total activity of the network. This is the reason why, once some ADs have been elicited, the rate of kindling is relatively insensitive to the amplitude of the stimulus.

The first few ADs are accompanied by a rapid increase in the number of synapses i.e. the excitability of the network. Hence, initially the AD threshold drops rapidly. Soon, the number of new synapses formed is so large that a small perturbation on the resting state tends to pull the network towards higher activity patterns. As the rate of learning saturates with increasing number of ADs, so does the rapid drop in the AD threshold (see Figure 7).

The drop in the AD threshold due to repeated stimulations is by about 50% in our simulations, whereas the experimentally observed drop is not so large (Racine 1972a). This difference is possibly due to the fact that the number of neurons participating in kindling in laboratory animals is much larger than the number of neurons (200) used in our simulations.

5. Frequency Dependence of Kindling

It has been experimentally observed (Cain 1981; Cain and Corcoran 1981) that the number of ADs needed to reach the kindled state is larger for high frequency stimuli than for low frequency ones. This type of frequency dependence was also observed in our simulations.

As mentioned earlier, time is measured in our modeling in the natural units of "time" needed to update the states of all the neurons once, i.e. in units of passes. Each biphasic pulse lasts for two passes (which corresponds to a few milliseconds in reality). The separation between the pulses is inversely proportional to the frequency. Hence, frequency is measured in units of $(pass)^{-1}$. The simulations consisted of administering a fixed number (35) of fixed amplitude (0.56) suprathreshold stimulations. The interpulse interval was varied from 6 passes to 20 passes. The highest AD amplitude (averaged over 20 subjects) obtained after 60 stimuli is plotted as a function of frequency (given by the inverse of the interpulse interval) in Figure 8. The results show a frequency dependence of kindling rate similar to that observed experimentally.

In our model, the cause of such a frequency dependence is the synaptic refractoriness, as discussed below. As we have seen, after a few suprathreshold

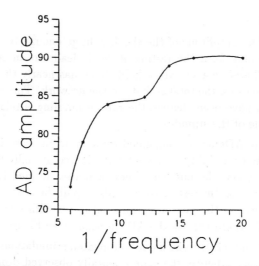

Figure 8 : The highest averaged (over 20 subjects each) AD amplitude after 60 suprathreshold stimulations ($s = 0.56$) is plotted as a function of the interpulse interval (i.e. $(frequency)^{-1}$).

stimuli, a large number of synapses are formed between the neurons near the electrodes (Figure 3). When the next session of pulses are applied, due to the increased excitability, most of the neurons near the electrodes are put in the firing state by the first few pulses, thereby setting up large activity oscillations. As these high activity oscillations continue, the afferent synapses of these neurons become refractory for a period t_{ref} according to Rule 2. Further, according to Rule 2, if another pulse activates these refractory neurons during this period, afferent synapses remain refractory for a further period t_{ref} from the instant of reactivation. Thus the effect of stimulating a refractory neuron is to keep the afferent synapses refractory for a longer time. Since most of the neurons near the electrodes fire simultaneously (due to suprathreshold stimulation), their afferent synapses become refractory simultaneously. The effect of an excitatory pulse is therefore largely shielded from the rest of the network by these refractory synapses. This in turn reduces the pulse induced excitation in the rest of the network, leading to a lower rate of synapse formation and a slower rate of kindling.

In our stimulations, the refractory period t_{ref} was chosen randomly between 6 and 12 passes. Hence simulations with interpulse interval less than 12 passes kindle slower than stimulations with larger interpulse interval (Figure 8). Further, the difference in the rate of kindling is not much for pulses with interpulse interval greater than t_{ref} (12) but the difference is large for pulses with interpulse interval less than t_{ref} (i.e. between 5 and 12). This confirms the above mentioned mechanism for the frequency dependence of kindling in our model.

In our simulations, we have observed that the number of (very low) subthreshold stimuli needed to produce the first AD is larger for low frequencies than for high frequencies. This is related to the rate of learning induced by the shocks. Before an AD is generated, as discussed in subsection 3.2, subthreshold shocks induce only small deviations in the average activity of the network and the network quickly relaxes to normal oscillations after the pulse is over. If another pulse arrives before these oscillations die out, it enhances the deviations thereby producing somewhat larger oscillations and hence a faster rate of synapse formation. These deviations last for a short time and there is no coherent firing of a large number of neurons. Hence the mechanisms related to the synaptic refractoriness are not operative in this situation. Since the interpulse interval is smaller for high frequencies than for low frequencies, the rate of learning is faster for high frequencies and lesser number of subthreshold stimulations are needed to get the first AD. Thus, for example, the number of stimuli (averaged over 20 subjects each) of amplitude 0.34 needed to produce the first AD is 24 for an interpulse interval of 6 (high frequency) and is equal to 28 for an interpulse interval of 16 (low frequency). Such a behavior should be experimentally observable. Further, the AD threshold has been observed to be much larger for very low frequencies for which the interpulse interval is much longer than the time scale of learning.

Subthreshold stimulations, unlike suprathreshold ones, do not immediately lead to a large amount of synapse formation near the electrodes. As the kindling progresses, more synapses are formed near the electrodes, but the total number remains less than the maximum possible value (see Figure 3). Hence, not all synapses can become refractory due to the small amplitude stimuli. Using the arguments presented in this section, it can be inferred that the kindling rate is likely to have a weaker dependence on the frequency for subthreshold stimuli than for suprathreshold ones.

The frequency dependence of kindling rate is quite sensitive to many model parameters. There are many time scales inherent to the phenomena we are trying to model. The relative value of some of these are quite important for our modeling. Such time scales are: τ, the average delay time of the slow synapses; t_{max}, the duration of time for which a synapse can be activated before it becomes refractory; t_{ref}, the duration of time for which such a synapse remains refractory and the average time for which a pattern has to persist before it is learned via synaptic modifications. We have assumed (as it seems reasonable) that τ is much shorter than the other three time scales. The value of τ used in our simulations corresponds to a few milliseconds in reality. In our model, each spike lasts for a period τ and the periods t_{max} and t_{ref} determine the duration of the spiky and the wavy part of the AD respectively.

If the actual value of the delay period τ is much longer, then the structure of AD obtained in our model will change. For example if τ is much longer than the other time scales, then the duration of the spike and the wave parts of the AD will be of the order of τ. Refractoriness can now set in a spiky period of duration $\sim \tau$. Due to the absence of delayed inhibition and spontaneous neuronal activity, a new set of neurons will then fire simultaneously, leading to a different rate of synapse formation and kindling. Since the frequency dependence of kindling in our modeling is due to the synaptic refractoriness, this too will change when different time scales are used.

Unlike the results for the frequency dependence of kindling rate, the rest of the results presented here are fairly insensitive to changes in parameters and hence are quite general (see Mehta *et al* 1993 for details).

6. Chemical Kindling

Kindling can also be generated by chemical stimulations (Prince 1968). The chemicals suppress the activity of some of the inhibitory neurotransmitters in a localized region of the brain. Unlike biphasic electrical stimulations, chemical stimulations affect a large number of neurons, continuously, for a long time.

Chemical kindling was also observed in our simulations. The chemical stimuli were modeled by a reduction in the weight of inhibition from the resting value of 0.6 to 0.36 throughout the network for 100 passes. (All the other parameters for the network are the same as the ones used for electrical kindling.) Such a stimulus is suprathreshold and is immediately followed by an AD. The AD amplitude versus the number of stimuli is plotted in Figure 9. The graph is similar to that obtained using electrical stimulations (Mehta *et al* 1993). The saturation value of the AD amplitude is larger in the case of chemical stimuli than for electrical stimuli because a larger number of neurons are directly affected by chemical stimuli.

The mechanism involved in chemical kindling is the same as that for electrical kindling, described earlier. That is, the reduction in the relative weight of inhibition leads to excess simultaneous firing of neurons, leading to excitatory

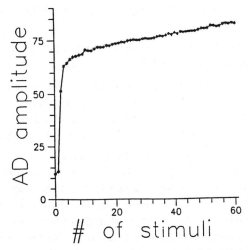

Figure 9 : The AD amplitude (averaged over 20 subjects) is plotted as a function of the number of suprathreshold chemical stimuli of amplitude 0.24.

synapse formation and increased excitability.

7. Discussion and Conclusions

We have modeled and explained a number of kindling related phenomena using a neural network model. The qualitative results and explanations are robust against small changes in some of the model parameters such as the weight of inhibition, strength of the delayed signal, number of patterns stored in the initial (normal) network etc. In this work we have not incorporated biophysical details of individual neurons. Such work will make it possible to have quantitative comparisons of the predictions of our model with results of laboratory experiments. Also, we have not incorporated "forgetting" in our model. This can be modeled by a slow withering of unused synapses. However, the rate of "learning" or synapse formation during kindling is much faster than the normal rates of learning or forgetting. Hence, over the time scale for which we are modeling kindling, "forgetting" is unimportant. Of course, many results will change if the time scale of learning is changed relative to the other time scales in the model.

The work presented here predicts the following observable consequences which in turn could shed light on mechanisms of the functioning of the brain and of epilepsy.

Our model of subthreshold kindling due to linking of the attractors leads to the following interesting and verifiable predictions.

The post-stimulus EEG amplitude should show a sudden increase at the time of occurrence of the first AD, corresponding to the linking of attractors. A related phenomenon has been observed by Lothman *et al* (1991) where 'behavioral seizure score' shows a sudden increase after a few stimulations.

It is known that the hippocampal pyramidal neurons in rats fire in a place specific fashion and are called place cells (O'Keefe and Dostrovsky 1971). Consider for simplicity a rat walking on a nearly one dimensional track, as is often the case in the experiments. The place cells would then fire in a sequence and the nature of the environment could be stored in the hippocampus by a mechanism similar to the model presented here. It is also known that sometimes a neuron fires at more than one distinct locations, i.e. these neurons have multiple place fields. These neurons can therefore be thought of as belonging to more than one pattern. Our model would then imply that the AD threshold for a rat should be a decreasing function of the highest number of place fields per neuron.

Further, if a few subthreshold stimuli are given to the hippocampus and an AD elicited, some of the attractors would get linked. This would mean that such rats would have larger than normal number of neurons with multiple place fields, and consequently, a larger than normal value of the average number of place fields per neuron.

If the kindled state is indeed similar to focal epilepsy, our model makes the following two distinct predictions. First, the subjects suffering from focal epilepsy would make a larger than normal number of errors in cognitive tasks involving identification of objects belonging to the same category or class. This is because the existing models of storage of hierarchies of memories have the property that the patterns belonging to the same category have the largest overlaps, i.e. the largest number of common active neurons. Our model suggests that such patterns may become linked together in the epileptic state, so that the activation of one of these patterns may lead to a simultaneous activation of the others. If this happens, then the subject would not be able to distinguish between the objects represented by the patterns which become linked together.

The next prediction is regarding the treatment of focal epilepsy. As we have seen, during kindling there is a large increase in the strength of the fast excitatory synapses J_{ij} while the strength of all the other synapses remains the same. In order to keep the kindled network close to the normal low activity state, merely increasing the strength of inhibition is not enough. One should either administer drugs which reduce the strength of fast excitatory neurotransmitters or use drugs which *increase* the strength of slow and fast inhibition *and* of fast excitation. This would, to some extent, restore the balance of relative strengths of various synapses which is a necessary condition for the normal functioning of the network.

Finally, the AD in our model terminates when the kindled network gets trapped in the low activity attractors. As we have shown, this always happens when the network is evolving out of the very low activity state that occurs during the AD. This implies that the EEG would return to the normal pattern from the same direction.

To conclude, we have studied various features of kindling using a neural network model. Kindling in our model occurs due to the formation of fast excitatory synapses, which corresponds to a linking of the original low activity attractors. We have argued that the afterdischarge threshold is a decreasing function of the largest number of neurons which are common to more than one pattern. As is observed in experiments, the AD threshold in our model drops with repeated stimulations due to the formation of new synaptic connections corresponding to high activity patterns. The same mechanism is also responsible for the insensitivity of the rate of kindling to the amplitude of the stimulus. The rate of kindling in our model exhibits a frequency dependence similar to that observed in experiments. This, we believe, is the first theoretical modeling of the process of kindling. We hope that our work will stimulate the development of more detailed and biologically realistic models incorporating the basic ingredients of our model. Experimental investigations of some of the predictions derived from our study would be most welcome.

References

D. J. Amit, *Modeling Brain Function* (Cambridge Universigy Press, 1989).

Y. Ben-Ari and A. Represea, *Trends in Neuroscience* **13** (1990) 312.

D. P. Cain, in *Kindling 2*, ed. J. A. Wada (Raven Press, 1981) p. 49.

D. P. Cain and M. E. Corcoran, *Experimental Neurology* **73** (1981) 219.

J. M. R. Delgado and M. Sevillano, *Electroencephalography and Clinical Neurophysiology* **13** (1961) 722.

J. C. Eccles, *The Physiology of Synapses* (Springer-Verlag, Berlin. 1964).

Y. Geinisman, F. Morrell and L. de Toledo-Morrell, *Proceedings of the National Academy of Sciences, USA* **85** (1988) 3260.

W. G. Gibson and J. Robinson, *Neural Networks* **5** (1992) 645.

G. V. Goddard, D. C. McIntyre and C. K. Leech, *Experimental Neurology* **25** (1969) 295.

D. Golomb, N. Rubin and H. Sompolinsky, *Physical Review A* **41** (1990) 1843.

B. Gustafsson and H. Wigstrom, *Trends in Neuroscience* **11** (1988) 156.

C. A. Guyton, *Textbook of Medical Physiology* (W. B. Saunders Co, 1986) p. 505.

D. O. Hebb, *The Organization of Behavior* (Wiley, New York, 1949).

J. R. Hotson and D. A. Prince, *Journal of Nurophysiology* **43** (1980) 409.

S. R. Kelso, A. H. Ganong and T. H. Brown, *Proceedings of the National Academy of Sciences USA* **83** (1986) 5326.

D. Kleinfeld and H. Sompolinsky, *Biophysical Journal* **54** (1988) 1039.

W. D. Knowles, R. D. Traub, R. K. S. Wong and R. Miles, *Trends in Neuroscience* **8** (1985) 73.

E. W. Lothman, E. H. Bertram and J. L. Stinger, *Progress in Neurobiology* **37** (1991) 1.

D. Marr, *Philosophical Transactions of the Royal Society of London B* **262** (1971) 23.

W. S. McCulloch and W. A. Pitts, *Bulletin of Mathematical Biophysics* **5** (1943) 115.

J. O. McNamara, *Epilepsia* **30 (Suppl. 1)** (1989) S13.

M. R. Mehta, C. Dasgupta and G. Ullal, *Biological Cybernetics* **68** (1993) 305; M. R. Mehta, C. Dasgupta and G. Ullal, *International Journal for Neural Systems* **6 (Suppl. 1)** (1995) 107.

J. O'Keefe and J. Dostrovsky, *Brain Research* **34** (1971) 171.

D. A. Prince, *Experimental Neurology* **21** (1968) 467.

J. P. J. Pinel and L. I. Rovner, *Experimental Neurology* **58** (1978) 190.

R. J. Racine, *Electroencephalography and Clinical Neurophysiology* **32** (1972a) 269-279.

R. J. Racine, *Electroencephalography and Clinical Neurophysiolgy* **32** (1972b) 281.

M. Reiss and J. G. Taylor, *Neural Networks* **4** (1991) 773.

D. E. Rumelhart and J. L. McClelland, eds. *Parallel Distributed Processing* (MIT Press, Cambridge, Mass. 1986).

L. R. Squire, A. P. Shimamura and D. G. Ameral, in *Neural Models of Plasticity —Experimental and Theoretical Approaches*, eds. J. H. Byrne and W. O. Berry, (Academic Press, New York, 1989) 208.

T. Sutula, H. Xiao-Xian, J. Cavazos and G. Scott, *Science* **239** (1988) 1147.

J. D. Willshaw, O. P. Buneman and H. C. Longuet-Higgins, *Nature* **222** (1969) 960.

A NEURAL NETWORK MODEL OF MOVEMENT PRODUCTION IN PARKINSON'S DISEASE AND HUNTINGTON'S DISEASE

JOSE L. CONTRERAS-VIDAL, HANS L. TEULINGS AND GEORGE E. STELMACH

Laboratory of Motor Control, Arizona State University
Tempe, AZ 85287-0404, USA
E-mail: pepe@cacaphonix.la.asu.edu

ABSTRACT

A network model of basal ganglia-thalamocortical relations during movement production is used to provide a mechanistic account for the motor deficits seen in Parkinson's disease (PD) and Hungtinton's disease (HD) subjects. The model is based on the anatomical, neurophysiological and pharmaco-logical opponent interactions seen in the basal ganglia internal and external loops. Simulations of single-joint and multi-joint arm movements in PD and HD support the notion that the basal ganglia are involved in movement initiation and execution. Simulated lesions in the globus pallidus and sub-thalamic neurons suggest that although these focal lesions may improve some PD motor deficits such as rigidity and tremor, they may further reduce the movement modulatory capabilities in these patients. It is suggested that an approach that both reduces the tonic level of pallidal activity and restores the phasic modulatory capabilities of pallidal neurons may be an optimal strategy for the management of PD.

1. Introduction

A neural network model of movement production in Parkinson's disease (PD) and Huntington's disease (HD) patients is presented. The model is based on anatomical, neurophysiological, and neurochemical evidence that support the notion of segregated basal ganglia-thalamocortical motor systems. Parkinson's disease, which results predominantly from nigrostriatal pathway damage, and Huntington's disease, which results predominantly from a differential loss of striatal projection neurons, are used as a window to study basal ganglia function[1,2]. We illustrate through simulations how dopamine depletion in PD produces motor impairments consistent with motor deficits observed in PD patients such as akinesia, bradykinesia and hypometria. Furthermore, simulations of HD deficits are consistent with hyperkinesia observed in HD patients.

The network model aims to unify hypo- and hyper-kinetic disorders seen in PD and HD within a single comprehensive mechanistic account of the neu-ropathology of these diseases. It is hypothesized that PD produces smaller-than-normal pallido-thalamic gating signals that cause slower and smaller-than-normal movements. It is also postulated that highly variable and larger-than-normal basal ganglia gating signals are responsible for the choreic form of HD.

The goals of our modelling efforts are to hopefully provide a mechanis-tic account for these movement disorders, evaluate current surgical and/or pharmacological interventions, and make suggestions (or predictions) about alternative procedures that may restore some of the movement capabilities in patients with PD and HD.

2. Neurobiology of normal basal ganglia interactions

The striatum serves as a major target for inputs to the basal ganglia. It is comprised of medium spiny neurons that provide efferent projections to the globus pallidus internal (GPi) and external (GPe) segments, and the substantia nigra pars reticulata (SNr) (Figure 1A). Striatal neurons form compartments that can be distinguished on the basis of neurotransmitter and receptor density[3]. Their main neurotransmitter γ-aminobutyric acid (GABA) co-exists with several neuropeptides forming two main subpopulations: One subclass of neurons projects exclusively to GPe (also refered to as the indirect pathway) and primarily contains the neuropeptide enkephalin (ENK), while a second class projects to GPi and SNr (also known as the direct pathway), and primarily expresses substance P (SP)[4]. In the direct pathway, excitatory (glutamate) cortical activation of the striatal neurons results in inhibition of the GPi, which produces disinhibition of the thalamic nuclei. Therefore, the direct pathway works as a normally-closed movement gate (e.g., non-movement state), that is opened by corticostriatal activity (e.g., movement state). The indirect pathway has the opposite effect on GPi neurons: Corticostriatopallidal activity in the indirect pathway tends to increase the activity of GPi cells via the subthalamic nucleus, therefore inhibiting movement (Fig. 1A).

The anatomical and neurochemical differentiation in the striatum supports the view that dopamine differentially affects neurons in the direct and indirect pathways through the differential expression of D1 and D2 dopamine (DA) receptors[5]. This means that the striatal output neurons can be differentiated not only by their target neurons, but also by the expression of neuropeptides and DA receptor subtypes[6]

3. Neurobiology of Parkinson's disease

The differentiation of the direct and indirect pathways is also observed during degeneration of the dopaminergic nigrostriatal tract in PD. In particular, it has been shown that in the 1-methyl-4-phenyl-1,2,3,6-tetrahydropyridine (MPTP) model of PD, there is a tonic increase of activity in neurons in GPi/SNr, whereas the activity in the GPe decreases[7]. Overactivity of the glutamatergic projection neurons from STN resulting from a decrease in GPe output combined with the increased activity of GPi/SNr produce a pathological level of excess tonic activity in the basal ganglia output pathways. This is consistent with increases in ENK and decreases in SP that induce increases and decreases in activity of the indirect and direct pathways, respectively[4]. This differentiation in neural activity is enhanced by mutual inhibition between GPi and GPe neurons.

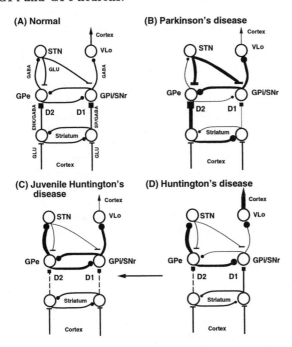

Figure 1. Neural network depicting the anatomical, neurophysiological, and neurochemical relations of the basal ganglia, and their activity under normal conditions (A); following damage of the substantia nigra pars compacta in PD (B); after damage of both direct and indirect pathways in juvenile HD (C); and in adult-onset HD (D). Abbreviations: GPi, GPe, internal and external segments of the globus pallidus respectively; STN, subthalamic nucleus; SNr, substantia nigra pars reticulata; VLo, ventrolateral thalamus; DA, dopamine; GABA, γ-aminobutyric acid; GLU, glutamate; ENK, enkephalin; SP, substantia P; D1, D2, DA receptor subtypes. Symbols: black circles and squares indicate inhibition; black squares indicate neurotransmitter/neuropeptide dynamics; bars indicate excitation; thin lines indicate reduced activity; and thick lines indicate overactivity.

Furthermore, damage of the DA subsystem in PD (see Figure 1b) causes differential expression of D1 and D2 dopamine receptor mRNA in the two subpopulations of striatal neurons[5]. In this regard, administration of DA antagonists results in decreases in SP expression and increases in ENK mRNA levels, and alternations in endogeneous DA release differentially modulate the level of both neuropeptide mRNA and peptide expression. Furthermore, this differential expression occurs in different temporal scales[8]. Additionally, changes in sensitivity to decreased DA release also co-occur. In particular, the affinity of the D2 receptor for dopamine is 100-1000 fold greater than that of the D1 receptor so that small changes in DA release would likely affect D1 receptor-mediated processes prior to D2 receptor mediated processes[8].

Current views of hypokinetic disorders point to a loss of striatal dopamine that leads to overactivation of pallidal neurons that in turn inhibit thalamocortical neurons influencing the frontal lobe[9]. However, some experimental observations of motor activity related to basal ganglia function have produced divergent results: (1) Behavioral and neurophysiological data investigating the involvement of the basal ganglia do not always show an effect on motor initiation[10]; (2) Focal basal ganglia lesions or inactivations do not consistently impair reaction time, only movement time and amplitude[11,12]; and (3) Stereotaxic lesions directed at the globus pallidus, which improve rigidity and tremor, do not always influence hypokinesia, bradykinesia, or dyskinesias[13].

4. Neurobiology of Huntington's disease

Movement disorders in Huntington's disease (HD), which usually co-occur with psychiatric and cognitive dysfuntion, could be caused by selective neurotransmitter deficits in the basal ganglia similarly to PD. In particular, the GABA levels in the caudate and putamen are markedly decreased in HD patients[14] (Figure 1C and 1D). This results from the prominent loss of medium spiny projection neurons in the caudate and putamen (but no striatal interneurons[15]), although other brain regions also show fewer neurons (e.g. thalamus, cerebral cortex, and cerebellum) that may contribute to the behavioral deficits.

The behavioral and neurobiological characteristics of HD and the progression of the disease depend on age. Early onset or juvenile HD patients (less than age 15 years) show akinesia, bradykinesia, dystonia, and rigidity. Adult-onset HD (average onset age between 35 and 45 years) is characterized by chorea, decreased coordination, rigidity, dystonia, abnormal eye movements, and progressive cognitive decline[16]. In adult-onset cases of HD, the medium-spiny projections to the lateral globus pallidus (GPe) and substantia nigra

(SNr) appear to be affected earlier than those projecting to the medial globus pallidus (GPi)[17]. However, in juvenile HD, all the three projections are affected at the same time[18]. The adult-onset HD patients eventually become akinetic as in juvenile HD (Fig. 1C and 1D).

The behavioral motor deficits in both adult-onset and juvenile HD can be explained in terms of the effects of the disease in the direct and indirect pathways. The choreic symptoms in the adult HD may result from the disinhibition of GPe neurons that lead to inhibition of the subthalamic nucleus that project with excitatory sign to the GPi neurons (Figure 1D). The reduced activation of GPi cells disinhibits the ventrolateral thalamic neurons producing chorea. In juvenile HD, the loss of both striatal pathways to the globus pallidus and substantia nigra causes overactivation of GPi and SNr and inhibition of thalamic neurons, resulting in rigidity and akinesia (Figure 1C).

5. A network model of basal ganglia-thalamocortical relations

Contreras-Vidal and Stelmach (1995) have proposed a neural network model of basal ganglia-thalamocortical relations in normal and Parkinsonian movement (Fig. 2)[19]. This model is based on anatomical, neurophysiological, and neurochemical interactions in the basal ganglia internal and external loops. In this chapter, it is shown how the model can explain some of the symptoms of PD and HD described above.

In the model of Figure 2, medium spiny striatal neurons receive segregated GLUergic inputs from motor, premotor cortex, and supplementary motor areas (SMA). These striatal neurons in turn are differentially organized and neurochemically differentiated in terms of their target neurons and the neuromodulators in their output pathways. In particular, striatal neurons projecting to GPe coexpress GABA/ENK, while neurons projecting to GPi and SNr coexpress GABA/SP. GABAergic pallidal output neurons are shown projecting to ventrolateral thalamus (VLo), and GLUergic thalamic neurons project back to premotor and supplementary motor areas[1,20,21]. Therefore this cortico-striato-pallido-thalamo-cortical direct pathway is activated by cortical input resulting in facilitation of premotor and SMA areas. Differential loss of striatal output projection neurons in adult-onset HD would facilitate in excess motor, premotor and SMA areas; loss of both types of striatal projection neurons in juvenile HD would remove basal ganglia modulation of premotor areas; and dopamine depletion in PD would reduce basal ganglia activation of cortical motor areas. It is hypothesized that the basal ganglia loops are associated with a movement gating network that modulates a cortical trajectory formation network (VITE model)[19,22].

382

The VITE model computes the desired kinematics of the movement. It compares a target position vector (TPV) delivered from premotor and SMA areas containing the movement plan with a Present Position Vector (PPV) to compute a Difference Vector (DV) that codes desired movement direction and amplitude. The dynamics of the trajectory formation network are modulated by the gating module such that the outflow command from the DV stage is gated by the movement gating signals from the basal ganglia-thalamus circuit. Therefore, these signals modulate movement onset and speed of movement. This system may be represented as a proportional and derivative controller with time-varying position and velocity gains. It is hypothesized that these position and velocity gains are impaired in PD and HD[23].

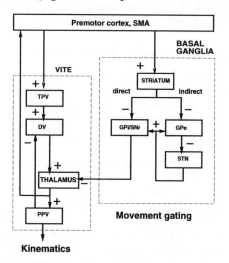

Figure 2. Schematic diagram depicting a basal ganglia-thalamocortical loop formed by the basal ganglia network of Fig. 1 and the neural network for trajectory formation (VITE) of Bullock and Grossberg (1988)[22]. The VITE model specifies the desired kinematics of the movement in terms of position and velocity in motor coordinates. The basal ganglia outputs gate or modulate the dynamics of the trajectory generated by VITE. Keys: TPV, target position vector; DV, difference vector; PPV, present position vector. Other keys as in Figure 1. The VITE model computes the difference between the TPV and the PPV at the DV stage. The DV carries instantaneous information about the direction and amplitude of the movement. As the PPV approaches the TPV, the DV approaches zero. The pallido-thalamic gating signal has the dual purpose of gating movement initiation and scaling movement.

Figure 3 depicts a simulation of a single joint movement of a PD network where the level of DA depletion is varied from zero to less than 40% (See the Appendix). The inset shows the increase in reaction time (RT) with DA depletion level. The figure illustrates that the network goes from a state of normal RT and movement time (MT) to bradykinesia (slow movement) and increased RT, to finally akinesia (i.e., inability to initiate movement). Note also that the network shows hypometria at extreme levels of DA depletion. The simulations suggest that small movement amplitudes, increased MTs, and increased RTs may be produced by neurochemical imbalances in the direct and indirect basal ganglia pathways that produce smaller than normal gating signals that modulate movement production.

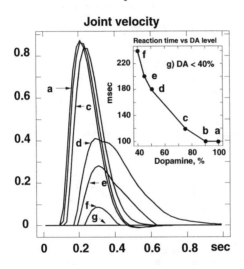

Figure 3. Parametric simulation of a simple movement when dopamine (DA) resources are varied from normal (a) 100, (b) 90, (c) 75, (d) 50, (e) 45, (f) 40, and (g) less than 40 % of DA. As the amount of DA decreases, the output of the network shows an increase in reaction time, slowness in movement (bradykinesia), and finally akinesia. Note the subtle effects for small percentages of DA depletion. From Contreras-Vidal and Stelmach (1995)[19].

Current experimental and theoretical data on the basal ganglia loops suggest a segregation or compartmentalization of these systems at the anatomical, neurophysiological and neurochemical levels[4,19–21,24]. The neurochemical imbalance in PD is supported by non-uniform spatiotemporal distribution of neurotransmitters in the basal ganglia. Uneven DA distributions have been documented in patients with PD[25]. This neurochemical segregation is paralleled by an anatomical segregation provided by multiple output channels in the basal ganglia[21]. The anatomical and neurochemical segregation may be responsible for the large motor variability seen in PD and HD patients, and for the apparent uncorrelation between MT and RT data in PD[10-12].

As reviewed in section 4, Huntington's disease can also be seen as a neurotransmitter disorder as GABA levels are severely decreased in the striatum. This disease is simulated in Figure 4 for both the adult-onset and the juvenile variants of HD by removing the GABAergic projections in the indirect and in both indirect and direct pathways, respectively.

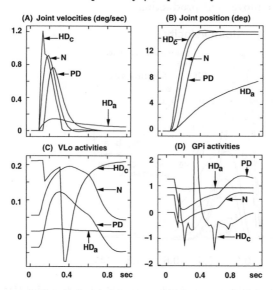

Figure 4. Joint velocity (A), joint position (B), thalamic (VLo) activity (C), and GPi activity (D) generated by the model during normal (N), Parkinson's disease (PD), juvenile HD (HD$_a$), and adult-onset HD (HD$_c$) simulations of a single joint movement. The simulations show that PD causes slower and smaller-than-normal movements due to overactivation of GPi neurons that inhibit VLo neurons. In contrast, adult-onset HD causes faster-than-normal movements due to disinhibition of VLo neurons.

Figure 4 compares the simulated joint velocities (A), joint positions (B), VLo activities (C), and GPi activities (D) corresponding to a normal (N), Parkinson's disease (PD), juvenile Huntington's disease (HD$_a$), and adult-onset HD (HD$_c$) networks. The control simulation depicts normal joint position and velocity profile with normal RT and MT, as well as normal VLo and GPi activities. However, the PD simulation shows that MT and RT is increased and that GPi activity is larger-than-normal causing smaller-than-normal VLo gating signals. In the case of the juvenile HD simulation, movement rate is greatly reduced and can be labelled as rigid/akinetic; VLo activity is depressed and GPi activity is larger-than-normal. Therefore bradykinesia appears to be a fundamental feature of the motor deficits of juvenile cases of HD[26]. Note that the GPi activity in juvenile HD differs from that in PD in that the range of GPi modulation is almost non-existent in the former as expected from damage to both the direct and indirect pathways. Also reaction time is increased in both the rigid HD simulation and the PD simulation (Fig. 4B). The similarities and differencies between PD and HD motor deficits may be explained (according to the model) in terms of the effects of DA depletion in PD and the loss of striatal projection neurons in HD. Figure 2B shows that the activity of the direct (indirect) pathway is decreased (increased) in PD leading to overactivation of GPi; however, in juvenile HD both pathways are damaged. This leads to overactivation of both GPe and GPi. Thus, the common feature is that in both diseases, GPi activity is increased. This may explain the hypokinetic features in both PD and juvenile HD. In contrast, in adult-onset HD peak velocity is larger-than-normal due to disinhibition of VLo neurons. This hyperkinetic movement is reminescent of HD chorea. This behavior is expected as only the indirect pathway is damaged in adult-onset HD, which results in disinhibition of VLo neurons.

Figure 5 shows a handwriting simulation using a finger-wrist system with three degrees of freedom (DOF): vertical finger flexion/extension; local horizontal displacement using wrist rotation; and left-to-right progression using radial flexion/ulnar extension wrist angle. Each DOF is controlled by a model basal ganglia-thalamocortical system of Figure 2. The motor plan consisted of a series of target position vectors (TPV_k) that are sequentially delivered to the trajectory formation network at times of zero or peak velocity in any DOF[27].

In the model, the production of a stroke is modulated by the thalamic (VLo) gating signals from the basal ganglia network. Deficiencies in neurotransmitter DA dynamics or loss of striatal output projection neurons in HD produce characteristic handwriting impairments. Figure 5 depicts the X-Y spatial handwriting path, the vertical finger velocity, and the thalamic (VLo) activities for (A) normal, (B) PD, (C) juvenile HD, and (D) adult-onset HD simulations respectively.

The PD simulation (Figure 5B) shows longer movement duration (15 sec), smaller-than-normal handwriting or micrographia[19,23,28] as well as smaller-

386

than-normal pallido-thalamic gating signals. This is in agreement with observations of overactivation of GPi neurons in PD which results in inhibition of VLo neurons. Figure 5C shows that juvenile HD, in which both projections from striatum to globus pallidus are destroyed, produces subtle changes in VLo activities that do not impair handwriting production. However, these activities are highly regular due to the lack of modulatory action from striato-pallidal projections. Finally, adult-onset HD, in which only the indirect striato-pallidal projection is damaged, produces faster-than-normal (e.g. chorea or ballism) movement speed, as well as distortion of the handwriting trajectory[29]. Also the variability in VLo activities is increased in adult-onset HD.

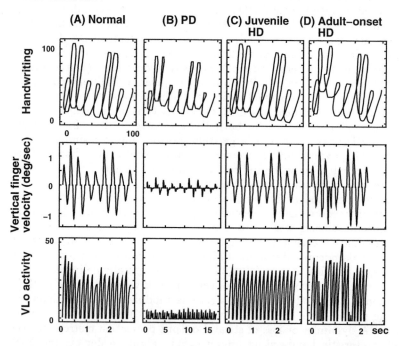

Figure 5. Handwriting simulations of normal (A), PD (B), juvenile HD (C), and adult-onset HD (D). The handwriting, vertical finger velocity, and thalamic (VLo) gating activities are shown. PD was simulated by 70 % DA depletion. Juvenile HD was simulated by removing both striatal projections to GPe and GPi, while adult-onset HD was simulated by removing only the striatal projection to GPe. Note different time scale for the PD simulation.

6. Intervention studies

Based on the identification of rather selective neurochemical pathways in the basal ganglia, pharmacological therapies have been developed that aim to restore the balance of specific neurotransmitters in the Parkinsonian brain by administrating DA agonists (e.g. Levodopa). However, early pharmacological attempts to restore the striatal GABA deficiency in HD with GABA agonists were not as successful as those interventions in PD. The reasons were that (1) the role of GABA in the striatum is not modulatory as in the case of DA; (2) the effects of GABA are not as pathway-specific as those of DA; and (3) GABAergic agents affect other nonstriatal pathways causing other deficits[16]. It is proposed that other neurotransmitter systems that are more specific to the striatal projection neurons, which are impaired in HD, could be manipulated to increase striatal activity.

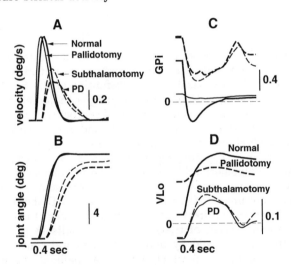

Figure 6. Simulated lesion studies. (A) joint velocity, (B) joint position, (C) GPi activity and (D) VLo activity for normal, PD, subthalamotomized PD, and pallidotomized PD networks. Pallidotomy produces the most improvement in PD restoring reaction time, movement time, and movement amplitude. Subthalamotomy was total and pallidotomy destroyed only 70% of pallidal output. From Contreras-Vidal and Stelmach (1995)[19].

It is suggested that acetylcholine (ACh) may be manipulated as giant cholinergic interneurons, which are not affected by HD, have an excitatory effect on medium spiny projection neurons. The model suggests that increasing the level of ACh in the striatum will increase the levels of GABAergic activity of the remaining medium spiny neurons in HD.

An alternative procedure to reduce the pathological levels of GP activity in PD involves stereotaxic surgeries in the subthalamic nucleus, globus pallidus, or thalamic nucleus[30]. The reasoning is that damaging STN or GPi neurons would decrease the level of excess inhibition upon thalamic target neurons therefore disinhibiting motor cortical areas[31,32]. However, simulations of sterotaxic surgeries depicted in Figure 6 suggest that although these types of interventions may reduce the tonic level of inhibitory activity and reduce the PD symptoms of rigidity and tremor, they cannot restore the normal range of modulatory striato-pallidal activity in the direct pathway. It is predicted that PD patients treated with stereotaxic surgeries would have reduced movement modulation capabilities.

7. Conclusions

The computational neural network studies of movement control deficits in specific brain disorders presented attempts to provide a unified account of basic mechanisms responsible for basal ganglia dysfuntion in PD and HD. Recent data and simulations suggest that the basal ganglia-thalamocortical motor loops are functionally segregated on the basis of neurochemically specified subsytems and anatomical differentiation of inputs and output basal ganglia neurons[21,24]. Computational modeling of these systems in single and multiple joint tasks suggest that in PD, gating signals that modulate movement production through the thalamus are inhibited due to an imbalance in the basal ganglia direct and indirect pathways. This results in slower and smaller-than-normal (hypokinetic) movements. On the other hand, in HD the differential loss of striatal neurons of the indirect pathway leads to reduced activation of GPi and therefore overactivation of thalamus. This results in hyperkinetic movements which are characterized by poor spatiotemporal control and increased variability. Juvenile HD, in which both striatopallidal pathways are damaged, results in PD-like hypokinetic deficits. The simulation results are consistent with the observations that HD increases variability of movement parameters and causes problems in producing smooth movements[29].

The model suggests that stereotaxic surgeries, albeit reducing some PD deficits such as tremor and ridigity, may further reduce the ability to modulate movement parameters. It is suggested that this technique reduces only the overall activation level of pallidal or thalamic areas but cannot restore the striato-pallidal modulation of movement which is also impaired in PD. Pharmacological interventions in PD should aim to restore both tonic and phasic levels of pallidal activity. This strategy may also help to improve the motor performance in patients with HD by increasing the level of cholinergic striatal activity. In particular, the dynamic range of pallidal and nigral activities may be crucial for the kinematic trajectory profile of movement.

8. Acknowledgements

This research has been supported by grant NINDS NS33173.

9. References

1. J. B. Penney and A.B. Young, *Ann. Rev. Neurosci.* **6** (1983) 73.

2. A. Reiner, R. L. Albin, K. D. Anderson, C. J. D'Amato, J. B. Penney, A. B. Young, *Proc. Natl. Acad. Sci. USA* **85** (1988) 5733.

3. A. M. Graybiel, C. W. Ragsdale Jr., *Proc. Natl. Acad. Sci. USA* **75** (1978) 5723.

4. C. R. Gerfen, *Ann Rev Neurosci.* **15** (1992) 285.

5. C. R. Gerfen, *Soc Neurosci Abst* **19** (1993) 133.

6. J.S. Fink, *Clinical Neurosci.* **1** (1993) 27.

7. M. R. DeLong, *Trends Neurosci.* **13** (1990) 281.

8. L. K. Nisenbaum, S. T. Kitai, W. R. Crowley and C. R. Gerfen, *Neuroscience* **60** (1994) 927.

9. R. L. Albin, A.B. Young and J.B. Penney JB, *Trends Neurosci.* **12** (1989) 366.

10. E. B. Montgomery, D. S. Gorman, J. Nuessen, *Neurology* **41** (1991) 1469.

11. J. W. Mink and W. T. Thach, *J Neurophysiol.* **65** (1991a) 301.

12. J. W. Mink and W. T. Thach, *J Neurophysiol.* **65** (1991b) 330.

13. C. D. Marsden and J. A. Obeso, *Brain* **117** (1994) 877.

14. T. I. Perry, S. Hansen, D. Lesk, M. Kloster, in *Huntington's chorea 1872- 1972. Advances in neurology*, ed. A. Barbeau, T. N. Chase and G.W. Paulson (Raven Press, New York 1973), p. 609.

15. R.J. Ferrante, M.F. Beal, N.W. Kowall et al., *Brain Res.* 411 (1987) 162.

16. A. B. Young, *Progress in Clinical Neuroscience* 1 (1995) 51.

17. R. L. Albin, A. Reiner, K.D. Anderson, J.B. Penney, A.B. Young, *Ann Neurol.*, 31 (1992) 425.

18. R. L. Albin, A. Reiner, K.D. Anderson, J.B. Penney, A.B. Young, *Ann. Neurol.* 27 (1990) 357.

19. J.L. Contreras-Vidal and G.E. Stelmach, *Biological Cybernetics* 73 (1995) 467.

20. G.E. Alexander, M. R. DeLong, P.L. Strick, *Ann. Rev. Neurosci.* 9 (1986) 357.

21. J. E. Hoover, P. L. Strick, *Science* 259 (1993) 819.

22. D. Bullock and S. Grossberg, *Psychol. Rev.* 95 (1988) 49.

23. J.L. Contreras-Vidal, H.L. Teulings and G.E. Stelmach, *Proc. 7th International Graphonomics Society Conference* (London, Ontario, August 1995), p. 38.

24. A. M. Graybiel, in Functions of the Basal Ganglia (Ciba Foundation Symposium 107) (Pitman, London, 1984), p. 114.

25. S. J. Kish, K. Shannak and O. Hornykiewicz, *New England J. Med.* 318 (1988) 876.

26. P. D. Thompson, A. Berardelli, J. C. Rothwell, B. L. Day, J. P. R. Dick, R. Benecke, C. D. Marsden, *Brain* 111 (1988) 223.

27. D. Bullock, C. Mannes, S. Grossberg, *Biological Cybernetics* 70 (1993) 15.

28. D. I. Margolin and A. M. Wing, *Acta Psychologica* 54 (1983) 263.

29. J. G. Phillips, J. L. Bradshaw, E. Chieu, J. A. Bradshaw, *Mov. Disorders* 9 (1994) 521.

30. H. Bergman, T. Wichmann and M. R. DeLong, *Science* **249** (1990) 1436.

31. J. Guridi, M. R. Luquin, M. T. Herrero and J. A. Obeso *Mov. Disorders* **8** (1993) 421.

32. L. V. Laitinen, A. T. Bergenheim and M. I. Hariz, *J. Neurosurgery* **76** (1992) 53.

10. Appendix

The trajectory formation network (VITE) is specified by,

$$\frac{d}{dt}V_k = 200(-V_k + TPV_k - PPV_k) \tag{1}$$

$$\frac{d}{dt}PPV_k = \gamma * V_k * P_k \tag{2}$$

where V_k is the difference vector for the k degree of freedom; TPV_k is the target position vector specifying the motor program; PPV_k is the present position vector; and P_k is the pallido-thalamic gating signal. The basal ganglia-thalamus circuit is described by,

Striatum

$$\frac{d}{dt}S_k = -A_sS_k + (B_s - S_k)(\sum_n I_n + I_{ACh} + f(S_k)) - (D_s + S_k)\sum_{n \neq k} S_n \tag{3}$$

Globus Pallidus, internal segment (GPi)

$$\frac{d}{dt}G_k = 2[-A_gG_k + (B_g - G_k)(10J_k + f(G_k)) - (D_g + G_k)(50S_kT_k + .2H_k)] \tag{4}$$

Globus Pallidus, external segment (GPe)

$$\frac{d}{dt}H_k = -A_hH_k + (B_h - H_k)(10J_k + f(H_k)) - (D_h + H_k)(50S_kU_k + .2G_k) \tag{5}$$

Dopamine (DA) dependent Transmitter dynamics

$$\frac{d}{dt}T_k = b(B_{SP/DYN}(DA) - T_k) - cS_kT_k \tag{6}$$

$$\frac{d}{dt}U_k = b(B_{ENK}(DA) - U_k) - cS_kU_k \tag{7}$$

Subthalamic nucleus (STN)

$$\frac{d}{dt}J_k = -A_jJ_k + (B_j - J_k)(I_k + I_s + f(J_k)) - 10(D_j + J_k)H_k \tag{8}$$

Ventrolateral Thalamus (VLo)

$$\frac{d}{dt}P_k = 5[-A_pP_k + (B_p - P_k)I_{tonic} - 0.5(D_p + P_k)G_k] \tag{9}$$

where (A_*) is a decay rate, B_* and D_* are upper and lower bounds of neural activity, I_n is an input from premotor areas, I_{ACh}, I_s, I_{tonic} are baseline tonic inputs, I_k is an excitatory input from cerebral cortex, b is an accumulation rate, c is a depletion rate, $B_{SP/DYN}(DA)$ and $B_{ENK}(DA)$ are maximum amounts of neurotransmitter available for signalling, which depend on dopamine DA levels, and the term $f(x) = x^3/(0.25+x^3)$ represents positive feedback. Equations (3-5, 8-9), which model neuronal average firing rates, contain a neural decay term and shunting excitation and inhibition terms. Equations (6-7) model the dynamics of neurotransmitter expression in the direct (T_k) and indirect (U_k) pathways. The amount of neurotransmitter available in these pathways depend on DA which modulates differentially the expression of peptides (e.g. SP and ENK).

The parameters used in the simulations were: $A_s = 10.0$, $A_g = 3.0$, $A_h = 3.0$, $A_j = 10.0$, $A_k = 2.0$, $b = 2.0$, $c = 8.0$, $I_{tonic} = 0.2$, $I_s = 0.4$, $I_{ACh} = 0.5$, $I_k = 0$, $\gamma=0.7$ (0.3 in handwriting simulations).

The spatial coordinates of the pen tip are derived from the internal present position vector (PPV_k) as follows:

$$x = PPV_x * cos(PPV_z) + (400 + PPV_y) * sin(PPV_z) \tag{10}$$

$$y = -PPV_x * sin(PPV_z) + (400 + PPV_y) * cos(PPV_z) \tag{11}$$

The sequence of relative target position vectors (TPV_k) for the 3 DOF hand used in the simulations of Figure 5 was: $\{\{12.5, 50, 0\}, \{0, 0, -.02\}, \{-5, -50, 0\}, \{0, 0, .03\}, \{12.5, 100, 0\}, \{0, 0, -.02\}, \{-5, -100, 0\}, \{0, 0, .03\}, \{12.5, 100, 0\}, \{0, 0, -.02\}, \{-5, -100, 0\}, \{0, 0, .03\}, \{12.5, 50, 0\}, \{0, 0, -.02\}, \{-5, -50, 0\}, \{0, 0, .03\}\}$.

MODELING CORTICAL DISORDERS USING NESTED NETWORKS

JEFFREY P. SUTTON

Neural Systems Group
Massachusetts General Hospital
Harvard Medical School
Building 149, Thirteenth Street
Charlestown, MA 02129, USA
E-mail: sutton@nmr.mgh.harvard.edu

ABSTRACT

An approach to modeling normal and altered neural networks within the neocortex is described in this chapter. The approach is motivated by accumulating evidence that groups of neurons and networks functionally cluster together in the neocortex to encode cognitive and behavioral information. The clustering traverses many levels of spatial organization and operates on a multiplicity of time scales. This chapter reviews some of the evidence for, and theoretical modeling of, nested networks, and it postulates how simulated lesions in nested networks may provide insight into some disorders affecting the neocortex.

1. Introduction

In neuroscience, model building has a long tradition (e.g., Freud, 1895; McCulloch, 1965), and it has helped to characterize mechanisms at several levels, including individual cells (Hodgkin and Huxley, 1952; McKenna et al., 1992), small networks (Koch and Segev, 1989) and large brain regions (Koch and Davis, 1994). Models have been useful in examining psychological phenomena (Rumelhart et al., 1986; Parks and Levine, in press), and they are beginning to be taken seriously as a means to complement experimental approaches to studying brain dysfunction.

Physiological based modeling, like experimentation, has tended to focus on one, or at most two, level(s) of phenomenology. There have been few attempts to bridge multiple levels of analysis and to elucidate the mutual inter-dependence of activities at each scale of investigation. This chapter presents a modest attempt to model networks across different scales of neural organization. The approach is somewhat atypical in that it looks at common principles underlying how neurons and networks cluster together throughout the neocortex, and attempts to extract the general manifestations which might occur when disease processes affect the system. This modeling strategy is complementary to the more common technique of specifying a particular disease and constructing a model to better understand its detailed mechanisms.

Although somewhat counter-intuitive, the neocortex may possess general computational features which apply to networks that span many orders of magnitude and that mediate a spectrum of functions. These features may provide clues for modeling certain disease processes, and it is in this spirit that nested neural networks are examined here. Section 2 introduces the basic ideas, and a computational model that attempts to integrate parallel and hierarchical properties is described in Section 3. The effects of simulated lesions in a model system are discussed in Section 4. In attempting to give a general overview of the topic, many of the mathematical and simulation details have been omitted, but ample references are provided for the interested reader.

2. The Neocortex as a Dynamic Nested Network

2.1. Evolving Perspectives

Historically, the cortex was conceptualized as a highly sophisticated neural structure sitting atop a stack of evolutionarily lower structures. The influence of Darwin (1859) was evident, and the serial stacking idea of the neuroaxis was elaborated upon by such eminent scholars as Spencer (1855), Hughlings Jackson (1884) and Sherrington (1906). The notion extended into the cortex with the phylogenetically based subdivisions of paleocortex, archicortex and neocortex. Furthermore, structural divisions within the neocortex were characterized based on evolutionary grounds (Pandya and Selzer, 1982), and feedforward and feedback connections within and between neocortical regions allowed for local processing as well as for coordinated processing at more global levels (Abeles, 1991; Van Essen et al., 1992).

With the discovery of the microelectrode and other technologies in the 1950's to the present, a complementary view of the neocortex that included but transcended the phylogenetic view began to emerge. Collections of neurons appeared to form functional units that were delineated, to large measure, on physiological grounds. Cytoarchitectonic differences existed from region to region within the neocortex, but similarities in functional organization across the neocortex were greater than the differences. Cortical columns, for example, were identified as one type of functional unit (Hubel and Weisel, 1959; Szentágothai, 1977). Oriented perpendicular to the surface of the neocortex, they measured 200 to 300 μm in diameter and contained on the order of 10^2 to 10^4 neurons. Columns could be demarcated based on the collective activity of neurons associated with particular tasks, even though no obvious structural boundaries existed.

Developmentally, individual columns were shown to arise from single clone cells which projected radially outwards from the periventricular region (Rakic, 1981). The cells generated a column with the inner aspects being constructed before the outer aspects, and the neocortex appeared to be built up from these columns. Increases in neocortical size across species were the result of more columns, rather than an increase in columnar size (Rockel et al., 1974).

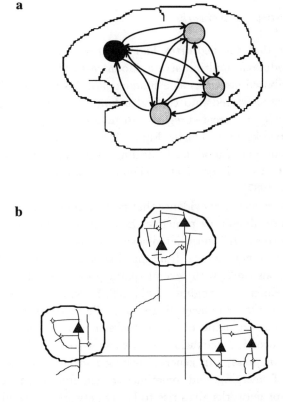

Figure 1. (a) Schematic lateral view of the human brain depicting an inter-connected network of four brain regions. The linkages represent fiber pathways. (b) Within a region [e.g., the black region in (a)], there are nested sub-regions, or networks, down to the level of cortical columns. Three columns are represented with connections among neurons that are both intra-columnar and extra-columnar. Modified from Sutton (1995) and Sutton and Anderson (1995).

As functional anatomy advanced, it became increasingly apparent that neurons and networks, including columns, were linked together in ways that mediated parallel and overlapping processes (Goldman-Rakic, 1988). There was both diversity and specificity in connection patterns, and many different types of networks were identified at different scales using a host of technological probes. Moreover, many networks displayed adaptability, with plasticity occurring not only in development, but also in the context of adult learning (Karni et al., 1995) and injury (Merzenich et al., 1983).

2.2. Nested Distributed Networks

Recognizing that the neocortex had features of parallel distributed and overlapping modules at multiple strata, Mountcastle (1978) posited the notion of nested distributed networks as a fundamental design principle of the neocortex. Neurons clustered into cortical columns, which were nested within cytoarchitecturally demarcated regions. Regions connected with each other to form larger networks, and so forth (Figure 1). The arrangement had similarities to other concepts of modularity dealing with brain function, psychology, categorization and social organization (Fodor, 1983; Gazzaniga, 1985; Minsky, 1985; Edelman, 1987).

Recently, there has been evidence that nesting among neocortical networks might be a more ubiquitous principle than initially realized. For instance, Phillips and Porter (1977) postulated several levels of network nesting in the motor cortex. It is now known, from multiple unit recordings, that complex motor subdivisions exist, with several spatially distinct networks subserving particular movements (Donoghue et al., 1992). Small networks coalesce to form larger networks. Similarly, there are preliminary data from functional magnetic resonance imaging of motor tasks in humans demonstrating the simultaneous neocortical activation of networks nested within larger networks (Sutton et al., in press). In general, nesting and network boundaries have different ways of emerging, and sometimes the simultaneous activation of adjacent neurons or networks gives rise to larger networks. Several studies support a recurring theme that functional networks linked to behavioral tasks are spatially localized within the neocortex, and that these networks consist of and comprise parts of other networks (Ts'o et al., 1986; Vaadia et al., 1995).

3. A Model of Nested Neural Networks

3.1. General Architectural and Dynamic Principles

Enormous simplifications are required to model aspects of the neocortex and nested networks, with the aim of emulating features of biological computation. It is therefore fitting to recall that all models are inherently limited in that they are not the actual systems themselves. They are models, and as such they are subject to simplifications to make their analysis tractable.

In the case of nested neural networks, there are several approaches which have been taken (Sutton et al., 1988a; Sutton and Anderson, 1995). All of the approaches are in their early stages of development. It is not an area that has been well explored, from either a basic computational perspective or from the view of modeling disease processes.

The basic architecture of the model is illustrated in Figure 1b. There are two ways of conceptualizing the structure, and they are equivalent. In the bottom-up view, neurons are linked together to form functional networks, such as cortical columns. Populations of networks join together to form larger networks, which are nested together within still larger networks, and so on. In the top-down view, the neocortex is subdivided into large overlapping networks based on anatomical and functional criteria. Smaller networks are nested within one or more of these large networks, and there is progressive nesting down to the level of individual cells. The scaling between levels of nesting is, in principle, continuous, although discrete levels do exist (e.g., columns).

For convenience, a bottom-up view will be adopted here. Small networks of neurons link to encode distributed information, as in the case of attractor networks. The neurons in a network are joined together by synaptic connections such that certain firing patterns among the neurons are stable for specified periods of time. These stable or quasi-stable states of the network are the *memory states*. When the network is in a state that partially resembles a particular memory state, the network evolves, or is attracted, to that memory state.

The memory states represent biological responses, and they operate at multiple levels. Different networks encode different responses which depend, in part, on the inputs to the networks. One way to think about hierarchical memory is to consider the smallest functional networks (e.g., columns) as first level networks. Second level networks are formed by the groupings among different first level networks, and the corresponding second level memory is generated by select combinations of first level memories. Similarly, third level memories are formed by correlations among second level memories, and so on. The combinations of memory states scale exponentially with the number of nested networks, and this has advantageous features for high speed computing (Anderson and Sutton, 1995). It also has implications for adaptability within the neocortex (Singer, 1995). A key feature of the nested network architecture is that multi-level nesting of memory states is associated with relatively few connections between networks. There is no scalar averaging, and the individual properties of neurons are maintained within and between all levels. Some neurons only have connections to other neurons in their immediate vicinity, while other neurons propagate great distances and have many collateral connections. The heterogeneity among neurons is important for local functional clustering among neurons and for the overall sparseness of connections throughout the network.

Furthermore, the preservation of individual neuron properties means that all learning is local. The same synaptic rules mediate the boundary changes of networks throughout the nested hierarchy. Consequently, it is possible to tease out scaling rules that allow one to rigorously traverse levels of organization. The entire architecture has fractal-like properties. It is an adaptable vector computing model with rather unusual temporal characteristics that are not well understood. For instance, networks at different levels can appear over very short time scales, due to the synchronous activity among adjacent neurons and networks, and transient boundaries can rapidly propagate information across widespread distances (Sutton and Anderson, 1995). The role of altered dynamics in simulated pathological processes has not been explored, although dynamic issues are clearly important in disease modeling (Belair et al., 1995).

3.2. Implementations

There have been a variety of investigations concerning the mathematical and computational features of nested neural networks (Sutton et al., 1988b; Anderson et al., 1990; Sutton, 1991; Sutton, 1993; Anderson and Sutton, 1995). The models tend to use very simple neurons to emphasize the nesting aspects of the system. It is somewhat surprising how complex the analysis can be on nested structures despite enormous simplifications. Usually the analysis is restricted to a model with three levels: neurons, a network of neurons and a network of networks. The boundaries between the networks of neurons have an analogy, to first approximation, to the clustering involving short range (e.g., stellate) and long range (e.g., pyramidal) cells. Networks of neurons contain both stellate and pyramidal cells, but only pyramidal cells project between networks.

Using Hebbian learning, adaptive nested architectures have been explored with particular emphasis on the multi-level memory performance as a function of inter-network connectivity and of the temporal delays between levels. Recently, nested neural networks have been shown to have unusually rapid and adaptable information processing capabilities (Guan et al., submitted). A growing body of work on nested networks complements other neural computation studies involving small networks that are arranged into larger networks (e.g., Jacobs et al., 1991).

From the perspective of modeling pathological processes, a three layer version of a nested network will be described in Section 4. The remainder of this section highlights some of the *qualitative* properties of nested neural networks. *Quantitative* details concerning neurobiologically motivated simulations can be found in the references. There are also applications of the approach which address complex signal processing (Anderson et al., 1990), real time imaging (Guan, 1994) and semantic networks.

3.3. Main Findings and Assertions

The concept of nested networks as a means to model some aspects of the neocortex are summarized below.

• The neocortex uses nested networks of neurons as an organizing principle. Network boundaries are initially determined by structural and functional criteria laid down in development. However, they are also plastic and governed by experience.

• The same rules dictating individual neuron and synaptic changes can alter boundaries at all levels. The boundaries are also determined by the simultaneous activation of linked networks.

• Patterns of neuron activity within a network are stored in stable ways. The stability endows the network with multi-leveled memory properties. Memory states or responses are manifest by particular dynamic patterns distributed among different networks. This property is ubiquitous and may challenge well accepted maps of cortical localization.

• Higher level memories are spatio-temporal correlations among lower level memories. Memory storage scales exponentially with the number of levels. However, the speed of computation is linearly related to the number of neurons.

- The model is massively parallel, with scaling between levels that is vector valued. This is a result of preserving individual neuron properties across all levels. Traversing levels does not necessitate scalar averaging, wherein a network of neurons is mapped onto a single large "neuron".

- In principle, the boundaries between networks do not have to be discrete. They vary in time and may be continuous in space.

- Within a level of network organization, stable memory states may represent information that has *meaning* at different levels. For example, states (i.e., responses) in the dorsolateral pre-frontal cortex, which are important in working memory, may perform more sophisticated tasks relative to similarly sized networks in primary sensory cortex.

- The model is readily testable using current techniques which record spatio-temporal signals across different scales (e.g., multiple unit recordings, functional magnetic resonance imaging).

3.4. Limitations and Open Questions

More detail must be built into the model to elevate it from an impressionistic stage to an explanatory stage. Other shortcomings include the following:

- Considerable anatomical detail at all levels of description is ignored.

- The evidence for nested clustering is limited to relatively small regions of the neocortex.

- It is not clear what constitutes intermediate levels of nesting. Spatial and temporal properties are clearly important, but it is difficult to delineate the relationship between these properties and levels of neural nesting.

- The approach is hard to validate and refute, despite being a simple postulate of brain organization.

4. Simulated Neocortical Lesions using Nested Networks

4.1. Overview

Pathology, the study of disease, encompasses perturbed physiology. Studying the response to perturbation generally gives insight into the normal workings of a system, as well as into the possible mechanisms that underlie disease. This is related to the fact that normal homeostatic processes attempting to drive a system back to equilibrium are often the very same mechanisms involved in the development of disease.

Within the context of artificial neural networks, perturbations afford an opportunity to test the resilience of a model to destructive forces, as well as to simulate pathological processes (Sutton et al., 1988a; Ruppin and Reggia, 1995). The more accurate the model is neuroanatomically and neurophysiologically, the more likely it is that the simulated disturbances give rise to biologically meaningful information.

Simulated lesions on nested networks, which are representative of some neocortical features, fall into three main categories (Sutton, 1995). There are lesions affecting the flow of information to and from the neocortical system. There are lesions intrinsic to the neocortical networks, and there are combinations of these two lesions. The discussion in this section will be restricted to *intrinsic lesions* of nested neural networks. Lesions of this type may be localized or generalized. A representative localized effect destroys part of the system, which may result in the focal loss of neurons and connections. Local effects may be compounded by distant effects, since regions project to, and receive projections from, other regions. Generalized alterations build on this notion and affect different levels of nesting through the diffuse loss of neurons and synapses.

4.2. Example Lesions

A simple version of a nested network model containing three networks is shown in Figure 2. More complicated networks are required to adequately portray pathological features, but some of the principle characteristics can be outlined. Each network in Figure 2 contains two populations of neurons. Each network also has a repertoire of first level memory states. Select combinations of these states form triplets, where each component of the triplet is a memory state from a different network. The triplets comprise memories at a second level, which consists of a network of networks. In modeling the effects of brain lesions on this architecture, the goal is to relate structural damage to a breakdown in the performance of memory at the first and second levels. The breakdown may manifest itself as decreased accuracy of memory recall or as slowing of memory association.

Four sample lesions are outlined below. The first three are treated in a cursory manner, and the fourth is described in more detail in the next two sub-sections.

1. *Local lesions which disrupt connections between some networks and not between other networks.* This is shown by line B in Figure 2. The result is

that first level memories are preserved throughout the system, but second level information is destroyed locally. In Figure 2, network 2 does not receive inputs from networks 1 and 3, and this effectively isolates network 2. Some minimal impact on its first level memory performance may occur. However, the second level memories will be altered significantly, since correlated activities between networks 1 and 3 do not have the benefit of input from network 2. Thus, at the site of the lesion, local function is maintained only at the lowest levels and distant effects occur but they are small. This highly simplified scenario might be representative of some processes occurring in *multiple sclerosis*, which is characterized by focal white matter lesions that vary in space and time.

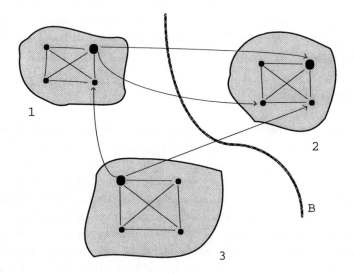

Figure 2. Three levels of simplified nesting are shown. Two populations of neurons cluster into three networks. One population of neurons (small dots) forms connections only within a network; whereas, another population of neurons (large dots) forms connections within and between networks. Simulated lesions can affect either one or both populations directly (gray matter lesions) and/or connections between networks (white matter lesions). Modified from Sutton (1995).

2. *Local lesions which destroy a circumscribed region of networks.* This type of lesion destroys neurons within nested networks, and all levels of memory are affected. In the example in Figure 2, the loss of one of the networks destroys its first level memory and its contribution to memory at the second level. Consequently, distant networks are altered by a local lesion, since there is a loss of connections emanating to and from the affected regions. This scenario is not unlike the picture seen in *cerebrovascular accidents.*

3. *Generalized lesions which diffusely destroy neurons.* The destruction of all neurons in the model leads to a rapid and progressive deterioration of memory function at all levels simultaneously. As in *Creutzfeldt-Jacob disease,* where there is a spongiform degeneration of the gray cells in the neocortex, a progressive and massive destruction of function occurs.

4. *Generalized lesions which appear to randomly but preferentially destroy select neuron populations.* When large neurons projecting between the networks in the model are selectively but randomly destroyed, the second level memory deteriorates, while preserving first level memory function. This is discussed more fully in the next two sub-sections concerning *Alzheimer's disease* as a prototype disorder of altered connectivity.

4.3. A Model of Associative Memory Loss

Alzheimer's disease is a degenerative condition afflicting more than four million individuals in North America. Evidence of neuropathological changes in the disease dates back to a landmark case report early in this century which described the autopsy findings of a 55 year old woman who died with a history of progressive dementia (Alzheimer, 1907). Newly available silver stains at the time demonstrated the presence of abnormal cortical neurons containing tangles of fibers, known as *neurofibrillary tangles.* Collections of degenerating nerve endings, or *neuritic plaques,* were also observed. To this day, a definitive diagnosis requires histopathological evidence obtained from a biopsy or autopsy.

The neuropathological mechanisms are complex and include genetic alterations, β-amyloid deposits, deficits in acetylcholine release from affected neurons in the basal forebrain and disruptions in the pathways between the hippocampus and the neocortex (Lamour, 1994). Synaptic loss is a key factor determining the severity of the disease. This loss is correlated with neuron degeneration, which is somewhat selective for layer III cells larger than 90 μm^2 residing in the association cortices (Terry et al., 1981). These large cells comprise roughly 20% of all neurons in the association neocortex, and they are important in providing cortico-cortical fibers. In contrast to these large cells, small localized neurons remain relatively unaffected.

The clinical manifestations of Alzheimer's disease are complicated, and they encompass a progressive dementia characterized by intellectual deterioration, which is severe enough to interfere with occupational or social performance. The cognitive changes include not only disturbances in memory, but also disruptions of language, perception, praxis, learning, problem solving, abstract thought and judgment (Schwartz, 1990). One of the intriguing things about Alzheimer's disease is that despite a severe disruption of brain function, only about 10% of all neocortical neurons are actually lost in even the worst clinical presentations (Katzman, 1986).

One approach to modeling the effects of neocortical synaptic loss in disorders such as Alzheimer's disease is to construct artificial neural networks with associative memory capabilities that function at multiple levels (Sutton et al., 1988a). The progressive destruction of neurons and connections can then be simulated in the context of evaluating the deterioration of neocortical-like function. For instance, is it possible to model the loss of information due to the *random yet selective destruction* of large neurons? How do losses occur at high associative levels with minimal impact at low levels? These questions can be approached using models, and although they are impressionistic, the models can nevertheless shed insight into how large scale networks react to destructive forces. The techniques, as outlined in the next sub-section, complement other ways of modeling synaptic and neuromodulatory alterations in Alzheimer's disease (e.g., Hasselmo, 1994).

4.4. Simulation Results

Within the conceptual framework of nested networks and neocortical dysfunction, the loss of synapses in Alzheimer's disease can be simulated by percolation techniques [see, for example, Essam (1980) or Stauffer (1987)]. The loss of synapses associated with *partial* neuron destruction is achieved by decreasing the numbers and relative strengths of connections linking networks. Synaptic loss associated with *complete* neuron loss corresponds to a site percolation problem.

Sutton et al. (1988b) simulated the effects of random but selective neuron loss in a nested network similar to the one shown in Figure 2. Each network consisted of fifty model neurons and had associative memory capabilities that stored three stable memory states at the first level. Twenty percent of the neurons in each network projected to each of the other two networks. The synaptic density of the projection neurons was three times greater than the non-projection neurons. The connections between networks served to encode memory at a second level. Specifically, three of the 27 $(3 \times 3 \times 3)$ possible combinations of first level memories were stored at a second level. By initializing one of the networks in a first level memory state, and starting the other two networks in random states, the performance of the entire network could be evaluated. This was accomplished by observing whether or not the network of networks was able to correctly recall an entire second level memory state, given that it was partially cued into one of the second level memories.

The results from several simulations are summarized in Figure 3. Memory recall at a second level is plotted as a function of the relative strength of projection neuron linkages between networks. The shape of the curves shows that as the connection strength of the linkages between the networks increases, the performance of the second level memory also increases. It reaches a maximum and then falls off, due to the breakdown of first level memory stability when second level memory properties dominate.

In Figure 3, the formation of neurofibrillary tangles is analogous to the process of partially destroying projection neurons. The linkages between the networks diminish and become severed when neurons die. In Figure 3, this is represented by a transition from the solid response curve to the dotted response curve. The curves were generated from computer experiments, wherein the projection neuron population was decreased from 20% (solid line) to 10% (dotted line). A 10% loss of neurons in the network, coupled with a lack of biasing in the inter-network connection strength, resulted in an *enormous deterioration of second level memory performance*. The associative recall performance dropped from greater than 70% efficiency to approximately 10% efficiency (Sutton et al., 1988b). However, there was *no effect on first level memory performance*. Without network boundaries and neuron heterogeneity, a 10% random loss of neurons had minimal effects on memory loss at either level.

Similar findings have been observed in simulations of nested neural networks with four levels of nesting (Sutton et al., 1988b). The random but selective destruction of key neurons can have catastrophic consequences on network performance. This is rather obvious. However, what is more subtle is that the destruction may be the result of a uniform process that has the appearance of being selective because some neurons have a relatively high synaptic density. Moreover, the random and uniform destruction of neurons results in a deterioration of function that starts with the highest levels and progresses to the lowest levels. This progression is not accounted for by the lesioning process per se, but rather by the underlying structural and dynamic features of the system. It may be that some associative losses in Alzheimer's and other diseases are the result of disconnections within and between multiple levels of structural and functional organization. In the context of views postulated by Wernicke (1874) and Geschwind (1965), some of the neocortical changes may constitute disconnection syndromes *par excellence.*

Nested Network with Simulated Synaptic Loss

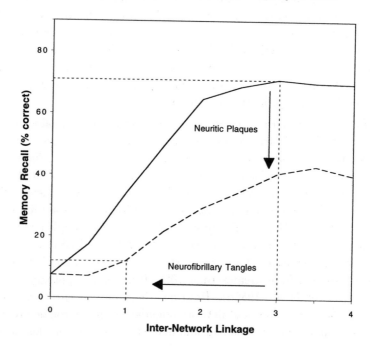

Figure 3. Plot of second level memory recall as a function of the strength of inter-network linkages. The solid line corresponds to 20% projection neurons and the dotted line corresponds to 10% projection neurons. The combined effect of simulated neurofibrillary tangles and neuritic plaques destroys second level memory performance, while essentially leaving first level memory performance unaltered. Modified from Sutton et al. (1988b).

5. Conclusions

As basic and clinical neuroscience move toward the next century, there will undoubtably be a need to develop new models to help integrate and illuminate our knowledge of the brain and mind. One of the fundamental challenges will be to link information about normal and altered function across different scales of organization. This chapter presents a modest attempt to look at this problem using nested neural networks. A theoretical framework, aided by computational and experimental ideas, has been described. Some links between structure and function in neocortical disease processes, including Alzheimer's disease, have examined. This work is only a beginning and is perhaps reflective of a renewed interest in developing physiologically based models of the brain and its disorders. With persistence and coordinated efforts using computer simulations, new experimental techniques and better clinical insights, the frontiers of integrative neuroscience of the neocortex and other structures will hopefully advance at an exciting pace.

6. Acknowledgements

The support of the NIH, Scientist Development Award MH01080, is gratefully acknowledged.

7. References

Abeles, M. *Corticonics: Neural Circuits of the Cerebral Cortex* (Cambridge U, Cambridge, 1991).

Alzheimer, A. *All Z Psychiatr* **64**, 146-148 (1907).

Anderson, J.A., Gately, M.T., Penz, P.A. & Collins, D.R. *IEEE Proceedings* **78**, 1646-1657 (1990).

Anderson, J.A. & Sutton, J.P. *World Congress of Neural Networks* **1**, 561-568 (1995).

Belair, J., Glass, L., an der Heiden, U. & Milton, J. *Dynamical Disease: Mathematical Analysis of Human Illness* (Am Institute of Physics, Woodbury, NY, 1995).

Darwin, C. *The Origin of the Species* (John Murray, London, 1859).

Donoghue, J.P., Leibovic, S. & Sanes, J.N. *Experimental Brain Research* **89**, 1 (1992).

Edelman, G.M. *Neural Darwinism* (Basic, New York, 1987).

Essam, J.W. *Rep Prog Phys* **43**, 833-912 (1980).

Fodor, J. *The Modularity of Mind* (MIT, Cambridge, 1983).

Freud, S. in Standard Edition of the *Complete Works of Sigmund Freud, Vol. 1* 281-397 (Hogarth (1953-1966), London, 1895).

Gazzaniga, M.S. *The Social Brain* (Basic, New York, 1985).

Geschwind, N.G. *Brain* **88**, 237-294, 585-644 (1965).

Goldman-Rakic, P.S. in *Annual Review of Neuroscience* (eds. Cowan, W.M., Shooter, E.M., Stevens, C.F. & Thompson, R.F.) 137-156 (Annual Review, Palo Alto, 1988).

Guan, L. in *Real time imaging: Theory, techniques and applications* (eds. Laplante, P. & Stoyenko, S.) (IEEE, New York, 1994).

Hasselmo, M.E. *Neural Networks* **7**, 13-40 (1994).

Hodgkin, A.L. & Huxley, A.F. *J. Physiol. (London)* **117**, 500-544 (1952).

Hubel, D.H. & Wiesel, T.N. *J. Physiol. (London)* **148**, 574-591 (1959).

Jackson, J.H. in *Selected Writings of John Hughlings Jackson, Vol. 2* (ed. Taylor, J.) 3-118 (Basic Books (1958), New York, 1884).

Jacobs, R.A., Jordan, M.I., Nowlan, S.J. & Hinton, G.E. *Neural Computation* **3**, 79-87 (1991).

Karni, A., et al. *Nature* **377**, 155-158 (1995).

Katzman, R. N. *Engl. J. Med.* **314**, 964-973 (1986).

Koch, C. & Segev, I. *Methods in Neuronal Modeling* (MIT, Cambridge, 1989).

Koch, C. & Davis, J.L. *Large-scale Neuronal Theories of the Brain* (MIT, Cambridge, 1994).

Lamour, Y. *Biomed Pharmacother* **48**, 312-318 (1994).

McCulloch, W.S. *Embodiments of Mind* (MIT, Cambridge, 1965).

McKenna, T., Davis, J. & Zornetzer, S. *Single Neuron Computation* (Academic, Cambridge, 1992).

Merzenich, M.M., Kaas, J.H., Wall, J., Nelson, R.J. & Sur, M. *Neuroscience* **10**, 639-665 (1983).

Minsky, M. *The Society of Mind* (Simon and Schuster, New York, 1985).

Mountcastle, V.B. in *The Mindful Brain* (eds. Edelman, G. & Mountcastle, V.B.) 7-50 (M.I.T., Cambridge, 1978).

Pandya, D.N. & Selzer, B. *J Comp Neurol* **204**, 196-210 (1982).

Parks, R. & Levine, D.S. *Fundamentals of Neural Networks for Neuropsychology* (MIT, Cambridge, In press).

Phillips, C.G. & Porter, R. *Corticospinal Neurones: Their Role in Movement* (Academic, London, 1977).

Rakic, P. in *The Organization of the Cerebral Cortex* (eds. Schmitt, F.O., Worden, F.G., Adelman, G. & Dennis, S.G.) 7-28 (MIT, Cambridge, 1981).

Rockel, A.J., Hiorns, R.W. & Powell, T.P.S. *Proc Anat Soc Gr Br Ire* **118**, 371 (1974).

Rumelhart, D.E., McClelland, J.L. & PDP, R.G. *Parallel Distributed Processing* (MIT, Cambridge, 1986).

Ruppin, E. & Reggia, J.A. *Neural Computation* **7**, 1105-1127 (1995).

Schwartz, M.F. *Modular Deficits in Alzheimer-Type Dementia* (MIT, Cambridge, 1990).

Sherrington, C.S. *The Integrative Action of the Nervous System* (Yale U, New Haven, 1906).

Singer, W. *Science* **270**, 758-764 (1995).

Spencer, H. *The Principles of Psychology* (Appleton, London., 1855).

Stauffer, D. *Introduction to Percolation Theory* (Taylor and Frances, London, 1987).

Sutton, J.P., Beis, J.S. & Trainor, L.E.H. *Mathl. Comput. Modelling* **11**, 346-350 (1988a).

Sutton, J.P., Beis, J.S. & Trainor, L.E.H. *J. Phys. A: Math. Gen.* **21**, 4443-4454 (1988b).

Sutton, J.P., Caplan, J.B. & Bandettini, P.A. *Human Brain Mapping* (abstract) In press (1996).

Sutton, J.P. *Intern. AMSE Conference on Neural Networks* **1**, 47-58 (1991).

Sutton, J.P. *World Congress on Neural Networks* **2** 536-539 (1993).

Sutton, J.P. *World Congress of Neural Networks* **1** 569-572 (1995).

Sutton, J.P. & Anderson, J.A. in *Neurobiology of Computation* (ed. Bower, J.M.) 317-322 (Kluwer Academic, Boston, 1995).

Szentagothai, J. *Proc. R. Soc. Lond. B.* **201**, 219-248 (1977).

Ts'o, D.Y., Gilbert, C.D. & Wiesel, T.N. *J Neurosci* **6**, 1160-1170 (1986).

Terry, R.D., Peck, A., DeTeresa, R. & et al. *Ann. Neur.* **10**, 184-192 (1981).

Vaadia, E., et al. *Nature* **373**, 515-518 (1995).

Van Essen, D.C., Anderson, C.H. & Felleman, D. *Science* **255**, 419-423 (1992).

Wernicke, C. *Der aphasische Symptomencomplex* (Breslau, 1874).

PSYCHIATRIC DISORDERS

Modeling Dysfunction of the Prefrontal Executive System

Daniel S. Levine
Departments of Mathematics and Psychology
Box 19528, University of Texas at Arlington, Arlington, TX 76019
b344dsl@utarlg.uta.edu

Abstract. The concept of executive function in the brain is given a new definition, as based in a distributed neural system whereby prefrontal cortex is interconnected with various other cortical and subcortical loci. Executive function is divided roughly into three interacting parts: affective guidance of responses; establishing linkage among working memory representations; and forming complex behavioral schemata. Neural network models of these parts are reviewed and fit into a preliminary theoretical framework.

1. Introduction

The prefrontal cortex has been called "the executive of the brain"[1,2]. This is because, based on lesion, electrophysiological, and imaging studies, this part of cortex seems to play a special role in coordinating and integrating plans of action based on a combination of sensory signals from the environment and visceral and motivational signals from the organism.

The variety of symptoms arising from lesions to different prefrontal subregions has led some researchers to doubt that prefrontal functions can be fit into a central "executive" role[3]. Their statements about lack of executive function, however, were made in opposition to the notion of a hierarchy under tight control of a single brain area (D. Stuss, personal communication). Rethinking based on neural network principles leads us not to reject but to reformulate the concept of executive function. We believe the brain has an executive *system* that is hierarchical and yet *distributed*. On the basis of both lesion and brain imaging studies, we argue that the frontal lobes perform an interrelated set of roles in cognition, and that the interrelations can be studied through a neural network model combining the frontal lobes with other regions (e.g., basal ganglia, thalamus, amygdala, hippocampus, cingulate cortex, cerebellum, temporal cortex, and parietal cortex). While lesions to dorsolateral, orbital, and medial areas of the prefrontal cortex tend to have different effects, the functions ascribed to these areas exert strong mutual influences, perhaps via frontal-to-frontal[4] or striatal-to-striatal[5] connections.

Various primary prefrontal functions have been proposed, including cognitive-emotional integration[6]; establishing flexibility of sets[7]; linking events across time[8]; and joining active working memory representations[9,10]. Model network studies suggest theory that can link all these different functions. Within this theory, emotional-cognitive integration, monitoring central sets, cross-temporal linking, and making working memory connections are all aspects of the overall "executive" role of calculating effective (although not always optimal) responses to a complex environment[11]. Before developing our models, we will review different components that various researchers and clinicians have identified as part of "executive function" or a "central executive."

413

1.1. What is Executive Function?

One of the best definitions of executive function (EF) was by Welsh and Pennington[13]: "EF is defined as ability to maintain an appropriate problem-solving set for attainment of a future goal" (pp. 199-230). These authors divided the maintenance of set for goal attainment into subfunctions such as inhibition (or deferral) of inappropriate responses; maintaining strategic plans of action sequences; and forming mental representations of tasks, including representations of both stimuli and the desired future goal state. Inhibition of inappropriate responses has been identified as an executive function by other authors[2,14-16]. The more "positive" components to EF, described by Welsh and Pennington as maintaining strategic plans and forming mental representations, were associated by Pribram[15] (Chapter 10) with three prefrontal subregions. Pribram called their functions *evaluating proprieties*, that is, deciding what actions are appropriate; *ordering priorities* among these actions; and *assessing practicalities*, that is, forming detailed subgoals and plans for performing appropriate high-priority actions. Lezak[14] enumerated clinical symptoms typically regarded as EF disturbances: decreased spontaneity and initiative; perseveration and rigidity of behavior; impulsiveness, and disinhibition of commonly suppressed responses; loss of sensitivity to one's role in social situations and one's errors on cognitive tasks; and concrete attitude, that is, inability to understand and plan around the abstract nature of situations.

Tranel, Anderson, and Benton[17] subsumed many common EF themes under planning, decision making, judgment, and self-perception. They reviewed neuropsychological tests widely used as measures of some aspect of EF and affected by damage to some prefrontal area. One is the *Wisconsin Card Sorting Test* (*WCST*), to be described in Section 1.4, used to test flexibility in shifting between cognitive categories. Another is the *Stroop Test*, whereby words for one color are presented in ink of another color and the subject asked to name the color. This is a test both of shifting cognitive set and inhibiting a habitual response (reading the word) in favor of a planned response (naming the color). There is also *verbal fluency*, whereby the subject produces words beginning with a certain letter, not allowing repetitions or proper names. This tests both spontaneity and ability to follow instructions, and is sensitive to left frontal lobe lesions; in its right frontal counterpart, *design fluency*, the subject generates drawings instead of words. Another is maze learning, used to test planning and executing a movement sequence. Planning movement sequences is also tested by the *Tower of Hanoi* puzzle or its variant, the *Tower of London*. More general planning ability is tested by cognitive estimation tasks, such as estimating the average length of a human spine, on which few people have rote knowledge but common sense reasoning leads to good guesses. Finally, there are tests of sensitivity to future consequences of behavior, such as a card game whose goal is to maximize long-term profit on a loan of play money — with strategies that may call for forgoing immediate rewards.

While these views of EF differ in details, all the above authors agree that EF is not needed for routine sensorimotor tasks or ordinary memory. This suggests a hierarchical "division of labor" whereby the executive system is connected in a feedback loop to lower-order systems in charge of routine behaviors. Under conditions that provide unambiguous signals to perform specific actions, the executive is inactive. Hence, the prefrontal cortex exhibits little neural activity in many simple motor, perceptual, and cognitive tasks (which is why for a long time it was called the "silent cortex"). When signals for action become ambiguous or weak, however, the executive is activated and regulates lower-order systems.

Our own theory of EF combines parts of functions posited separately by Nauta, Mishkin, Fuster, Goldman-Rakic and others. We suggest a computational theory of brain EF that encompasses and interrelates all these components. Broadly, these generic subfunctions include: (1) establishing links between working memory representations, which could represent sensory stimuli, potential motor actions, rewards or punishments, et cetera[9,10]; (2) creating, learning, and deciding among high-level schemata that embody repeatable, but often flexible action sequences[18-21]; (3) incorporating affective evaluations of sensory events or motor plans and using these evaluations to guide actions[6,22]. Another generic function suggested is linking events across time[8], which includes elements of both (1) and (2).

Kimberg and Farah[10] showed that a model of prefrontal (mainly dorsolateral) function based on working memory connections (our Subfunction (1)) could fit data on the WCST, Stroop Test, memory for context, and elementary aspects of motor sequencing. A variety of other tasks, used in either monkey or human experiments, involve some part of prefrontal cortex and are also related to forming working memory connections[23]. These include self-ordered pointing; learning serial order or relative recency of events; recognition memory; conditional learning; nonspatial conditional tasks; nonspatial delayed alternation; nonspatial matching; delayed matching to sample; delayed nonmatching to sample; and noun-verb transformation.

This shows that connecting working memory representations is a prominent part of what the prefrontal cortex does. Yet subfunction (1) of our list cannot account for *all* frontal lobe activity. There are other prefrontal tasks, such as the Tower of Hanoi, Tower of London, and stylus maze tests, which require deductive reasoning (see Section 1.2.2 below). This involves active creation of new rules based on sequences and recombinations of existing schemata, which comes under Subfunction (2) of our list. In fact, Kimberg and Farah's own model of the WCST involved creating nodes called "Color Sort," "Shape Sort," and "Number Sort." The existence of such nodes depends on some active reasoning or rule forming process based on environmental stimuli, not just connecting working memory representations of those stimuli. This kind of rule formation can be treated as a classification problem among remembered or potential sequences of motor acts[19,20,24].

Subfunction (2) includes learning a new motor pattern, such as driving a car, which makes new combinations from both innate reflexes and previously learned movements. It also includes developing strategies for games such as the Tower of Hanoi. It even includes learning by a monkey of appropriate rules in tasks such as delayed alternation (see Section 1.2.2). These situations differ in how much forming new schemata is externally or internally directed. All have in common, though, that contextually dependent sequences and combinations of existing schemata are newly encoded. In some cases, two or several new schemata are either tested or mentally imagined, and a choice made between them. As Grafman[18] described, the process can go on indefinitely, with elementary sequences (apparently stored in either the basal ganglia or supplementary motor area), then chunks of these sequences, then chunks of chunks, and so forth. At some point, the complexity becomes such as to require first the orbital, then the dorsolateral, prefrontal cortex[23]. As high-level chunks become more flexible, they eventually become representations of motor plans or goals, regardless of the exact method of implementing them[24].

Many connections between working memories in cognitive tasks are strengthened *by reward* or weakened *by punishment*. In monkeys, rewards are related to primary reinforcers such as food, whereas in humans rewards may, as in the WCST and Stroop Test, be related to secondary reinforcers such as approval. Hence limbic affective structures play an important role in executive function, as per our Subfunction (3). Interactions between current internal states, mediated in part by the amygdala, and the current external environment, mediated in part by the hippocampus, bias mental representations of sensory and motor events through modulation by other neural systems. Weakening this biasing mechanism due to prefrontal damage means that affect could be as strong as in a normal person but not guide actions. An example is the frustration felt by frontal patients on the WCST, which does not change their perseverative incorrect responses[25]. However, in other cases the patient's *uncontrolled* affect guides action, and because of frontal damage it is not moderated by normal intuitive perception of contextual appropriateness. In those situations[6,26], it is the *restraints* on raw emotional expression that have broken down, restraints also mediated by limbic system interactions.

Executive function also includes setting goals, which are determined in part by the person's or animal's basic drives and mediated by the cingulate cortex, as indicated by the lack of will in people with cingulate damage. Once the overall goals of the current situation have been arrived at, Subfunctions (1)-(3) of the executive are all involved in choosing subgoals. A similar "subgoaling" process in our own work has motivated our choice of subfunctions. We take the approach of breaking larger cognitive functions into smaller components, and using similar modeling principles repeatedly for the same components as they appear in different combinations[27]. This does *not* mean that these components are separate, rather that they interact dynamically and each has some structural and functional autonomy.

The distinction between working memory, affective guidance, and complex schema selection is analogous to the distinction between basic maintenance, emotion, and reasoning in the "triune brain." MacLean[28] located these three functions in different brain regions, but we believe the prefrontal executive system is involved in all of them. This makes the frontal lobes the best communicator between the "man, horse, and crocodile" inside us that MacLean lamented. However, this communication is often suboptimal. Visceral and affective systems elude executive control in some situations, such as crimes of passion or toxic relationships. The rational system eludes executive control in other situations, such as efficient fascism. This is because the executive remains silent when other brain systems have arrived at unambiguous decisions on how to act. Lower-level autonomy frees the organism to respond automatically, but its "down side" is that powerful subsystem signals can drown out important information. Yet the cortical-subcortical executive system works remarkably well much of the time. Section 2 explores network architectures for parts of this system, some of which have been simulated and some of which are in progress. To prepare for our theory, we first review data on cognitive effects of prefrontal lesions. Our general conclusions are also supported by extensive evoked potential and brain imaging data, not reviewed here for space reasons but discussed elsewhere[29].

1.2. Cognitive and Psychological Data from Lesion Studies

1.2.1. Effects of Lesions on Cognitive Flexibility

The Wisconsin Card Sorting Test (WCST) calls for changing classification rules when external reinforcement signals are altered. A sequence of cards is given, each displaying a number, color, and shape. The subject must match the card shown to one of 4 template cards, and is told whether the match is right or wrong, no reason given. After ten straight correct matches based on color, the criterion is switched to shape without warning. Then if ten correct matches are made to shape, the criterion shifts to number, then back to color, and so on. Patients with damage to the dorsolateral prefrontal cortex (DLPFC) can learn the color criterion as fast as normals but tend to perseverate in color choices even after the criterion is changed. By contrast, normals tend to change criteria 3 or 4 times over 128 trials. Though some recent results have been equivocal, it is still generally accepted that patients with DLPFC damage do worse than normals or patients with other cortical damage on the WCST[25,30]. Moreover, the nature of these frontal patients' errors is largely perseverative, that is, persisting in a classification rule after the context changes so that the rule is now inappropriate.

Petrides[31] studied conditional associative learning in humans with frontal surgical excisions, that is, part of all of prefrontal cortex (usually including DLPFC) removed to treat epilepsy. Subjects were shown six white cards in a row and six blue lamps in an irregular, but constant, pattern. They were told that each card corresponded to a different lamp, and asked to point to the correct card when a lamp was lit. Petrides found that frontal excisions impaired learning the mapping between lamps and cards. This task taxes the ability to choose the correct context for each response and inhibit previously learned responses that do not fit the current context. Excisions including the right hippocampus also interfered with learning this task. (The laterality seemed to be related to the spatial nature of the task. Another task, whereby required responses were hand postures rather than pointing to fixed locations, was impaired by left hippocampal damage.) To locate the crucial subregion of the prefrontal cortex, Petrides[32] taught a simpler conditional association task to monkeys with various lesions. Monkeys were rewarded for touching a stick when a green bottle cover was presented, but touching a button when a toy truck was presented. He found that the key cortical areas for this task in monkeys were Area 8 and the rostral part of Area 6: regions that are ambiguous, sometimes considered as posterior DLPFC, and other times considered "premotor" and not properly prefrontal.

1.2.2. Effects of Lesions on Inductive or Deductive Reasoning

Inductive reasoning has been studied in many monkey experiments. These involve monkeys who are rewarded with food for certain sequences of behaviors and try to discern what is the rule for sequences that are rewarding. A variety of evidence indicates that prefrontal lesions interfere with the ability to reliably learn rules above a certain level of complexity. In the classical delayed alternation test[33], a monkey has a choice of two places to go for food after a short pause, and is rewarded for alternating between the two locations on successive trials. Animals with lesions to the DLPFC have trouble learning this task.

Brody and Pribram[34] lesioned juvenile macaque monkeys in the DLPFC and assessed postoperative retention in two types of test. In the first type, known as the *externally ordered* or *invariant sequence* test, subjects had to respond in an exact order by pushing a series of panels based on given cues. In the second type of test, the *internally ordered* or *flexible sequence* test, subjects had to push all of several cued panels without repetitions but could push them in any order. There were three separate externally ordered sequences consisting of two or three panels the monkeys had to press in order. On each trial in the externally ordered case, the stimuli appeared in randomly placed locations on the four-by-four panel array. In order to receive a reward the monkey, in the two-stimulus case, pressed first a red and then a green panel irrespective of their location. The trial ended if the first panel pressed was not red, if the second press was incorrect, or if the subject was successful. The internally ordered sequence was presented in exactly the same manner except that the monkey was permitted to choose different orders from trial to trial as long as any given sequence contained no repetitions.

Pribram[35] tested rhesus monkeys in an environment where the number of objects rose successively from 2 to 12. Each time a new object was added, a peanut was placed under it. In the early stages of the experiment, monkeys with orbital frontal damage came to the novel object sooner than normals (though not reliably) because their tendency to go to the site of previous reward was not strong enough to overcome their attraction to novelty. As the number of objects increased to about 10, however, the performance of normal monkeys improved and overtook that of frontal monkeys. It has been suggested[22] that normal monkeys learn a high-order rule of "novelty is rewarding," and that this is a reasoning process unlike the simple emotional attraction to novelty. As in the delayed alternation and internally ordered sequence cases, frontal damage (though now in a different subregion) impairs the ability to learn such a rule.

Deductive reasoning tasks can only be effectively studied in humans. Unlike monkeys where lesions can be deliberately confined to a particular subregion, human patients rarely have lesions that are cleanly localized. Often, they have sustained frontal lobe damage due to head wounds from, for example, automobile accidents or gunshots, or else the damage is due to a tumor or a stroke. In any of those cases, their lesions may well cover more than one of the three canonical subregions (DLPFC, orbital, and medial). Hence, we usually can say with certainty only that some part of what we call the "executive network" is damaged. The "cleanest" cases are patients who have had surgical excisions to treat intractable epilepsy[36]; the areas removed typically include the DLPFC, but may also include parts of the orbital and medial frontal areas.

Some tasks involve devising puzzle solving strategies. Shallice[37] found patients with left frontal lesions deficient in his Tower of London, a simplification of the Tower of Hanoi which is popular in artificial intelligence circles. In the Tower of London, three beads of different colors are stacked up on one of three sticks of different sizes. The subject is given initial and goal positions, and must move from one position to the other in the fewest moves. This requires anticipating future consequences, because the short-term oriented algorithm of moving one specific bead to its target position is often not optimal. Karnath, Wallesch, and Zimmermann[38] studied frontal patients and controls on a maze, only part of which was in view at a time. They found that frontal patients do much worse than normals until they have learned enough about the environment to find the maze steps routine. Alivisatos[36] compared patients who had undergone frontal (largely DLPFC) or temporal surgical excisions with normals on a mental rotation task. Subjects were shown rotated alphanumeric characters, and asked if these characters when upright were in a correct or mirror-reversed position. Normals and temporal patients, but not patients with DLPFC excisions, could benefit on this task from advance viewing of the upright character.

Shallice and Evans[39] asked subjects questions whose answers they would be unlikely to know from memory but they could deduce from common knowledge. Some questions might be answered by calculations; for example, "How long is an average man's spine?" could be estimated by knowing the average man's height and subtracting plausible fractions for head and legs. Others might be answered by comparisons with better-known facts; for example, "How fast do race horses gallop?" might be inferred from typical walking speeds and typical car driving speeds. On this type of questions, frontal lobe patients made significantly more guesses outside the normal range than patients with other brain lesions.

2. Neural Network Models of Frontal Dysfunction

We now discuss modeling the three parts of executive function — first, affective guidance of behavior; second, schema and sequence formation; third, working memory — and their typical dysfunctions. The neural modeling principles we use are suggested by a combination of behavioral and neural data. The units or nodes in the networks typically correspond to groups of neurons rather than including detailed processing of single neurons. Rather than adopting a "one size fits all" approach to neural network modeling, we employ suitable combinations of existing network architectures, each previously designed for a somewhat different function.

2.1. Modeling of Cognitive-Motivational Linkages

Because the frontal lobes link cortical semantic processing areas with motivational areas of the limbic system and hypothalamus[6], frontal lesions often produce behavior that lacks affective guidance. Such dissociation between affect and action can lead to perseveration in behavior that was once, but is no longer, rewarding — even in the face of emotional frustration at the lack of reward. It can also lead frontally damaged humans or monkeys to respond more quickly than normals to novel stimuli in preference to rewarded stimuli. Finally, weakened affective guidance impairs performance of complex motor sequences or learning of rules that classify which sequences are rewarding. Perseveration and novelty preference are discussed in this section, and sequence learning in Section 2.2.

2.1.1. Perseveration

Leven and Levine[40] modeled the Wisconsin Card Sorting Test (WCST) as an example of perseveration due to dorsolateral prefrontal lesions. Their network (Figure 1) simulates the result that patients with DLPFC damage learn the first sorting criterion of the WCST but are often unable to switch when the criterion changes[25]. The network adds selective attentional modulation to the adaptive resonance theory network (ART) for pattern classification[41] (Figure 2). Classification of both sensory and motor patterns is important to models of frontal lobe function in many ways. In the WCST, the subject must classify sensory patterns in a way that may be dependent on external reinforcement contingencies. In various tasks that a monkey performs to obtain food reward (see Section 1.2.2), the monkey must classify together all motor patterns associated with reward and discern the rule they fit in order to generalize to other patterns.

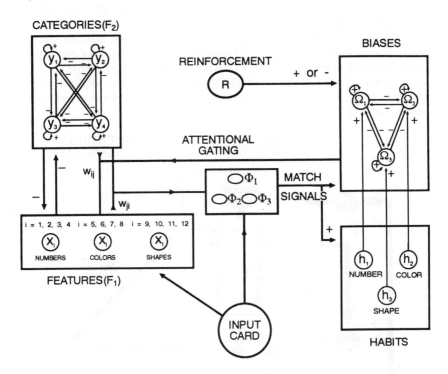

Figure 1. Network used to simulate card sorting data. Frontal damage is modeled by reduced gain from the reinforcement node to bias nodes λ_i (i=1 for number, 2 for color, 3 for shape.) "+" means excitation; "-" means inhibition; an arrow means the connection is unmodifiable. (Adapted from Leven and Levine, copyright © 1987 IEEE; reprinted with permission of the publishers.)

Since ART is also a basis for our sequence models, it is worth discussing its basic features and possible biological substrates. ART networks include nodes that respond selectively to novel stimuli and that may make either fine or coarse categorizations; Desimone[42] found similar properties in some neurons of visual association (inferotemporal) cortex. The original ART (Figure 2) is an unsupervised network that self-organizes natural "clusters" in a stream of incoming sensory patterns. This involves two layers of nodes, often identified with two layers of sensory cortex or with cortex and thalamus, whereby "higher" level nodes encode classes of "lower" level node activity patterns. Standard ART dynamics lack executive function, but "executive" nodes can modulate a two-layer ART network.

422

First, the executive system can mediate attentional biases in favor of the input attributes most relevant to current goals. This is done in the model of Figure 1 using "bias nodes" that modulate inter-layer synapses. Since affective values of stimuli are mediated by the amygdala[43], the effects of such bias nodes could be analogous to some type of amygdalar modulation of signals between layers of sensory cortex. Second, there can be learnable connections between two separate ART classifying networks, as in ARTMAP[44] (Figure 3). In particular, Bapi and Levine[45] used a simplified version of ARTMAP combined with a sequence learning network to model how a monkey learns to associate a class of motor sequences with a reward, as will be discussed in Section 2.2.

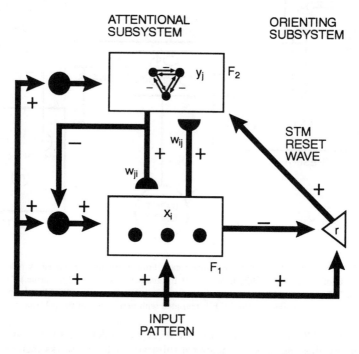

Figure 2. An adaptive resonance theory (ART) network. When an input pattern arrives at F^1, it sends bottom-up signals to F_2, where nodes compete for storage of the pattern. The orienting system causes testing or creation of a new category if the input sufficiently mismatches the prototype (stored at top-down synapses) of the current one. Semicircle means a connection is modifiable. (Adapted from Carpenter and Grossberg, 1987, with permission of Academic Press.)

In the modified ART of Figure 1, a card is presented to the feature layer (F_1) as a binary vector encoding its features. The category layer (F_2) classifies the input card with one of the templates depending on similarity. Nodes representing template categories compete via lateral inhibition. Corresponding to each feature class (color, number, shape) is a habit node and a bias node. The habit node for a feature class keeps track of the frequency of classifications using that attribute. Bias nodes gate signals from the feature to the category layer so as to emphasize one of the criteria. The bias strength for a given criterion is influenced both by the corresponding habit and by the (positive or negative) reinforcement signal.

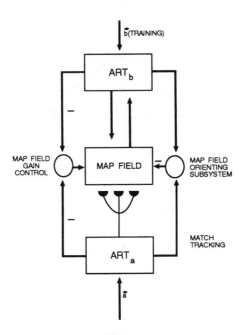

Figure 3. ARTMAP, consisting of two ART modules (ART_a and ART_b), with detailed structure not shown but as in Figure 2, and a "map field" that forms associations between categories learned in each ART module. (Reprinted from Carpenter et al., 1991, with permission of Elsevier Science Publishing Company.)

Suppose the network learns to classify cards based on color. Then color habit and color bias are increased relative to habits and biases for shape and number. If the criterion changes to shape, and reinforcement is strong, color bias eventually decreases and shape bias increases, leading to classification based on shape. But if reinforcement is weak, it cannot overcome the positive feedback leading to color habit perseveration. The network with strong reinforcement is assumed to mimic a normal subject, and the network with weak reinforcement is

424

assumed to mimic a patient with DLPFC damage. Interpreting frontal damage as weak reinforcement signals is based on the fact that prefrontal is the area of cortex with the strongest connections to reward areas such as the amygdala and hypothalamus[6,9]. Suggestive anatomical analogues can be found for other parts of the network: the bias signals might be somewhat like noradrenergic innervation of the amygdala[46] and the habit signals like activity of some part of basal ganglia[47].

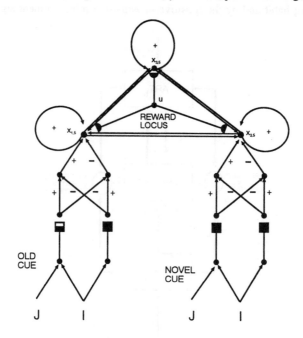

Figure 4. Network to simulate novelty data. Two gated dipoles (see text) shown correspond to an old cue and a novel cue; their outputs $x_{i,5}$ represent tendencies to approach each cue. $x_{3,5}$ is the output of a third dipole, the rest of which is not shown. Competition among $x_{i,5}$ nodes is biased both in favor of rewarded cues, by Hebbian synapses with u, and in favor of novel cues, by transmitter depletion (indicated by smaller dark area) at "square" synapses. Relative strength of biases depends on gain of reward signals to $x_{i,5}$'s, which frontal damage lowers. (Adapted from Levine & Prueitt, 1989, with permission of Pergamon Press.)

2.1.2. Modeling Novelty Preference

Weakening connections between cognition and reinforcement also explains the paradoxical result that monkeys with lesions of a different prefrontal area, the orbital prefrontal cortex, are excessively attracted to novel cues[35]. Levine and

Prueitt[22] simulated this effect using the network of Figure 4. This network consists of a field of *gated dipoles*[48] each of which represents the approach behavior of monkeys to a different cue. The gated dipole was introduced as a general circuit for opponent processes (e.g., fear-relief, novel-familiar, on-off) using habituating (depletable) neurotransmitters. In this network it accounts for approach to novelty. This tendency competes with the tendency to approach previously rewarded cues, due to associative learning of connections between cue representations and a reward locus. In normal monkeys it is assumed that the gain on the reward is high so that the monkey approaches a previously rewarded cue even when a novel cue is introduced. For frontally damaged monkeys, the reward signal gain is low so approach to cues is now based more on novelty than on previous reward.

2.2. Schemata and Motor Sequences

Shallice[49] (p. 332) described two premises of his model: "The first ... is that routine selection of routine operations is decentralised. The second is that non-routine selection is qualitatively different and involves a general-purpose supervisory System, which modulates rather than dictates the operation of the rest of the system." In his theory neural systems operate by means of discrete programs for thought or action called *schemata*. There is, for example, a schema for driving a car, or cutting a slice of bread, or saying the word for a digit. Deciding which schema to use is based on what Shallice called *contention scheduling*: competition among existing, determined, courses of action. If contextual information is clear, contention scheduling suffices. If the context is more complex or ambiguous, however, the *supervisory system* is required to decide which of the previously developed schemata to activate in the current situation.

Shallice's evidence includes data indicating that frontal patients often activate the "wrong" schema based on a single contextual cue, without evaluating the rest of the context. In one example, a patient was given a written arithmetic problem: find the combined age of a son and his two parents, given that the son is 15, his father is 25 years older, and his mother is 5 years younger than the father. In addition to arithmetic errors leading to a wrong answer, this patient said that 40 was the total age of "the father, the son and the Holy Ghost." It appeared that hearing himself talk about the father and son triggered a prevailing schema in the patient's mind that included the contextually irrelevant association "Holy Ghost."

Schemata have varying degrees of flexibility. An example Shallice uses is the distinction between driving, which calls for well-defined and invariant actions in certain situations (although they can be overridden), and paying a bill, which can be done in different ways (e.g., by check or credit card). The more flexible schemata he called *memory organization packets* or *MOPs*. The boundary line between schemata and MOPs, however, is fuzzy, as Shallice[49] (p. 333) notes.

Shallice's schema theory is a useful starting point for theories of EF, but leaves unanswered questions: (1) If a schema has many variations, how does the brain decide which variation to use when the context does not strongly bias the choice? Some patients with orbitofrontal damage have trouble with such decisions, even minor ones such as what restaurant to eat at[26], suggesting that non-forced choices require the orbitofrontal part of the executive system. (2) How are new schemata created, and how does the executive modulate their creation? Children, whose frontal lobes are not fully developed until the age of about 15, learn repeatable behavior patterns, so the executive seems not to be needed for all new schemata, only the more complex ones (MOPs). Grafman[18] suggested that commonly activated behavior patterns should be less sensitive to frontal damage than rare ones. Does this mean that even some MOPs are eventually coded outside prefrontal cortex if activated often enough? (3) What signal triggers control transfer from contention scheduling to the supervisory system? Does some measure of ambiguity in lower-level circuits pass a threshold? Several model networks include some such measure[41], but no theory yet exists of how the brain computes this measure. (4) How is the hierarchy of schemata structured? Grafman[18] defined a *structured event complex* (SEC) as a "set of events, actions, or ideas that ... form a knowledge unit (e.g., a schema)" (p. 194). He defined a subclass of SECs called *managerial knowledge units (MKUs)* which are the SECs "specifically involved with planning, social behavior, and the management of knowledge." For example, high in the hierarchy there is an MKU for eating a meal in general, followed a step down by the MKU for eating a meal in a restaurant, then by eating lunch at McDonald's, finally by eating French fries with a fork. Where are such nested structures "located" in the brain and how do they interact? (5) How do schemata relate to motor sequences? Several of Shallice's examples of planning involve novel sequences of previously learned behaviors. Yet as noted in Section 1.2, frontal lobes are not required to learn a rote sequence of behaviors based on reward[34] but are required to learn rules bringing together variations of a sequence.

Answers to these questions are in progress. How they relate to prefrontal cortex can be deduced from what sorts of actions require frontal lobes. In general, the data discussed in Section 1.2 suggest that frontal lobes are needed to express flexible schemata, to create complex new schemata, and to decide which existing schema to use in a complex context, but not to keep performing invariant schemata in unambiguous contexts. Yet frontally damaged behavior is not always more rigid than normal behavior; in some cases (e.g., the "Holy Ghost" example) frontally damaged patients behave in unpredictable ways. This is when partial contextual cues retrieve an inappropriate schema; Shallice[37] calls this a *capture error*.

Prefrontal damage also impairs sequential task performance (see Section 1.2.2). Monkeys with DLPFC damage can perform a sequence of movements (touching specific objects) when the order of items is fixed but not when the order is variable[34]. If there are several available cues and the monkey must touch a certain set of cues, without repeats but in any order, intact frontal lobes are required. Bapi and Levine[45,50] simulated this sequence task[34] with a network (Figure 5) that combines the *avalanche*[51] for sequence storage and recall with a simplified version of ARTMAP for associating two sets of patterns[44]. The ARTMAP module associates particular spatiotemporal patterns with a reward. In this network, a vector of sequence items is presented to the F_1 layer. Interactions among F_2, F_3, and F_4 layers enable the order of item activations at F_1 to be in a primacy distribution (that is, the first item has highest activity and the last item the least, leading to recall of items in the correct order for performance). This order is also stored in the weights between F_3 and F_4. Thus the avalanche combined with the sequence detector F_4 layer can store sequence order information for subsequent recall.

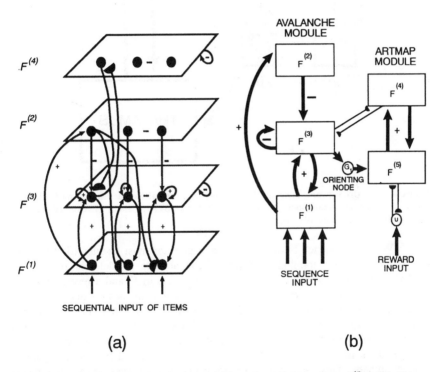

(a) (b)

Figure 5. (a) Motor sequence learning network. A sequence detector layer, $F^{(4)}$, is joined to an avalanche module consisting of the other layers, that forms conditioned associations between items at $F^{(1)}$. (Adapted by permission of the publisher from Bapi & Levine, *Neural Networks*, 7, 1167-1180. Copyright 1994 by Elsevier Science Publishing Company.) (b) Network for sequence classification, combining the avalanche of part (a) with ARTMAP. (Reprinted from Levine, 1995, with permission of the Psychonomic Society.)

428

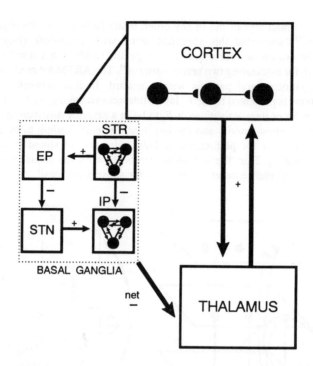

Figure 6. ACTION network, including learning between cortical modules and learned effects of cortex on striatal lateral inhibition; see text for more details. STR=striatum, EP=external pallidum, STN=subthalamic nucleus, IP=internal pallidum.

When a sequence is first presented, a detector must be identified to learn that sequence. After training, a sequence can activate its detector in F_4. The ARTMAP module consists of a copy of the detectors in F_5 and a reward node, to classify sequences as rewarded or unrewarded. Now assume the network has learned sequences ABC and ACB but only ABC is rewarded. If A is presented as the first item, both sequences are activated at F_4. However, since only one has been rewarded, only the ABC detector is recalled in the avalanche module. Frontal damage is, as in the WCST and novelty models, mimicked by lowered gain of reward signals. This sequence learning network may have some anatomical analogues. The avalanche module might be analogous to some part of corpus striatum, as indicated by data showing that striatal, but not neocortical, damage interferes with a stereotyped grooming sequence in rats[52]. The network can learn independently that ABC and CBA are both rewarding, but cannot infer from what it has learned that another arrangement of A, B, and C (ACB, BAC, BCA, or CAB) will be rewarding. Models of general rule-learning (inductive reasoning) will be considered in Section 3.

2.3. Working Memory and the ACTION Network

The ACTION network of Taylor and his colleagues[21,53] mimics anatomy of frontal cortex, basal ganglia, and associated thalamic nuclei. It decomposes at least into five main loops of motor action, frontal eye fields, limbic activity, object and position working memory, and strategy working memory). These correspond to the cortico-thalamo-striatal loops described by Alexander, DeLong, and Strick[54] (see Figure 6). The network has a feedback loop between cortex and thalamus whose threshold is modulated by a disinhibitory feed from cortex through basal ganglia to thalamus. Thus activity arriving at a cortical region from posterior cortex (parietal or temporal) connections to frontal cortex may cause the cortico-thalamic loop to be activated, and stay on. Such persistence may crucially require support from the basal ganglia disinhibition, which may be achievable by means of cingulate activation (as "drive")[55] from some set point detector, or from some goal memory set up there or on another portion of the network.

ACTION, combined with the modulated ART networks described in Section 2.2, can support the EF functions of working memory, sequence learning (schema construction), and learning affective values of inputs. Storing flexible representations on frontal cortex requires representations of posterior activity both by lateral connections within frontal cortex and by cortico-striatal connections that can modify thresholds. Lateral connections turn the cortices into feedback networks, and can be trained so as to lead to particular attractor states. Cortico-striatal connections sculpt the sizes of the basins of attraction around these memory fixed points so as to allow one or other of them to be accessed (and be persistent as a working memory) according to signals from other regions, such as limbic cortex.

2.4. Work in Progress: Modeling Executive Function as a Whole

Executive function as a whole should utilize some network that combines the ACTION and modified ART modules described above, connected by other yet unknown architectures.

2.4.1. Value Driven Learning

Valuation arises from bodily responses to rewards, via the hypothalamus, signaled to the amygdala at about the same time as a representation of the rewarded input. The resulting signal can be modifiable by either reinforcement learning or Hebbian associative learning. The former might arise via circuitry whereby differences between desired and actual responses are part of the signal modifying connection weights. Yet neither amygdala nor cortex seems to possess that type of circuitry. Moreover, Taylor and Alavi[56] showed that Hebbian and reinforcement learning can both fit equally well some data on amygdalar reward-association learning[57]. Hebbian learning seems to occur with the presence of NMDA receptors, which are common in both cortex and amygdala. Thus we assume that learning consists of Hebbian association of reinforcing signals and input representations. Reinforcing signals need not only be arriving at the amygdala (as primary signals) but also in output regions of the amygdala (for secondary reinforcement).

2.4.2. Modeling Active Working Memory

The ACTION network architecture includes both lateral connections on the cortical sheet and vertical connections from cortex to basal ganglia and thalamus. Their dynamics can be described as flow of states toward cortical attractors, with striatum guiding and modulating which attractor is being approached. This network structure facilitates forming connections between working memory representations via feedback resonance between cortex and thalamus, leading to a growth of activity unless there is a cutoff due to inhibition or adaptation. Taylor and Alavi[58] discussed this and fit their model to growth patterns of population vectors in motor cortex[59]. Lateral connections between cortical neurons sculpt basins of attraction so as to make the frontal cortex like a "blackboard" on which any input determining a desired direction can be written. Striatal modulation both facilitates fine control of these basins of attraction and gives other regions the power to modify the basins.

The five frontal loops of Alexander et al.[54] receive inputs from cortical and limbic areas relevant to the current task. For example, superior and inferior temporal gyri feed to lateral orbitofrontal cortex, and parietal cortex and arcuate premotor cortex to DLPFC, while limbic structures (hippocampus, amygdala, subiculum, superior temporal gyrus) feed to ventral striatum, a part of the orbitofrontal loop. Thus both posterior cortex and limbic system modulate striatal effects on cortical attraction basins. These combine with learned cortico-cortical effects between the frontal networks. Active memory combines a pattern arriving from posterior cortex with a value signal from amygdala. This signal is received by both cortical and striatal regions in the appropriate ACTION network. Response from cells sensitive to the input combines with Hebbian learning at relevant synapses so as to develop an active memory record of the input. This corresponds to persistence of joint cortical-striatal input to the network, hence to active memory of the most recent posterior inputs or of those from other ACTION networks.

2.4.3. Schema Learning, Selection, and Execution

As for how schemata develop, many models have been developed for learning temporal sequences[45,50,60]. A specific approach via the ACTION network[21] uses reinforcement learning to allow a basin of attraction of the network to be modified by activation of other cortical neurons. These newly activated neurons then send activity to the striatum and are assumed to cause, by lateral inhibitory connections there, a modification of the previous cortical activity so as to send it to a new basin of attraction. The learning process is assumed to be supported by a reinforcement signal from the amygdala acting on a Hebbian learning substrate, as described earlier. Further steps in the schema are learned similarly.

Selection between complex schemata seems to have two components. The first involves competition, via lateral inhibition, between striatal nodes impressed by these schemata. That may occur through inputs to striatum from given cortical nodes, so only short range inhibition is needed. The second component uses amygdalar input similar to that used in Hebbian learning. Limbic modulation could affect the process at multiple loci. First, as in the model of Figure 1, it can selectively enhance perception of certain attributes of incoming stimuli, thereby biasing categorization toward one that stresses salient attributes. As discussed in Section 2.3, such a mechanism could involve amygdalar modulation of connections between levels of sensory cortex, such as between striate and inferotemporal cortices[42]. As in the WCST model and a related decision model[61], such selective categorization influences relative values attached to different schemata and thereby biases selection among schemata. The medial orbital frontal cortex (MOBFC) seems to be required when the salient attribute shifts during the course of the task[62].

Now suppose a complex schema is being run. Then premotor, supplementary motor, and motor cortices generate sequences corresponding to this schema. This translates to continuous striatal modification of cortical basins of attraction. A valued input may then modify this sequence processing. This could occur at the beginning of the schema, in which case the value signal determines which schema is activated. Or it could occur at a later stage, causing a change in schema. What has been said for a single value signal can be extended to a self schema, which may be used to give guidance at a set of later decision points as various possible ACTION schema have to be chosen between at each of these points in time. Such higher order guidance would make for a highly flexible system of response. This also gives a mechanism to fuse affective value with action responses, since the valuation schema stored in the MOBFC can interact with ACTION schema in the other four frontal loops — possibly by means of the ART-related architectures described in Section 2.1. The construction of affective schemata themselves in the MOBFC also involves structures in the limbic system and ventral striatum[63].

3. Work in Progress: Rule Formation and Analogical Reasoning

Some cognitive scientists have argued that the connectionist approach is *inherently unsuitable* for modeling some kinds of high-order cognitive processing[64]. Fodor, Pylyshyn, and others believe connectionist networks are good for modeling pattern recognition and classification, but not processes involving learning semantic relationships and rules. Against that, it has been argued that the human brain is a connectionist system, being composed of neurons and synapses with continuously varying electrical and chemical activities[65]. And we are able to perform semantic reasoning, learn inference, and do arithmetic, though probably not in an optimal manner. Hence, our brains are an existence proof that neural networks *can* perform high-order rule learning and encoding. This process is likely to involve numerous brain regions, but three seem particularly important: the frontal lobes, hippocampus, and amygdala.

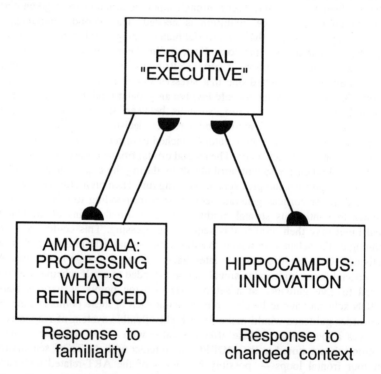

Figure 7. Schematic of connections between three brain regions and their functions in rule formation.

High-level concepts ("move to the right," "green plastic," "the number 4") correlate with brain activity at many loci. At this stage of modeling we assign network nodes to concepts without specifying the nodes' exact location in the brain (though we often have rough guesses), how many neurons each consists of, or how the nodes arose. Single cell data from prefrontal cortex[66], however, partially support the existence of such concept nodes as distinct cell groups. In the course of one behavioral task (delayed matching to simple), specific prefrontal cells became selectively tuned to significant stimuli or rewards related to the task.

Sections 2.1 and 2.2 discussed three rules that require intact frontal lobes to be learned well[33,34,35]. These rules can be summarized as (a) "do A, B, and C once each, in any order, with no repeats"; (b) "alternate A and B": (c) "go to the most novel object." In general, the prefrontal cortex seems necessary to learn any complex rule about which classes of stimuli or motor actions lead to reward. Can some network model how the prefrontal cortex, along with limbic motivational regions and neocortical sensory and motor regions, extracts the regularity from the organism's experience of reward or nonreward, thereby "deciding" the rule for obtaining reward? Supervised neural network algorithms, such as back propagation and ARTMAP, can learn to associate any arbitrary subset of spatial or spatiotemporal pattern space with reward. However, such algorithms learn only examples they have seen and cannot generalize to those they have not seen. Without this generalization capacity, these networks cannot yet be said to infer rules[45].

An intelligent rule learner must consider many possible levels of rule complexity. The prefrontal cortex is implicated in this search because it forms mental images of possible states[67]. So is the hippocampus because it processes inputs from all areas of sensory and association cortex for memory storage[68], and the amygdala because it does affective evaluation of sensory stimuli[43].

3.1. The "Trilogy" of Frontal Lobes, Amygdala, and Hippocampus

Pribram[15] (Chs. 8 and 9) reviewed data implicating amygdala and hippocampus in complementary roles. The amygdala produces a sense of familiarity, whereas the hippocampus is involved in innovation. More specifically, amygdalar lesions impair processing of parts of the environment that are currently being reinforced (positively or negatively). Monkeys with amygdalar damage, for example, are less prone than normals to avoid locations of earlier punishments. Hippocampal lesions, by contrast, interfere with processing of parts of the environment that are not currently reinforced. Hence the hippocampus is required to process currently irrelevant "background," which needs to be stored in case contextual changes make such background information necessary; for example, when approach to a previously neutral object is rewarded. As shown in Figure 7, the frontal lobes somehow "supervise" which of the other two systems (hippocampal or amygdalar) should be engaged in a particular context.

The hippocampus is required for orienting to novel events. Since the hippocampus deals with storing new associations in short-term memory[68], it has been suggested that it can also orient to novel *beliefs* such as rules[19]. If rules based on currently attended attributes lead to incorrect predictions, the frontal lobes could suppress their signals to the amygdala and enhance their signals to the hippocam-

434

pus. The hippocampus then engages a search over perceptual dimensions to which the amygdala has previously suppressed attention. If a rule based on one of these dimensions, which could have been encoded at any of several brain levels, turns out to predict what is reinforcing, attention shifts to that dimension. Selective attention then engages the amygdala. We still lack a complete theory of how the frontal lobes, limbic system, and related areas extract rules from the rewarded set of motor patterns. However, the three rules we list — delayed alternation, flexible sequence learning, and novelty discrimination — all involve time and novelty dimensions. We now present a tentative theory for extracting rules of this sort.

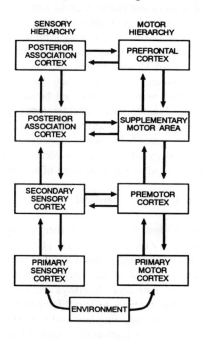

Figure 8. Parallel hierarchies of sensory and motor areas in the cerebral cortex. (From Fuster, *Current Opinion in Neurobiology*, 1993, with permission.)

3.2. Rules Involving Novelty and Time Dimensions

The paradigms of delayed alternation[33], flexible sequence learning[34], and pairing novelty with reward[35] are all impaired by frontal lobe damage, though the first two mostly involve DLPFC and the third orbitofrontal cortex. (Pairing *familiarity* with reward is also impaired by orbital damage[62].) All three paradigms involve rewarding a class of movement patterns that is somehow defined by novelty. In delayed alternation, the rule is: go to the location not where you were most recently. In flexible sequence learning, it is: touch a set of stimuli without repeating, which at each choice point is: move toward an object you have *never* moved to before. In pairing novelty with reward, it is: move toward an *object* that is novel. The difference between delayed alternation and the flexible sequence task is one of time scale: in one case the rewarded movement is novel over two trials, in the other it is novel over the whole task. The difference between both these tasks and the third task is one of rewarding "motor novelty" versus "sensory novelty." We assume that in the course of a task, any relevant object develops its own sensory representation. We propose that each object also develops a *motor* representation of movement toward that object.

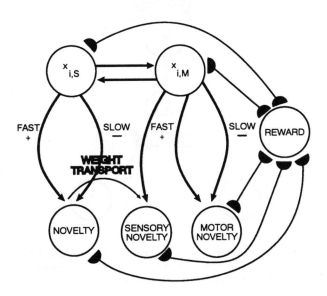

Figure 9. Weight transport model. Each input activates a novelty detector quickly then shuts it off slowly. Weights from $x_{i,s}$ to "novelty" are transported to weights from $x_{i,m}$ to "sensory novelty."

Such motor representations are supported by the hierarchy of brain motor areas that is roughly parallel to the sensory hierarchy in reverse order[24] (Figure 8). Primary motor cortex codes specific muscle movements; high-level motor areas code more abstract movement commands such as "move to that green triangle."

436

Since monkeys learn to associate certain movements with reward, the distinction between motor and sensory novelty must be drawn at nodes coding movements. But for a *motor* node to code *sensory* novelty, it must somehow inherit that property from its related sensory node. This suggests *hard wired* coupling between, say, the "green triangle" sensory node and the "move toward green triangle" motor node. Such a constitutive relationship has been considered hard to achieve in a connectionist network[64]. The hard wiring answers Fodor and Pylyshyn's[64] plaint that in neural networks all relationships are equally easy to learn.

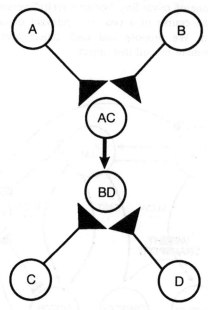

Figure 10. Scheme for weight transport. *AC* is a matching neuron, represented by filled triangles, that responds to the conjunction of signals from *A* and *C*; node *BD* is analogous. Hard-wired signal from *AC* to *BD* means that one association is transferred to the other.

If, as Fuster[24] says, the highest level of the sensory hierarchy is parietal cortex and the highest level of the motor hierarchy prefrontal, this fixed connection has implications for parieto-frontal signals. It suggests that while sensory neuron groups learn in the course of a task whether to code, say, green triangles or polka dotted bunnies, once they are committed to objects they commit the related motor neurons. Hence, learning at low levels of abstraction is followed by hard wiring at high levels. Figure 9 shows how if a sensory node x_{iS} has a fixed connection with a motor node x_{iM}, then x_{iM} can inherit a property of x_{iS} (e.g., sensory novelty). The mechanism proposed is *weight transport*: synaptic weights from $x_{i,S}$ to a node encoding an attribute are translated to weights from $x_{i,M}$ to a node encoding a corresponding attribute. This same property inheritance mechanism might also support a connectionist model of analogical reasoning.

Weight transport seems biologically implausible, which is a common objection to back propagation[69]. Yet its essence might be captured by another mechanism that seems more plausible: the *matching neuron* (Figure 10), a type of neuron that responds to converging signals from two other neurons. That is, a weight is encoded at a neuron instead of at a synapse. This idea is used in another model of prefrontal tasks[70]. If such neurons are found in frontal lobes, it will be one of many cases (others being Hebbian learning, lateral inhibition, and opponent processing) whereby a neural network principle is first suggested by cognitive data, and much later verified physiologically. Hence the words "biologically implausible" need not be taken as a death blow to a theoretical idea.

Acknowledgment. Raju Bapi, Guido Bugmann, and John Taylor are collaborators on some of the work in progress.

References

1. A. R. Luria, *Human Brain and Psychological Processes* (Harper and Row, New York, 1966).
2. K. H. Pribram, in *Psychophysiology of the Frontal Lobes*, eds. K. H. Pribram and A. R. Luria. (Academic Press, New York, 1973).
3. D. T. Stuss, T. Shallice, M. P. Alexander, and T. W. Picton, *Ann. N. Y. Acad. Sci.*, in press
4. H. Barbas and D. N. Pandya, *J. Comp. Neurol.* **286** (1989) 353-375.
5. J. C. Houk, J. L. Davis, and D. G. Beiser, eds., *Models of Information Processing in the Basal Ganglia* (MIT Press, Cambridge, MA, 1994)
6. W. J. H. Nauta, *J. Psychiat. Res.* **8** (1971) 167-187.
7. M. Mishkin, in *The Frontal Granular Cortex and Behavior*, eds. J. M. Warren and K. Akert (McGraw-Hill, New York, 1964).
8. J. M. Fuster, *The Prefrontal Cortex* (2nd Ed.) (Raven, New York, 1989).
9. P. S. Goldman-Rakic, in *Handbook of Physiology* (Vol. 5), ed. F. Plum (American Physiological Society, Bethesda, MD, 1987).
10. D. Y. Kimberg and M. J. Farah, *J. Exp. Psychol.: Gen.* **122** (1993) 411-428.
12. A. R. Damasio, in *Frontal Lobe Function and Dysfunction*, eds. H. S. Levin, H. M. Eisenberg, and A. L. Benton, p. 404 (Oxford, New York, 1991).
13. M. C. Welsh and B. F. Pennington, *Devel. Neuropsychol.* **4** (1988) 199-230.
14. M. Lezak, *Neuropsychological Assessment* (Oxford, New York, 1983).
15. K. H. Pribram, *Brain and Perception* (Erlbaum, Hillsdale, NJ, 1991).
16. D. T. Stuss and D. F. Benson, *The Frontal Lobes* (Raven, New York, 1986).

438

17. D. Tranel, S. W. Anderson and A. Benton, in *Handbook of Neuropsychology* (Vol. 9), eds. F. Boller and J. Grafman (Elsevier, Amsterdam, 1994).

18. J. Grafman, in *Handbook of Neuropsychology* (Vol. 9), eds. F. Boller and J. Grafman (Elsevier, Amsterdam, 1994).

19. D. S. Levine, *Behav. Res. Meth., Instr., and Comp.* **27** (1995) 178-171.

20. R. E. Passingham, *The Frontal Lobes and Voluntary Action* (Oxford University Press, Oxford, 1993).

21. N. Taylor, and J. G. Taylor, in preparation.

22. D. S. Levine and P. S. Prueitt, *Neur. Netw.* **2** (1989) 103-116.

23. M. Petrides, in *Handbook of Neuropsychology* (Vol. 9), eds. F. Boller and J. Grafman (Elsevier, Amsterdam, 1994).

24. J. M. Fuster, *Memory in the Cerebral Cortex* (MIT Press, Cambridge, MA, 1995).

25. B. Milner, in *The Frontal Granular Cortex and Behavior*, eds. J. M. Warren and K. Akert (McGraw-Hill, New York, 1964).

26. A. R. Damasio (1994). *Descartes' Error* (Grosset Putnam, New York, 1994).

27. D. S. Levine, *Introduction to Neural and Cognitive Modeling* (Erlbaum, Hillsdale, NJ, 1991).

28. P. D. MacLean, In *The Neurosciences Second Study Program*, ed. F. Schmitt. (Rockefeller University Press, New York, 1970).

29. R. S. Bapi, G. Bugmann, D. S. Levine and J. G. Taylor, in preparation.

30. E. A. Drewe, *Cortex* **10** (1974) 159-170.

31. M. Petrides, in *Frontal Lobe Function and Dysfunction*, eds. H. S. Levin, H. M. Eisenberg, and A. L. Benton (Oxford University Press, New York, 1991).

32. M. Petrides, *Behav. Brain Res.* **16** (1985) 95-101.

33. P. S. Goldman and H. E. Rosvold, *Exp. Neurol.* **27** (1970) 291-304.

34. B. A. Brody and K. H. Pribram, *Brain* **101** (1978) 607-633.

35. K. H. Pribram, *Exp. Neurol.* **3** (1961) 432-466.

36. B. Alivisatos, *Neuropsychologia* **30** (1992) 145-159.

37. T. Shallice, *Phil. Trans. Roy. Soc. London, Ser. B* **298** (1981) 199-209.

38. H. O. Karnath, C. W. Wallesch and P. Zimmermann, *Neuropsychologia* **29** (1991) 271-290.

39. T. Shallice and M. Evans, *Cortex* (1978)

40. S. J. Leven and D. S. Levine, *IEEE First International Conference on Neural Networks* (IEEE/ICNN, San Diego, 1987).

41. G. A. Carpenter and S. Grossberg, *Comp. Vis., Graph., and Image Proc.* **37** (1987) 54-115.

42. R. Desimone, in *Neural Networks for Vision and Image Processing*, eds. G. A. Carpenter and S. Grossberg (MIT Press, Cambridge, MA, 1992)

43. D. Gaffan, in *The Amygdala*, ed. J. P. Aggleton (Wiley-Liss, New York, 1992).

44. G. A. Carpenter, S. Grossberg and J. H. Reynolds, *Neur. Netw.* **4** (1991) 565-588.

45. R. S. Bapi and D. S. Levine, *Neur. Netw. World*, to appear (1996).

46. D. G. Amaral, J. L. Price, A. Pitkänen and S. T. Carmichael, in *The Amygdala*, ed. J. P. Aggleton (Wiley-Liss, New York, 1992).

47. M. Mishkin, B. Malamut and J. Bachevalier, In *Neurobiology of Learning and Memory*, eds. G. Lynch, J. McGaugh, and N. Weinberger (Guilford, New York/London, 1984).

48. S. Grossberg, *Math. Biosci.* **15** (1972) 39-67.

49. T. Shallice, *From Neuropsychology to Mental Structure* (Cambridge University Press, New York, 1988).

50. R. S. Bapi and D. S. Levine, *Neur. Netw.* **7** (1994) 1167-1170.

51. S. Grossberg, *J. Math. and Mech.* **19** (1969) 53-91.

52. K. C. Berridge and I. Q. Whishaw, *Exp. Brain Res.* **90** (1992) 275-290.

53. O. Monchi and J. G. Taylor, *World Congress on Neural Networks, Washington, DC* (Vol. 3).

54. G. E. Alexander, M. R. DeLong and P. L. Strick, *Ann. Rev. Neurosci.* **9** (1986) 357-381.

55. M. I. Posner and M. E. Raichle, *Behav. Brain Sci.* **18** (1995) 327-383.

56. J. G. Taylor and F. N. Alavi, *Biol. Cybernet.*, in press (1996).

57. D. Gaffan, E. A. Gaffan and S. Harrison, *J. Neurosci.* **9** (1989) 558-564.

58. J. G. Taylor and F. N. Alavi, in *Lateral Interactions in the Cortex*, J. Sirosh, R. Miikkulainen and Y. Choe, eds. (Hypertext, ISBN 0-9647960-0-8).

59. A. P. Georgopoulos, M. D. Crutcher and A. B. Schwartz, *Exp. Brain Res.* **75** (1989) 173-194.

60. M. Reiss and J. G. Taylor, *Neur. Netw.* **4** (1991) 773-788.

61. S. J. Leven and D. S. Levine, *Cognit. Sci.* (1996), in press.

62. E. T. Rolls, *Cognit. and Emot.* **4** (1990) 161-190.

63. Y. Kubota and M. Gabriel, *Behav. Neurosci.* **109** (1995) 258-277.

64. J. A. Fodor and Z. W. Pylyshyn, in *Connections and Symbols*, eds. S. Pinker and J. Mehler (MIT Press, Cambridge, MA, 1988).

65. M. Aparicio, IV, and D. S. Levine, in *Neural Networks for Knowledge Representation and Inference*, eds. D. S. Levine and M. Aparicio, IV (Erlbaum, Hillsdale, NJ, 1994).

66. J. M. Fuster, R. H. Bauer, and J. P. Jervey, *Exp. Neurol.* **77** (1981) 679-694.

67. D. H. Ingvar, *Hum. Neurobiol.* **4** (1985) 125-136.

68. N. J. Cohen and H. Eichenbaum, *Memory, Amnesia, and the Hippocampal System* (MIT Press, Cambridge, MA, 1993)

69. D. G. Stork, *International Joint Conference on Neural Networks, Washington, DC, June 18-22, 1989* (Vol. II, pp. 241-246) (IEEE, Piscataway, NJ, 1989).

70. E. Guigon, B. Dorizzi, Y. Burnod and W. Schultz, *Cerebral Cortex* **5** (1995) 135-147.

NEURAL NETWORKS, CORTICAL CONNECTIVITY AND SCHIZOPHRENIC PSYCHOSIS

Ralph E. Hoffman, M.D.
Yale Psychiatric Institute
Box 208038
New Haven CT 06520-8038
email hoffman@biomed.med.yale.edu

Abstract

Recent studies have suggested that reduced corticocortical connectivity is associated with schizophrenia. Using neural network simulations we have explored parallel, distributed processing systems with reduced connectivity. These systems often behaved in a "schizophrenic-like" manner. Excessively pruned attractor networks became functionally fragmented, suggesting "loose associations," and produced recurrent, intrusive representations suggestive of delusions. Pruning backpropagation simulations of speech perception networks produced spontaneous outputs which provided a model of hallucinated speech or "voices." This model also suggested how dopamine-blocking drugs might reduce positive symptoms, and why negative symptoms arise in the wake of positive symptoms.

Approximately one out every 150 persons living in the United States will be diagnosed as having schizophrenia during his/her adult life. The personal pain and functional disability caused by this disorder has led to intensive efforts to understand its pathogenesis and to develop better treatments. The cause(s) of schizophrenia remain poorly understood, however.

1. Clinical Manifestations of Schizophrenic Patients

For readers in non-psychiatric fields, I begin with some basic clinical information to anchor the later discussion. Signs and symptoms of schizophrenia are now broken down into "positive" and "negative" groups. The former consists of thought disorder, hallucinations and delusions. Thought disorder is often referred to as "loose associations" because the patient, when speaking, shifts idiosyncratically from one topic to another (Andreasen 1979). A majority of schizophrenic patients will also report "hearing voices" consisting of hallucinated spoken speech. Delusions are more or less unwavering false beliefs which are often bizarre and are invulnerable to invalidation. "Negative" signs and symptoms consist of emotional blunting, social withdrawal and curtailed production of speech. Positive symptoms seem to wax and wan while negative symptoms are more enduring and often worsen in the wake of an episode of positive symptoms (McGlashan & Fenton 1993).

2. Searching for Models

A major limiting factor imposed on this research endeavor is our own imagination. We tend to view schizophrenia in terms of diseases that we already know. For instance, focal neurological lesions are often invoked, either explicitly or implicitly, as a model for schizophrenia. This "lesion" model assumes that particular areas of the brain (for instance, the frontal lobes or the hippocampus) are functionally disabled. Studies of schizophrenia based on this model seek regional brain impairments using technologies such as positron emission tomography and neuropsychology. The second dominant paradigm consists in a "neurotransmitter disturbance." Increased functional availability of dopamine has often been hypothesized as causing schizophrenia. This hypothesis arose from the observation that amphetamine, a dopamine agonist, can induce a schizophrenic-like psychotic state (Angrist & Gershon 1970; Bell 1973), and that dopamine-blocking drugs are known to reduce certain schizophrenic symptoms. More recently, other neurotransmitter systems (involving, for instance, serotonin, glutamate and GABA) have been invoked as being possibly altered in schizophrenia, but the basic conceptual paradigm is the same. The "lesion" model is limited by the fact that no discrete anatomic lesion induces characteristic positive symptoms nor a waxing and waning course. The second, "neurotransmitter" paradigm does provide a defensible model for fluctuating psychotic illness. However, little evidence of a primary alteration of the dopamine system – the focus of most research of this sort – has been produced (Reynolds 1989). These largely negative findings suggest that the dopamine-blocking agents currently used to treatment schizophrenia reduce consequences of a pathogenic process rather than reverse a primary etiology.

We need new disease models to stretch our ability to imagine what schizophrenia could be. The work that I will summarize below uses computer models of parallel, distributed processing (PDP) neural networks (Amit 1989; McClelland & Rumelhart 1986). These simulations have enabled us to explore possible pathological effects of a novel form of brain dysfunction involving reduced *connectivity* within complex neural networks.

3. Excessive Cortical Pruning in Schizophrenia

The frontal cortex is the brain region responsible for higher cognitive processes that so often seem to be altered in schizophrenia (Weinberger et al. 1994). One clue regarding the etiology of schizophrenia is its characteristic age of onset, namely late adolescence or early adulthood. There is a significant decline in the density of synapses in frontal areas during adolescence (Huttonlocher 1978). These developmental findings suggest that abnormal pruning of frontal synapses might play an etiological role in schizophrenia (Feinberg 1982/1983; Hoffman & Dobscha 1989).

Supporting this view are two postmortem studies demonstrating reduced frontal dendritic spines in schizophrenia (Garey et al. 1995; Glantz & Lewis 1995). Although these studies do not directly count synapses, dendritic spines are microanatomic structures which receive axonal inputs and are therefore markers of connectivity. In addition, Selemon et al. (1995) have demonstrated that frontal tissue of schizophrenic brains has reduced neuropil volume. Neuropil is the complex entanglement of dendrites and axons surrounding cell bodies. Reduced neuropil volume is also likely to be a marker of reduced connectivity.

The primary source of input to cortical neurons is the thalamus. However, only about one percent of all synaptic inputs to cortical neurons are thalamic in origin (Braitenberg 1978). Therefore it is safe to conclude that the great majority of projections to neurons in the cerebral cortex derive from other cortical neurons. Reductions in synaptic density are likely to reflect reductions in corticocortical projections. Other studies suggesting reduced corticocortical connectivity in schizophrenia are reviewed in Hoffman and McGlashan (1993).

I have used two types of simulations to explore the "psychotogenic" effects of reduced connections within complex neural networks. The first relies on so-called attractor systems (Hoffman 1987; Hoffman & Dobscha 1989). These networks were heavily inspired by a branch of physics known as statistical mechanics. A second research strategy utilizes a "backpropagation" neural network architecture (Hoffman et al. 1995) which has emerged from a cognitive research tradition. These two research strategies will be briefly summarized and contrasted in terms of their usefulness in modeling schizophrenic disturbances.

4. Attractor Models of Reduced Corticocortical Connectivity

Attractor networks have a special appeal in terms of their usefulness in simulating schizophrenia given that they provide a model of "associative processes." As suggested above, the thought disorder of schizophrenia reflects abnormalities in how one representation is associated with another, especially during conversational speech. It therefore seems natural to attempt to use attractor systems to explore such language disturbances.

A network architecture originally described by Hopfield (1982) was used. Assumptions of a Hopfield network include the following:

(1) The network consists of a set of "neurons" which send projections to each other. The time delay is assumed to be the same for transmission of information from any one neuron to another.
(2) The activation of a neuron at any particular time has one of two states, active and inactive. The active state is coded by the number one, and the inactive state is coded as zero.
(3) Projections from one neuron to another are assigned a "synaptic weight" which can be either positive or negative.
(4) When a neuron re-assesses its state it does so by summing inputs from all neurons from which it receives synaptic projections. The result is called the "net synaptic input."

The readjustment of neuronal states can be represented as follows:

$$E_i = \sum_{j \neq i} w_{ji} (2*s_j - 1) \tag{1}$$

where E_i is the net synaptic input to neuron i, s_j is the state of neuron j projecting to neuron i, and w_{ji} is the synaptic weight of the projection from neuron j to neuron i. The net synaptic input, E_i, which can be either positive or negative, determines the state of the efferent neuron as by the following equation:

$$P_i = \frac{1}{1 + e^{-E_i/T}} \tag{2}$$

where P_i is the probability that neuron i will be activated (i.e., reset to an activation state coded by one) at the next time step in the simulation, and T is a "temperature" factor analogous to temperature of molecular interactions; in the latter case, heat induces increasingly random movement of individual molecules by reducing the effects of their interactive polarities. At higher T values, neuronal states are adjusted with increasing degrees of randomness or noise. For biological neural networks, it is likely that T is controlled by neuromodulatory processes (Servan-Schreiber, Printz & Cohen 1990). In general, a single neuron alone cannot activate or suppress activation of another neuron; simultaneous inputs from many neurons are required in order to induce a change in state.

Hopfield characterized the behavior of sets of such neurons (ranging from 30 to 100 elements) that were completely interconnected, i.e., where each neuron in the network provided a synaptic input to every other neuron. The critical discovery of Hopfield is that such networks can be made to flow into particular pre-determined "memories" by adjusting connection weights using a mathematical scheme referred to as the Hebb rule (Hebb 1949). There is some empirical evidence that cortical neurons actually modify the strength of their interconnections based on variants of the Hebb rule (Barrioneuvo & Brown 1983; Stanton & Sejnowski 1989). Memories stored according to the Hebb rule are *content-addressable*. Content-addressability implies that the network, when presented with a portion of a memory as a start-up state, will re-create that memory in its entirety. A simple model of perception is suggested if one assumes that activation of particular neurons indicates detection of particular features. A stored memory then would correspond to a gestalt consisting of a bundle of all relevant features which define it. It is well known that during actual perception only a portion of features needs to be discerned in order for the gestalt to be detected as a whole (Rock 1983). Similarly, Hopfield networks with content-addressable memories are able to re-create whole gestalts on the basis of small amounts of input information corresponding to a portion of the gestalt.

As noted above, the standard Hopfield system assumes that each neuron is connected to every other. What would happen if some of the connections were removed? In order to explore this question the neurons of a 100 neuron Hopfield system were deployed so that they occupied a 10×10 grid (Hoffman & Dobscha

1989). After memory/gestalts were stored using the Hebb rule, these systems were tested following removal of increasing numbers of neuronal connections. This was undertaken on the basis of a "pruning rule" based on a form of "neural darwinism" where neurons competed with each other for connections to other neurons; there is evidence that neural connectivity in actual brains is shaped by these competitive processes during development (Edelman 1987; Nelson et al. 1990). If a weak connection traversed a long distance, it was pruned away. Another way to think about the pruning rule is that the "cost" of maintaining long neuronal projections was weighed against the benefits of the amount of information it carried. If the "cost" was too great, the connection was eliminated. A schematic of pruning is illustrated in Figure 1.

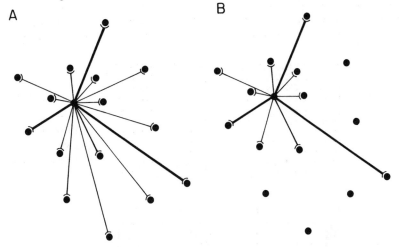

Figure 1. A schematic representation of axonal pruning (from Hoffman & Dobscha 1989, p. 483). Weak axonal projections that traverse longer distances in A are pruned away in B.

It turned out that these systems could function with up to 80% reductions in neuronal connectivity using this pruning rule (Hoffman & Dobscha 1989). However, connectivity reductions beyond this level caused the system to become dysfunctional. One consequence of excessive synaptic pruning was that the outputs became bizarre. Inputs would cause the system to flow into fragments of unrelated memories that were amalgamated together. This behavior provided a model for "loose associations" in schizophrenia. A second consequence of this pathology was that subpopulations of neurons episodically locked into a certain output configurations independent of information received from other parts of the system. These outputs arose de novo, i.e., *they did not reflect any particular memory previously stored in the system*, and relentlessly strove to reproduce themselves.

The emergence of this form of network pathology was referred to as a parasitic focus and is illustrated in Figure 2 (see following page). In this simulation, an excessively "pruned" network received as inputs parts of a memory and then

446

allowed to stabilize. When the system was functioning well it would stabilize in a state coding for the memory in its entirety. The amount of "missing information" in the input was quantified as Hamming units (HU). In the left column, the network received an input re-creating a portion of memory six. In the right column, the network received an input re-creating a portion of memory seven. The diagram demonstrates when missing information was relatively small (Hamming unit = 20), the network was quite successful in re-creating entire correct memories in response to input information. However, when inputs were more ambiguous due to missing information (Hamming unit = 30), the system began to fragment; in other words, different portions of the network converge on different memories. Moreover, the lower left-hand portion of the network tended to be co-opted by a parasitic focus that did not conform to any previously stored memory and repeatedly intruded into network processes. Parasitic foci therefore disregarded external inputs and re-created their contents. In short, they seem to have "minds of their own."

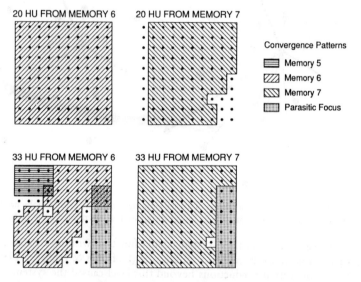

Figure 2. Behavior of a neural network where 92% of axonal connections have been pruned away (from Hoffman & Dobscha 1989, p. 483). HU = Hamming units and quantifies the level of input ambiguity.

If a parasitically produced activation pattern induces a belief orientation, a delusion could result. As is the case for overpruned networks, patients with this symptom repeatedly enter a particular state that disregards experiential input not consistent with it. The fact that a "parasitic focus" relentlessly re-creates particular representations also provides a model for understanding hallucinated voices. If a parasitic focus emerged in the language perception module of the brain, spontaneous linguistic representations with recurrent content would result. We have recently studied the content of hallucinated "voices" experienced by schizophrenic patients over time. As predicted by a "parasitic focus" model of psychotic systems, "voices" tended to re-create similar semantic content over time (Hoffman et al. 1994; Hoffman et al. 1995).

5. Pruned Backpropagation Networks and Hallucinated "Voices"

By modeling "associative disturbances" Hopfield networks offers interesting models of psychotic phenomenology. However, these simulations do not provide precise predictions regarding perceptual or cognitive abilities which could render them directly testable.

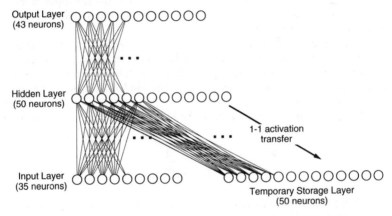

Figure 3. Backpropagation network with context module which stores a replica of the activation pattern of the hidden module (from Hoffman et al. [1995], p. 481, © MIT Press).

An alternative class of neural networks does provide such predictions. Referred to as backpropagation networks, they perform simulated perceptual or cognitive tasks which can be compared quantitatively to human performance on parallel, standardized tests. Models of normal and psychopathological information processing can then be critically evaluated.

Working memory plays a critical role in speech perception. Grammatical and semantic expectations based on prior speech inputs stored in working memory facilitate detection of the next word in a sentence (Jackendoff 1987; Elman 1990; Servan-Schreiber et al. 1990). Dominant hemisphere speech centers underlying speech perception are known to interact with brain areas underlying working memory (i.e., frontal cortex and hippocampus; see Goldman-Rakic 1987; Mesulam 1990).

Our strategy was to consider "voices" or hallucinated speech as a product of networks dedicated to speech perception. Consistent with this view are evoked potential and positron emission tomography studies suggesting endogenous activation of speech perception areas when patients experience this symptom

(Tiihonen et al. 1992; Suzuki et al. 1993). In particular, we wished to determine if overpruning the working memory module of backpropagation network models of speech perception could results in simulated "hallucinations." This would occur f perceptual expectations emerging from contextual memory became so pronounced that certain words are "detected" spontaneously, i.e., without *any* external input.

We consequently created a speech perception neural network similar to that described by Elman (1990). The architecture of our network is illustrated in Figure 3. The input layer consisted in 35 neurons, where each neuron coded for a portion of the "phonetic" information of a word. Along the lines of Elman, actual acoustic data were not used; instead our simplifying assumption was that the acoustic representation of each word corresponded to a "sparse" pattern of activation (roughly 25% of the neurons turned "on") distributed across the input layer. This yielded a 35-dimensional "phoneme" code consisting of zeroes and ones for each word in the system's vocabulary.

For each of fifty hidden layer neurons a weighted sum of inputs from all 35 input neurons was calculated. Each hidden layer neuron also received input from every neuron in the temporary storage module layer (also 50 neurons in size) which stored a replica of the pattern of activation of the hidden layer emerging from the preceding phonetic input.

The activation of each neuron in the hidden layer, $a_h(x)$, was then computed as follows:

$$a_h(x) = \frac{1}{1 + e^{-g(I(x)+M(x)+\beta)}} \tag{3}$$

where g (gain) and β (bias) together determine response profiles of simulated neurons. When combined input to any single neuron was very negative, its activation approached zero. When its combined input was very positive, neural activation approached a maximum level of one. Intermediate levels of firing were expressed as fractions. Each output layer neuron received inputs from all intermediate layer neurons. Output layer neurons coded for semantic and syntactic features of words.

Phonetic inputs corresponding to particular words were presented one word at a time in sequences corresponding to grammatical sentences (e.g., "Jane-love-small-child," "Bill-tell-old-man-story"). 256 sentences ranging between 2 and 6 words in length were used for backpropagation training. The system was trained to produce the appropriate output pattern in response to a particular "phonetic" input. During training, the network learned to use memory traces of prior information processing steps to facilitate recognition of new inputs presented to the hidden layer. The interaction of hidden and temporary storage layer neurons provided these memory traces. The network was 100% successful in detecting all words after 60 exposures to the training set of sentences. Following training, connection weights were fixed and a test input sequence was presented which consisted of 23 sentences distinct from those used during training but using the same vocabulary.

In order to force the system to rely on contextual memory to "disambiguate" phonetic input, the network was challenged using the same test input sequences with superimposed phonetic noise. Noise was created by activating random phoneme input neurons which were not part of the "phoneme code" for the current input word. The presence of noise forced the network to rely more on perceptual expectations (e.g., that certain types of verbs follow certain types of nouns) when decoding phonetic inputs.

In parallel, we undertook a human study of speech perception. Continuous spoken narrative was binaurally presented via headphones. Normal subjects were requested to "shadow" (i.e., to repeat while listening) spoken texts. The difficulty of this task was experimentally altered by electronically adding different levels of phonetic noise. Phonetic noise in human experiments consisted in "multi-speaker

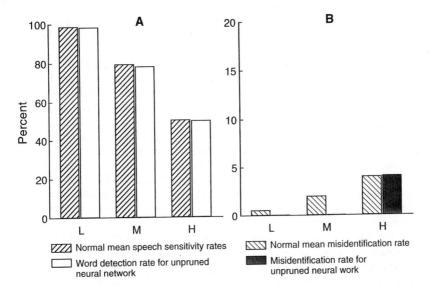

Figure 4. Comparison of normal human vs unpruned network speech perception performance (from Hoffman et al. [1995], p. 489, © MIT Press). L = Low noise; M = moderate noise; H = high noise.

babble," i.e., electronically superimposed speech of twelve persons. Babble-masking of actual speech was the empirical analogue of adding extraneous random phonetic activation to simulated speech perception neural networks.

This research strategy allowed us to compare neural network and human speech perception capacity when challenged with different levels of noise (Figure 4). In the Figure, hatched bars corresponded to mean performance of normal subjects. Speech sensitivity was a composite measure reflecting words perceived approximately or entirely correctly. Under higher noise conditions both neural networks and human subjects detected fewer words and made a larger number of word misidentifications relative to lower noise conditions. By adjusting noises levels of stimuli presented to the neural network, we were able to precisely mirror word detection rates and word misidentification rates by normal human subjects on the shadowing task.

We then experimented with this neural network to determine if it could be induced to "hallucinate" as defined above. As suggested by our pruned attractor network simulations, pruning projections from the context module to the hidden module produced spontaneous percepts. This phenomenon occurred when input sequences presented to the neural network consisted entirely of "null" inputs (all input neurons reset to zero). These "hallucinated" words were not random but were limited to a small number of words in the system's lexicon. In short, overpruning connections between the context and hidden module of the backpropagation simulation caused the system to be "parasitically attracted" to a small number of states analogous to "parasitic foci" in overpruned Hopfield networks.

We also attempted to induce "hallucinations" by altering the neuromodulatory parameters, bias and gain, of hidden layer neurons (see Eq. 3). This was prompted by reports that excessive dopamine, a neuromodulatory neurotransmitter, can induce a psychosis which includes hallucinated "voices" (Bell 1973; Angrist et al. 1970). In our simulation, "hallucinations" were induced by decreasing bias, which has the net effect deactivating hidden layer neurons. This finding was consistent with a hyperdopaminergic model of psychosis given that dopamine has been reported to have an inhibitory effect on cortical neurons (see, for instance, Bunney & Aghajanian, 1976; Thierry, Mantz, Milla, & Glowinski, 1988). Hallucinations induced by overpruning as well as a "hyperdopaminergic" state were also accompanied by impairments in the rate of correct word detection and elevated rates of word misidentifications.

We then studied the relationship between rate of simulated hallucinations and increases in hidden layer bias. This condition could arise from dopamine-blocking drugs or the brain's own down-regulation of the dopamine neuromodulatory system. Simulating a hypodopaminergic state reduced hallucinations and improved perceptual impairments induced by neuroanatomic pruning. It seemed that activating hidden layer neurons allowed them to make better use of their remaining inputs. However, if pruning was too severe, perceptual responsivity had to be sacrificed by in order to minimize hallucinations.

The relationship between hallucination rate, perceptual impairments and different bias settings is illustrated in Figure 5. On the left is performance of a 66% pruned network. Hallucinations were relatively prominent in the absence of bias adjustment. Increasing bias from zero to one was "therapeutic" as assessed by all three variables. Hallucinations diminished, word detection increased, and word misidentifications decreased, Further increasing bias to 2.5 was able to completely eliminate hallucinations but only by sacrificing word detection capacity (see inverted U for word detection). Word misidentifications were also reduced to zero by bias enhancement. For the more severely pruned network (pruning set at 75%), bias enhancement reduced but could not eliminate hallucinations. Again, the ability to

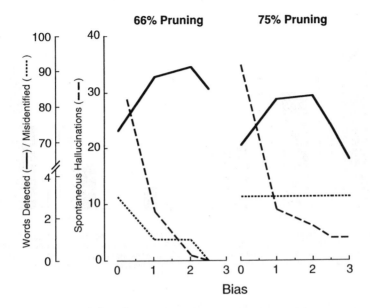

Figure 5. Effects of increasing bias on hallucinations, word detection rates and word misidentification rates in pruned networks.

detect words needed to be sacrificed in order minimize the positive symptom. Word misidentifications were also reduced by not eliminated. We suggest that decreased perceptual reactivity -- reflected by decreased word detection rates -- could be a model for negative symptoms in schizophrenia. These graphs illustrate how increased negative symptoms could reflect a compensatory adjustment to positive symptoms, which conforms to clinical observation (McGlashan & Fenton 1993).

Because different "hallucinogenic" speech perception networks also demonstrated speech perception impairments their validity as models could be tested by studying speech perception in actual hallucinating patients. Schizophrenic subjects underwent the same speech shadowing task described above for normal subjects. Noise levels of speech stimuli were also the same. As predicted from our network simulations, schizophrenic patients who heard "voices" demonstrated speech perception impairments not detected in nonhallucinating schizophrenics. Word detection rates of "hallucinogenic" overpruned and hyperdopaminergic networks were very close to that of actual hallucinating patients (Figure 6A). However, these simulations generated much greater rates of word misidentifications compared to human hallucinators (Figure 6B). An excellent fit between word misidentification rates of overpruned neural networks and actual hallucinating schizophrenics occurred if bias of hidden layer neurons in the overpruned network was enhanced (i.e., our simulated hypodopaminergic state).

Comparing human and neural network data suggest that the working

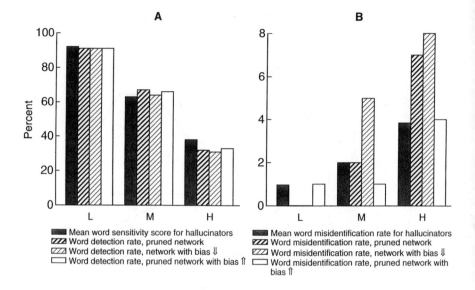

Figure 6. Comparing speech tracking by human hallucinators and performance of "hallucinogenic" neural networks. (from Hoffman et al. [1995], p. 490, © MIT Press).

memory networks of hallucinating schizophrenics have two alterations: (i) a primary pathology involving anatomic pruning of connections, and (ii) a compensatory adjustment of bias that reduces, in part, hallucinatory vulnerability. Insofar as most of our schizophrenic patients were maintained on dopamine-blocking antipsychotic medication, enhanced bias may model the mechanism of therapeutic action of these drugs. It is also possible that bias adjustments could be due to central feedback adjustment of the dopamine system by the brain itself.

6. Comparing Hopfield and Backpropagation Networks

One disadvantage of backpropagation training is that it is not realistic biologically. Insofar as learning is "supervised", there needs to be a monitoring system (or "trainer") that determines what the output of the neural network should be in response to particular input; such training also requires a very large number of learning trials. It is hard to imagine how such training could be undertaken in a biological network. In contrast, Hopfield systems do not require supervised training. The system learns "locally" and automatically; individual pairs of neurons examine their coactivation and automatically adjust their interconnectivity accordingly. Learning can take place on the basis of a single exposure to a new input rather than via repeated supervised learning. However, Hopfield systems are much more limited in terms of their information processing abilities. Hopefully new neural learning simulations will be developed that retain the biological plausibility of Hopfield systems while achieving the computational power of backpropagation systems. These models could then be used to study psychopathological conditions.

7. Closing comments

Even the relatively primitive models described above provide potentially useful insights into possible mechanisms of many of the symptoms of schizophrenia. Our findings indicate that additional studies of corticocortical connectivity in schizophrenia should be undertaken. A detailed assessment of effects of reduced and excessive dopamine levels on cortical neuron behavior in working memory systems is also indicated. We predict that this neuromodulator should specifically alter the bias of working memory neurons when responding to other inputs. An unanticipated finding based on the backpropagation model was that "negative symptoms" (viewed as decreased reactivity to stimuli) could be a compensatory adjustment (corresponding to dopamine down-regulation) to positive symptoms. This dynamic interplay of positive and negative symptoms can also be explored experimentally.

8. References

Amit, D.J. *Modeling Brain Function: The World of Attractor Neural Networks.* (Cambridge University Press, Cambridge, 1989).

Andreasen, N.C. Thought, language and communication disorders: I. Clinical assessment, definition of terms, and evaluation of their reliability. *Archives of General Psychiatry* **36** (1979) 1315-1321.

Angrist, B.M., Gershon, S. The phenomenology of experimentally induced amphetamine psychosis-preliminary observations. *Biological Psychiatry* **2** (1970) 95-107.

Barrioneuvo, G., Brown, T.H. Associative long-term potentiation in hippocampal slices. *Proceedings of the National Academy of Science USA* **80** (1983) 7347-7351.

Bell, D.S. The experimental reproduction of amphetamine psychosis. *Archives of General Psychiatry* **29** (1973) 35-40.

Bunney, B.S., Aghajanian, G.K. Dopamine and norepinephrine innervated cells in rat prefrontal cortex: pharmacological differentiation using microiontophoretic techniques. *Life Science* **19** (1976) 1783-1792.

Braitenberg, V. Cortical architectonics: general and areal, in *Architectonics of the*

Cerebral Cortex. eds. M.A.B. Brazier, H. Petsche (Raven Press, New York, 1978), pp. 443-465.

Crick, F., Mitchison, G. The function of dream sleep. *Nature* 304 (1983) 111-114.

Edelman, G.M. *Neural Darwinism: The Theory of Neuronal Group Selection* (New York, Basic Books, 1987).

Elman, J.L. Finding structure in time. *Cognitive Science* 14 (1980) 179-211.

Feinberg I. Schizophrenia: Caused by a fault in programmed synaptic elimination during adolescence? *J Psychiatric Res* 4 (1982/1983) 319-334.

Garey L.J., Ong, W.Y., Patel, T.S., Kanani, M., Davis, A., Hornstein .C., Bauer, M. Reduction in dendritic spine number on cortical pyramidal neurons in schizophrenia (abstract). *Society for Neuroscience* 21 (1995) 237.

Glantz, L.A., Lewis, D.A. Assessment of spine density on layer III pyramidal cells in the prefrontal cortex of schizophrenic subjects (abstract). *Society for Neuroscience* 21 (1995) 239.

Goldman-Rakic, P. Circuitry of primate prefrontal cortex and the regulation of behavior by representation knowledge, in *Handbook of Physiology*, Volume 5, eds. F. Plum, V. Montcastle (Washington DC, American Physiological Society, 1987), pp. 373-417.

Goldman-Rakic, P. Prefrontal cortical dysfunction in schizophrenia: the relevance of working memory, in *Psychopathology and the Brain*, eds. B.J. Carroll, J.E. Barrett (New York, Raven Press, 1991), pp. 1-23.

Hebb, D.O. *Organization of behavior* (New York, Wiley, 1949).

Hoffman, R.E. Computer simulations of neural information processing and the schizophrenia-mania dichotomy. *Archives of General Psychiatry* 44 (1987) 178-188.

Hoffman, R.E., Dobscha, S.K. Cortical pruning and the development of schizophrenia: A computer model. *Schizophrenia Bulletin* 15 (1989) 477-490.

Hoffman, R.E., Docherty, N., Oates, E., Walker, M., McGlashan, T.H. Semantic organization of hallucinated "voices" in schizophrenia: II. comparison with verbal thought samples. Under review (1995).

Hoffman, R.E., Oates, E., Hafner, R.J., Hustig, H.H., McGlashan, T.H. Semantic organization of hallucinated "voices" in schizophrenia. *American Journal of Psychiatry* 151 (1994) 1229-1230.

Hoffman, R.E., Rapaport, J., Ameli, R., McGlashan, T.H., Harcherik, D., Servan-Schrieber, D. A neural network simulation of hallucinated "voices" and associated speech perception impairments in schizophrenic patients. *Journal of Cognitive Neuroscience* **7** (1995) 479-496.

Hopfield, J.J. Neural networks and physical systems with emergent collective computational abilities. *Proceedings of the National Academy of Science* **79** (1982) 2554-2558.

Huttenlocher, P.R. Synaptic density in the human frontal cortex - developmental changes and effects of aging. *Brain Research* **163** (1979) 195-205.

Jackendoff, R. *Consciousness and the Computational Mind* (Cambridge MA, MIT Press, 1987).

McClelland, J.L., Rumelhart, D.E., eds. *Parallel Distributed Processing: Explorations in the Microstructure of Cognition, Volumes I and II* (Cambridge MA, MIT Press, 1986).

McGlashan, T.H., Fenton, W.S. Subtype progression and pathophysiologic deterioration in early schizophrenia. *Schizophrenia Bulletin* **19** (1993) 71-84.

Mesulam, M.M. Large-scale neurocognitive networks and distributed processing for attention, language and memory. *Annals of Neurology* **28** (1990) 567-613.

Nelson, P.G., Fields, R.D., Yu, C., Neale, E.A. Mechanisms involved in activity-dependent synapse formation in mammalian central nervous system cell cultures. *Journal of Neurobiology* **21** (1990) 138-156.

Reynolds, G.P. Beyond the dopamine hypothesis. The neurochemical pathology of schizophrenia. *British Journal of Psychiatry* **155** (1989) 305-316.

Rock, I. *The Logic of Perception* (Cambridge MA, MIT Press, 1983), pp. 12-13.

Selemon, L.D., Rajkowska, G., Goldman-Rakic, P.S. Abnormally high neuronal density in the schizophrenic cortex: A morphometric analysis of prefrontal area 9 and occipital area 17. *Archives of General Psychiatry* **52** (1995) 805-818.

Servan-Schreiber, D., Cleeremans, A., McClelland, J.L. Graded state machines: The representation of temporal contingencies in simple recurrent networks. *Machine Learning* **7** (1990) 161-193.

Servan-Schreiber, D., Printz, H.W., Cohen, J.D. A network model of catecholamine effects. *Science* **249** (1990) 892-895.

Stanton PK, Sejnowski TJ. Associative long-term depression in the hippocampus induced by hebbian covariance. *Nature* 339:215-218, 1989.

Suzuki, M., Yuasa, S., Minabe, Y., Murata, M., Kurachi, M. Left superior temporal blood flow increases in schizophrenic and schizophreniform patients with auditory hallucinations: a longitudinal case study using ^{123}I-IMP SPECT. *European Archives of Psychiatry Clinical Neuroscience* **242** (1993) 257-261.

Thierry, A.M., Mantz, J., Milla, C., Glowinski J. Influence of the mesocortical prefrontal dopamine neurons on their target cells. *Annals of the New York Academy of Science* **537** (1988) 101-111.

Tiihonen, J., Hari, R., Naukkarinen, H., Rimon, R., Jousmaki, V., Kajola, M. Modified activity of the human auditory cortex during auditory hallucinations. *American Journal of Psychiatry* **149** (1992) 255-257.

Weinberger, D.R., Aloia, M.S., Goldberg, T.E., Berman, K.F. The frontal lobes and schizophrenia. *J Neuropsychiatry Clin Neurosci* **6** (1994) 419-427.

DOPAMINE, FRONTAL CORTEX, AND SCHIZOPHRENIA: MODEL AND DATA

DAVID SERVAN-SCHREIBER

Clinical Cognitive Neuroscience Laboratory, Department of Psychiatry, University of Pittsburgh
University, 3811 O'Hara St., Pittsburgh , PA, 15213, U.S.A
E-Mail: ddss@pitt.edu

and

JONATHAN COHEN

Clinical Cognitive Neuroscience Laboratory, Department of Psychiatry, University of Pittsburgh
University, 3811 O'Hara St., Pittsburgh , PA, 15213, U.S.A and Department of Psychology, Carnegie
Mellon University, Schenley Park, Pittsburgh, PA, 15213, U.S.A
E-Mail: djc5e@andrew.cmu.edu

ABSTRACT

Schizophrenic patients show a variety of deficits in cognitive functions. These deficits have been difficult to understand in terms of a common unifying hypothesis. We describe a connectionist model of the function of prefrontal cortex and of neuromodulation of processing by dopamine. This model suggests that a single deficit may underlie poor performance in a variety of tasks: an impairment in maintaining contextual information over time and using that information to inhibit inappropriate responses. We tested schizophrenic on a new variant of the continuous performance test (CPT) designed specifically to elicit deficits in the processing of contextual information predicted by the models. The results confirmed the prediction.

Introduction

Psychiatric disorders are characterized by diffuse deficits that cannot be easily related to a single specific function. The clinical descriptions of psychiatric patients often appeal to terms such as "attention" or "inappropriate behavior" that are not well defined in information processing psychology.

Furthermore, psychiatric disorders typically have a fluctuating course with waxing and waning of symptoms — occasionally with complete remissions — and the symptoms often respond to drug therapies. These observations suggest that there is no simple structural lesion — such as damage to individual "units" or to "connection weights" — which can explain the nature of the deficits.

This state of affairs has left information processing theoreticians with no clear idea of exactly what should be modeled and even less clear ideas about how to model such disorders.

In this work, we have focused on how the modeling of neuromodulation can shed some light on impairments of attention and working memory that are particularly relevant to the deficits displayed by patients who suffer from schizophrenia.

1. Schizophrenia

Schizophrenia is a striking disorder of higher brain functions in which patients appear to have intact elementary information processing mechanisms but nevertheless display diffuse cognitive deficits — for example, in the ability to sustain attention or to solve problems or the concreteness in their interpretation of concepts — as well as gross impairments of social behavior (a familiar example of which is their tendency to address strangers in the street).

At the same time, biological research in schizophrenia has identified some salient abnormalities that can begin to constrain a model of such behavioral anomalies. Specifically, we will focus on the failure of schizophrenic patients to activate their prefrontal cortex during certain cognitive tasks, as documented by positron emission tomography (PET) [1], and a dysfunction of the dopaminergic system [2-5].

An important contribution of our modeling efforts has been to show how these behavioral and biological observations may be causally related in terms of specific neural mechanisms.

2. Function of Prefrontal Cortex

On the basis of empirical evidence accumulated over the last 30 years, the prefrontal cortex (PFC) has been assumed to support at least two critical higher functions: (1) active memory and (2) behavioral inhibition. The memory function refers to the ability to maintain information "on-line" in order to bridge the gap between the presentation of stimuli in the environment and the time when responses to such stimuli should take place [6, 7]. The inhibition function refers to the ability to prevent the expression of habitual responses when these are not appropriate to the present context [8].

Through our modeling work, we have come to believe that these two sets of observations can be described by a single function: the representation and maintenance of context information. [5]

3. Function of Dopamine

The cell bodies of dopamine neurons are grouped in small nuclei from which axons diffusely innervate other brain regions in a distributed fashion. The PFC is one of a several brain regions with an important dopaminergic innervation [9]. The effect of dopamine release on target neurons is not to excite or inhibit these neurons, but, rather, to modulate how the target neurons respond to other neurotransmitters. We have proposed that this modulation can be characterized as a change in the *gain* parameter of the activation function of target units [10], such that they are more sensitive to their excitatory or inhibitory inputs (figure 1.).

Hence, dopamine can be thought of as setting a state of information processing in target areas rather than as conveying a specific informational content.

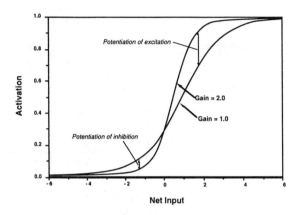

Figure 1.

4. A Minimalist Model of PFC Function

We have captured our hypothesis about the function of PFC with a simple model of selective attention and response selection (figure 2.) [5]. In this model, the flow of processing from an input to an output layer is influenced by the the pattern of activation in an additional module — the context module — which we associate with the function of the PFC. The pattern of activation over units in the context module can contain information about the processing of previous stimuli, or about task instructions, or anything else that captures the "context" in which current stimuli are being presented. This pattern interacts with the flow of activation from the input layer at the level of a "hidden" or associative layer. Through this interaction, it can bias processing of incoming stimuli and give rise to "selective attention."

We have implemented this model with a variety of different learning algorithms such as backpropagation ("Jordan Net" [11]), fully recurrent backpropagation [12] and LEABRA (a combination of associative and supervised learning [13]). The phenomena of selective attention and response selection can be observed in all of these implementations and we believe that they are independent of any particular learning algorithm.

Most importantly, explorations of this model allowed us to realize that the traditional PFC functions of "memory" and "inhibition" can be viewed as two aspects of the single mechanism mentioned above: the representation and maintenance of context information.

460

When the task involves maintaining information over time but no competition between stimuli, the context module appears to have a memory function. However, when the task assigned to this architecture does not involve maintaining the pattern of activation in the context module over time, but requires selective processing of some stimuli and not others based on context information, the context module appears to have an inhibition function.

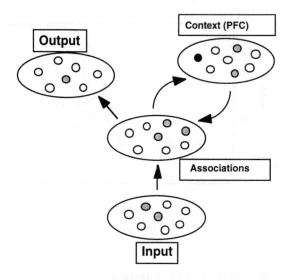

Figure 2.

5. Memory Function in Schizophrenia: The CPT Identical Pairs

The failure of the memory function in schizophrenic patients is well illustrated by the patients' performance on a variant of the continuous performance test called the CPT-Identical Pairs. In this task, subjects are instructed to respond when two consecutive letters in a sequence are identical. Only one letter is presented at any given time. An example of a sequence may be: A ... B ... C ... D ... C ... D ... D, where only the last pair of letters constitutes a target sequence.

In this task, individual stimuli are ambiguous and subjects need to keep in active memory the identity of the previous stimulus in order to respond appropriately. Previous stimuli therefore act as context for response selection.

Schizophrenic patients do not perform well in this task compared to controls, as illustrated in figure 3. [14]

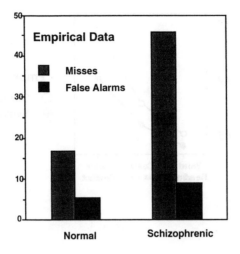

Figure 3.

6. Inhibition Function in Schizophrenia: The Stroop Task

The failure of the inhibition function can be illustrated with schizophrenics' performance in the Stroop task. In this task, subjects are asked to either read a word (the name of a color, such as 'green' or 'red') or to name the ink color in which the word appears. When the ink color and the word are in conflict (e.g., the word 'red' written in green ink), subjects need the context of the task instructions to select the appropriate response. However, for college-educated adults with average reading experience, reading the word is a much more natural (habitual) response than naming the ink color. The stimuli therefore have both a weak (the ink color) and a strong dimension (the word). Context information is critical when a conflict exists between the two dimensions and the strong response needs to be inhibited (i.e., in the color naming condition with conflict stimuli).

Schizophrenic patients perform particularly poorly in this color-naming conflict condition, as illustrated in figure 4. [15-17].

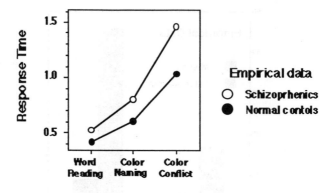

Figure 4.

7. Reduced Gain in PFC Module

After training a model such as the one described in Figure 2. to perform each of these two tasks, we simulated a deficit of dopamine in the prefrontal cortex by reducing gain selectively in the context module of both models (from 1.0 to 0.6).

This reduction of gain results in a decreased resistance to the cumulative effects of noise over time in the context module; which produces an impairment of "memory." Reduced gain also decreases the ability of the context module to selectively inhibit the strongest of two competing stimulus-response associations; which produces an impairment of "inhbition."

In both cases, the simulations reproduced the pattern of deficits of schizophrenic patients (figures 5 and 6).

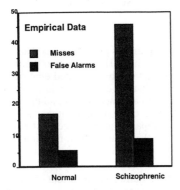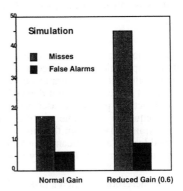

Figure 5.

It is important to note that only a reduction of gain in the context module produces these deficits. Reducing gain in other modules does not result in a deficit of memory or inhibition, unless the reduction includes the context module. Furhtermore, other manipulations (e.g., an increase in processing rate or a reduction of response threshold) fail to elicit the full patttern of effects, suggesting that such generalized deficits are not responsible for this particular phenomenon.

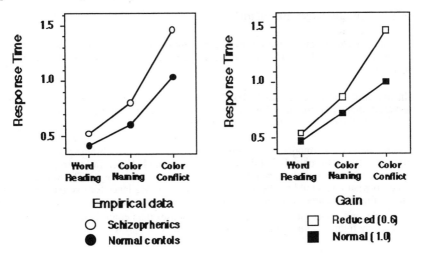

Figure 6.

8. New Predictions Derived from the Models: A New Variant of the A-X CPT

Our model of a dopamine deficit in the PFC of schizophrenics provides a good account of schizophrenic performance in the two tasks considered here. However, in order to test such models, it is important to derive new predictions that can be evaluated empirically. The most important insight derived from our models is that the context module supports both functions previously ascribed to the PFC — inhibition and memory — and that this is a consequence of its role in representing and maintaining context information. A direct prediction derived from this understanding is that an impairment of the context module should lead to a significantly heightened deficit in a task that requires both functions to be used at the same time ("memory-based inhibition").

We therefore designed a task that would have such a requirement: a variant of the A-X CPT. This task introduces a strong response bias (habitual response) as well as a variable inter-stimulus interval (ISI) to test the effect of long delays between stimuli [18].

Specifically, subjects are instructed to respond to the letter 'X' but only when it follows the letter 'A'. There are three conditions in the task:

- A-X: cue-target, 80% of trials

- A-Y: cue-distractor, 10% of trials

- B-X: distractor-target, 10% of trials

Because it is correct to respond to X eight out of nine times that it occurs, subjects develop a strong tendency to respond to X (habitual response), even when it does not follow an A.

In addition, the task includes two ISIs, 1 second and 5 seconds. With a 1 second interval, demands on memory for the previous stimulus are minimal; however, with a 5 second interval memory requirements are greater.

On the basis of the model, we therefore predicted that schizophrenic patients would be particularly likely to make B-X false alarms at the long ISI (i.e., fail to inhibit the strong response tendency when there is a greater requirement for memory). This prediction runs counter to what one would predict from the literature on vigilance for two reasons: First, in normal subjects, a longer ISI results in *improved* performance in continuous performance tests[19]. Second, schizophrenics make fewer responses than controls in vigilance tasks (as illustrated by figure 3), rather than committing more false alarms.

9. Results

We conducted an experiment with this new version of the CPT A-X in which we compared schizophrenic patients (medicated and unmedicated) to non-schizophrenic psychiatric patients. This experiment and related data analyses are reported elsewhere [18]. Only the main results are summarized here. For simplicity, we focus in this report on the comparison between patient controls and unmedicated schizophrenics.

9.1 Overall Performance (d')

Using the signal detection measure of performance known as d', we found that unmedicated schizophrenic patients performed overall more poorly than control psychiatric patients. Furthermore, whereas the performance of control subjects improved at the long ISI, the performance of schizophrenic patients did not (figure 7.).

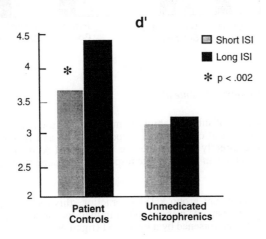

Figure 7.

9.2 False Alarms

Looking specifically at false alarms, we found that both groups made fewer A-Y errors at the longer ISI, confirming that the longer ISI is not simply a harder condition.

Furthermore, as predicted, unmedicated schizophrenic patients committed more B-X false alarms than controls at both ISIs, and this tendency was worse at the longer ISI (figure 8).

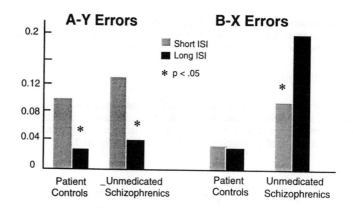

Figure 8.

9.3 Sensitivity to Context (d'-Context)

The most direct measure of subjects' ability to maintain and use context information in this task is a d' measure based only on A-X responses (hits) and B-X responses (false alarms). This measure directly reflects the use of context ('A' or 'B') to mediate an appropriate response or inhibit an inappropriate response to the same stimulus in both cases ('X').

As revealed by a significant group x ISI interaction, this measure confirmed that unmedicated schizophrenic patients were impaired in their use of context at the short ISI and that this impairment was worsened by a longer ISI (figure 9.).

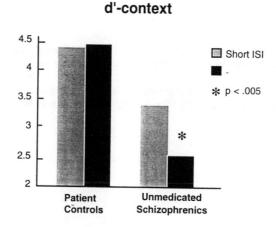

Figure 9.

10. Conclusion

We developed a model of PFC that captures both the memory and inhibition functions previously ascribed by different authors to this brain region. The model suggested that these two functions are supported by a single mechanism, the representation and maintenance of context in a module that interacts with processing between stimulus representation and response selection.

Schizophrenic patients are assumed to suffer from a disturbance of dopamine function in the PFC. In the model, the effect of reduced dopamine in the PFC was captured by reducing the gain parameter of the activation function of units in the context module.

Reducing gain produced a decreased resistance to the effects of noise over time — which induced a memory deficit — and a decreased resistance to the presence of a dominant response tendency — which induced a deficit of inhibition.

The model predicted a specific pattern of deficits for schizophrenic patients in a new task — a variant of the A-X CPT — that requires memory-based inhibition of a dominant response.

An empirical study of schizophrenic patients comparing them to non-schizophrenic patient controls confirmed the prediction.

11. References

1. Berman KF, Zec RF, Weinberger DR. Physiological dysfunction of dorsolateral prefrontal cortex in schizophrenia II: Role of neuroleptic treatment, attention and mental effort. *Archives of General Psychiatry.* 1986;43:126-135.

2. Crow TJ. Molecular pathology of schizophrenia: more than one disease process? *British Medical Journal.* 1980:66-68.

3. Mackay AVP. Positive and Negative Schizophrenic Symptoms and the Role of Dopamine. *British Journal of Psychiatry.* 1980;137:379-386.

4. Weinberger DR. Implications of normal brain development for the pathogenesis of schizophrenia. *Archives of General Psychiatry.* 1987;44:660-669.

5. Cohen JD, Servan-Schreiber D. Context, cortex and dopamine: A connectionist approach to behavior and biology in schizophrenia. *Psychological Review.* 1992;99:45-77.

6. Fuster JM, Alexander GE. Neuron activity related to short-term memory. *Science.* 1971;173:652-654.

7. Goldman-Rakic PS. Prefrontal Cortical Dysfunction in Schizophrenia: The Relevance of Working Memory. *Psychopathology and the Brain.* 1991:1-23.

8. Fuster JM. The prefrontal cortex. . New York: Raven Press; 1980.

9. Lewis DA, Hayes TL, Lund JS, Oeth KM. Dopamine and the Neural Circuitry of Primate Prefrontal Cortex: Implications for Schizophrenia Research. *neuropsychopharmacology*. 1992;6:127-134.

10. Servan-Schreiber D, Printz H, Cohen JD. A network model of catecholamine effects: Gain, signal-to-noise ratio, and behavior. *Science*. 1990;249:892-895.

11. Jordan MI. Attractor dynamics and parallelism in a connectionist sequential machine. . *Cognitive Science Society*; 1986:531-546.

12. Williams RJ, Zipser D. Gradient-based learning algorithms for recurrent networks and their computational complexity. In: Chauvin Y, Rumelhart DE, eds. *Backpropagation: Theory, architectures, and applications*. Hillsdale, NJ: Erlbaum; 1995:433-486.

13. O'Reilly RC. The LEABRA model of neural interactions and learning in the neocortex. . *Department of Psychology*. Pittsburgh: Carnegie Mellon University; 1995.

14. Cornblatt BA, Lenzenweger MF, Erlenmeyer-Kimling L. The Continuous Performance Test, Identical Pairs Version: II. Contrasting Attentional Profiles in Schizophrenic and Depressed Patients. *Psychiatry Research*. 1989;29:65-85.

15. Wapner S, Krus DM. Effects of Lysergic Acid Diethylamide, and Differences Between Normals and Schizophrenics, on the Stroop Color-Word Test. *Journal of Neuropsychiatry*. 1960:76-81.

16. Abramczyk RR, Jordan DE, Hegel M. "Reverse" Stroop Effect in the Performance of Schizophrenics. *Perceptual and Motor Skills*. 1983;56:99-106.

17. Wysocki JJ, Sweet JI. Identification of Brain Damaged, Schizophrenic, and Normal Medical Patients Using a Brief Neuropsychological Screening Battery. *An International Journal of Clinical Neuropscyhology*. 1985;7:40-44.

18. Servan-Schreiber D, Cohen JD, Steingard S. Schizophrenia Deficits in the Processing of Context: A Test of Neural Network Simulations of Cognitve Functioning in Schizophrenia. *Archives of General Psychiatry*. inpress.

19. Parasuraman R. Memory load and event rate control sensitivity decrements in sustained attention. *Science*. 1979;205:924-927.

MODELING UNIPOLAR DEPRESSION RECOVERY

JOANNE S. LUCIANO[†]

Department of Cognitive and Neural Systems
Boston University, Boston, MA 02215
Email: jluciano@nmr.mgh.harvard.edu

and

MICHAEL A. COHEN

Department of Cognitive and Neural Systems
Boston University, Boston, MA 02215

and

JACQUELINE A. SAMSON

Harvard Medical School, Depression Research Facility
McLean Hospital, Belmont, MA 02178

ABSTRACT

We describe how a neural network model based on a system of ordinary differential equations can be used to replicate and predict depression recovery in response to specific treatments. A method for examining detailed patterns of clinical recovery using systems of second order ordinary differential equations is presented. We discuss why this method was chosen and how it can be used to reveal new information about how symptom response patterns differ across treatments. These approaches may be more broadly useful in other areas of cognitive and brain disorder research.

1 Introduction

Our purpose in modeling the depression recovery process is to work towards establishing a basis for different patterns of response to antidepressant treatments. This study sought to advance our understanding of how these treatments alleviate symptoms and move a person's status from depressed to recovering to recovered. Relevant questions are: What symptoms do the treatments affect, when and how do they interact, and what characterizes the patterns of recovery?

A direct approach to fitting multiple patient recovery data over time has not previously been attempted for two major reasons. One major reason is the difficulty posed by the high level of noise and the seemingly idiosyncratic variations between patients in recovery. We claim that some of these variations are due to the lack of a detailed model which uses the patients' initial data as a starting point. We

---

[†] Present address: Neural Systems Group, Psychiatry Department, Harvard Medical School, Massachusetts General Hospital, Building 149, 13th Street, Charlestown, MA 02129

offer one such model here. Common sense indicates that the pattern of recovery should depend on the initial state of the patient. The second major reason why patient recovery progress has not been directly mapped and compared is the large amount of variance that remains after the best fitting model is constructed. Some of this variability is unavoidable given the noise inherent in the measuring instruments used. Luciano (1996) provides a more complete study of robust measures of recovery described fully therein.

In order to better understand depression, we sought an approach that could provide treatment specific information about the sequence, timing, and interaction of the symptoms of depression in response to a specific treatment.

Unlike previous approaches which used a global indicator (Quitkin et al., 1984; Quitkin et al., 1993), our neural network model could provide data regarding specific symptoms and their response to drug treatment. We therefore followed seven symptom factors (described below) over the first six weeks of treatment in data from six patients who recovered in response to desipramine and six patients who recovered in response to cognitive behavioral therapy. We also used our model to extend the response-trajectory information obtained from a few specific time points during recovery (Katz et al., 1987) and showing how these points relate to outcome, we estimated a set of parameters that governed the dynamics of recovery in these patients. The the evolution of the symptom profile during recovery is described in detail in (Luciano, 1996). The resultant model can reliably predict a more detailed treatment-dependent pattern of recovery than can be predicted from previous models. Our work also extended a time series study of an individual patient's response in which each symptom was modeled independently as an ARIMA process (Hull et al., 1993) by using a larger sample of patients than those reported in the literature and by allowing for interactions among symptoms.

2   Methods

Much of the individual pattern of recovery appears predictable from the patient's initial data notwithstanding the considerable idiosyncratic variation among patients. In order to capture the maximum individual variation within a treatment group and compare the responses across groups, we adopted the following approach.

We studied the histories of recovered patients from two treatment groups, desipramine and cognitive behavioral therapy, in order to compare specific symptom responses in the initial six weeks of treatment. Two sets of parameters, one for each treatment group, were estimated from the initial data in order to capture the differences in symptomatology between the two treatment groups. The changes in symptoms were modeled using differential equations and the models were fit to seven symptom factors derived from the Hamilton Depression Rating Scale (see Table 1). These factors corresponded to our clinical observations about which symptom groupings recovered in tandem. Three characteristics of the response pattern were studied: (1) Latency: when during the six week period do the symptoms start to respond, namely, what is the average time elapsed to reach a fifty percent improvement in severity from baseline to six weeks after treatment has begun; (2) Treatment intervention effects: both immediate and delayed effects are direct effects of a treatment on a symptom; and (3) Symptom interaction effects: direct effects between pairs of symptoms that are an indirect response to treatment.

We first specified an architecture, or network of connections among variables, corresponding to the symptoms, but independent of the treatment. Following the construction of the architecture, treatment-dependent parameter sets were estimated using a learning algorithm adopted from optimal control theory (Bryson & Ho, 1975; Luciano, 1996). The two resulting treatment–dependent models were compared for (1) goodness of fit, (2) parametric differences in latency, treatment effects (both immediate and delayed), and interactions between symptoms, and (3) differences between the trained models when initialized with individual patient's baseline data values. In this way, we were able to quantify the reliability of the predicted behavior within and across treatment groups. The architecture was specified to have one variable for each of the seven symptom factors. The direct effects of treatment and the interactions among symptoms were represented in two ways: as modifiable connections from treatment to symptom factor variables and between the symptom factor variables. A latency variable represented the varying time in which symptoms respond to treatment.

2.1 Recovery Pattern Characteristic Features

Three assumptions were made in order to highlight characteristic features of the recovery patterns for depression.

The first assumption was that treatments act directly on symptoms, possibly by affecting neuromodulatory pathways acting on brain regions that control the behavior manifested in the symptom. This *treatment effect* corresponds to the direct effect of weights in the model, which represents the strength of each symptom response to a specific treatment. Other possible causes, such as spontaneous recovery, sporadic fluctuations of symptoms, life events, and anticipatory anxiety about treatment termination, were not considered

The second assumption was that the direct treatment effect has two components: an component which acts directly on the symptoms without delay and a delayed, or *latent* component, which reflects the underlying processes that could delay the response. Latency is clinically defined as the response time of a symptom to a treatment. *Latency* was included because it has been observed in antidepressant drug response patterns (Quitkin et al., 1984; Quitkin et al., 1987) and clinically, where response to antidepressant drug treatments is known to take up to four weeks.

Table 1: Symptoms that were studied by category.

Symptom Factor	Hamilton Item(s)	Description
Physical		
E SLEEP	4	Insomnia, Early (Difficulty falling asleep)
M,L SLEEP	5	Insomnia, Middle (Restless or waking during the night)
	6	Insomnia, Late (Waking in early morning)
ENERGY	8	Retardation (involuntary) slowness
	13	Somatic Symptoms, General (Heaviness/Energy)
Performance		
WORK	7	Work and activities (voluntary) loss of interest in activity, hobby, or work, must push oneself
Psychological		
MOOD	1	Depressed Mood (helplessness, hopelessness, sadness, worthless)
COGNITIONS	2	Feelings of Guilt (having let others down, present illness is a punishment)
	3	Suicide (life not worth living, thoughts, attempts)
ANXIETY	10	Anxiety, Psychic (subjective tension, irritability, excessive worry)

Latency in this context is generally associated with a drug response. Latency in therapy response has not been studied. Latency as modeled, is due the effect of a fixed sigmoid which rises in time. This latency is assumed to be the same across all factors for a fixed treatment and is modeled by a fixed parameter θ.

The third assumption was that symptom changes affect other symptoms. For example, increased energy may increase productivity at work, possibly through interconnections among regions such as transcortical connections and through environmental and metabolic feedback responses to behavioral changes. These *interaction* effects are modeled by the coefficients (weights) of the links among symptom nodes.

2.2 Recovery Pattern Dynamics

Initial observations suggested that a second order system was needed to capture the oscillatory components observed in time series plots of many treatment–responsive patients' recovery. Oscillatory components can be captured naturally by second order or higher order equations. These qualitative observations were later quantitatively confirmed (Luciano, 1996).

2.3 Recovery Model

The architecture reflects the characteristic features (latency, treatment effects, symptom effects) of the response patterns. The equations reflect the dynamics of the recovery process, i.e., how the characteristic features change during recovery.

2.3.1 Architecture

The overall architecture is shown in Figure 1; details of the architecture are shown in Figure 2. The architecture is independent of treatment. The intensity of each symptom (it's HDRS score) is represented by a network *node* (shown as ellipses in Figure 1) which corresponds to the activity level of a node (x_i) in the system of differential equations which describes the behavior of the network. Treatment direct effects and interactions among symptoms correspond to weighted connections (arrows) in Figure 1. Connection weights (coefficients in the equations) in the architecture represent the strength of the direct treatment intervention effects (u_i for immediate effect, v_i for latent effect) and the strength of the interactions between pairs of symptoms (w_{ij} and w_{ji}). The overall latency of the response to treatment corresponds to the parameter (Δt) of the delay node transfer function. This node transforms elapsed time (linear) into an overall latent effect (nonlinear).

The intensity of a treatment effect on a symptom corresponds to the value of the coefficient of the connection from the treatment to a symptom factor. A direct effect is inferred for symptoms whose recovery is strongly affected by the treatment intervention. The recovery model's direct effects can occur through two treatment pathways: one immediate and one latent. To separate and thus capture both treatment effects, two nodes were added to the model. The pathway with latency is represented by a delay node that is a sigmoid function with two parameters: delay and steepness of the onset of the delayed effect. The pathway without latency is represented by a step function fixed to coincide with the onset of the treatment.

2.3.2 Dynamics

The dynamics of the recovery model are described by a linear second order differential equation with terms representing the three characteristic features of interest: the direct effects of treatment, the indirect effects of treatment (interactions among symptoms), and the timing of the response of the symptoms.

Overall latency (Δt) is defined as the time elapsed from the beginning of treatment to the time when the effect of the treatment achieves half of its full accumulated overall effect, which was measured at intervals after six weeks of treatment.

The immediate direct effect of treatment, represented by a step function, correlates linearly with the acceleration (second derivative) of symptom changes, through the immediate treatment effect coefficients. The latent direct effect of treatment, represented by a sigmoid function of time, correlates linearly with the acceleration

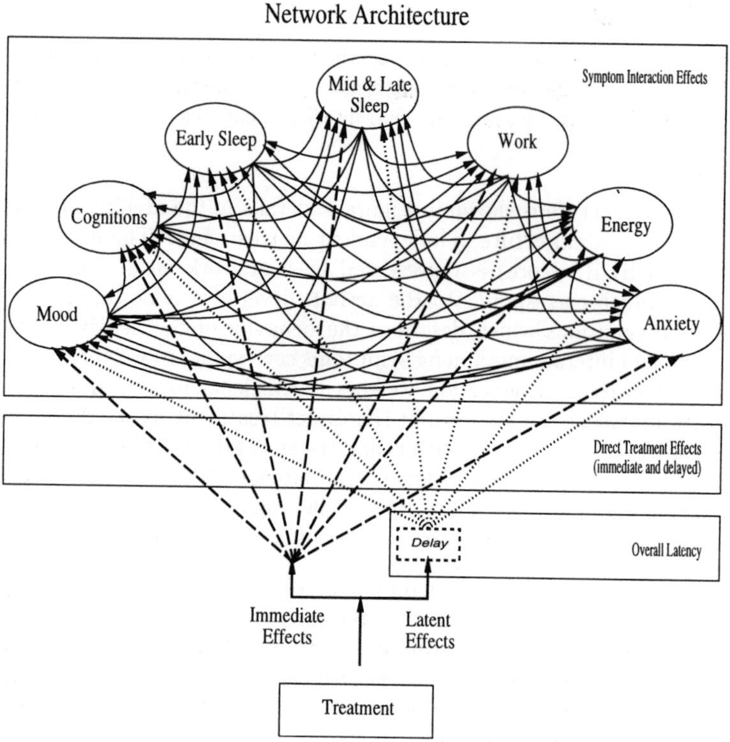

Network Architecture

Figure 1: Recovery model network architecture. Ellipses represent symptom factors; solid arrows between the symptom factors indicate symptom factor influences on other symptom factors. Short dashed arrows indicate delayed effects of treatment on symptoms; Long dashed arrows indicate immediate effects of treatment on symptoms.

(second derivative) of the symptoms, through the latent treatment effect coefficients.

The indirect effects of treatment, i.e. the effect symptoms have on each other, is modeled by a link from a source symptom to a target symptom (see Figure 2). A source symptom's intensity deviation correlates with the acceleration of target symptoms through the symptom interaction coefficients.

The scheme is formalized in:

$$\ddot{x}_i = -A_i\dot{x}_i + \sum_{j=1}^{N}(x_j - B_j)w_{ij} + s(t)u_i + h(\alpha, t - \Delta t)v_i \qquad (1)$$

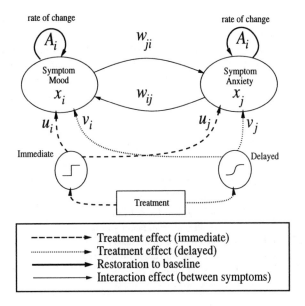

Figure 2: Direct effects and interactions in the recovery model. A_i represents damping; u_i represents the strength of the immediate effect of treatment on symptom node i; v_i represents the strength of the delayed effect of treatment on symptom i; and w_{ji} and w_{ij} represent the interaction between the symptoms: the strength of the effect of symptom i on symptom j and the strength of the effect of symptom j on symptom i, respectively.

$$s(t) \;=\; \begin{cases} 0 & t < 0 \\ 1 & \text{otherwise} \end{cases} \tag{2}$$

$$h(\alpha, t - \Delta t) \;=\; \frac{1}{1 + e^{-\alpha(t - \Delta t)}} \tag{3}$$

The meaning of each term in equation (1) is described in Table 2. The value of each variable x_i, (i=1,2,...,N; $N = 7$, the number of symptoms) is the predicted HDRS score of symptom i. Parameters are defined as follows: A_i is a damping coefficient which acts to slow down the rate of change of a symptom. B_j $(j = 1, 2, ..., N)$, is the baseline (pre-treatment) value of symptom factor x_j. w_{ij} is the coefficient of the interaction from symptom j to symptom i. Treatment intervention effects are represented by the outputs of two functions. The immediate effect is represented by a step function $s(t)$, with onset set to the beginning of treatment intervention. The latent effect is represented by a sigmoid function $h(\alpha, t - \Delta t)$, representing the delayed effects of treatment intervention. The sigmoid function uses two parameters to model the delayed onset of response: (1) overall latency (Δt [week]) *i.e.* the *delay* and (2) steepness (α), i.e. the *abruptness* of the response onset. It is possible to estimate overall latency from the data and was constrained to be the same for all factors. The intensity of the direct treatment intervention effect to a specific symptom factor i was determined independently by coefficients u_i (immediate) and v_i (latent).

Table 2: Recovery model parameters.

Parameter	Description
x_i	Activity of symptom factor i
A_i	Damping factor
B_i	Baseline (pre-treatment factor) value
w_{ij}	Interaction coefficient from factor j to factor i
u_i	Treatment Intervention (immediate) to factor i
v_i	Treatment Intervention (latent) to factor i
α	Steepness of latent onset of response
Δt	Overall Latency [weeks] of response

2.3.3 Training

The parameters used to fit the data were obtained through a training procedure (see Figure 3) that optimized the value chosen for each parameter. This section describes the training process, the data used and the optimization procedure.

The training algorithm was adopted from optimal control theory (Bryson & Ho, 1975; Luciano, 1996). The goal of training was to find model parameters that best fit the data. This method reduces the discrepancy between the prediction of the model and the actual data through a series of iterations over the data.

Prior to the optimization process, actual symptom values (ASV) were transformed into the same format as model symptom values (MSV). Thus, weekly patient data were linearly interpolated to yield daily data for training the model. The reason the data was transformed to be daily rather than weekly is because the theories of differential equations and optimal control are continuous, thus requiring finer time resolution than was available in weekly data from a six week study. The difference from each day to the next day was used as the training data for the first derivative of each day. For the last day, the first derivative was assumed to be the same as that of the previous day. In addition, Model symptom values begin one week prior to the onset of treatment, whereas actual symptom values begin at the onset of treatment. Based on the premise that the symptoms are at equilibrium before the onset of treatment, seven days of data were added before the beginning of treatment. The

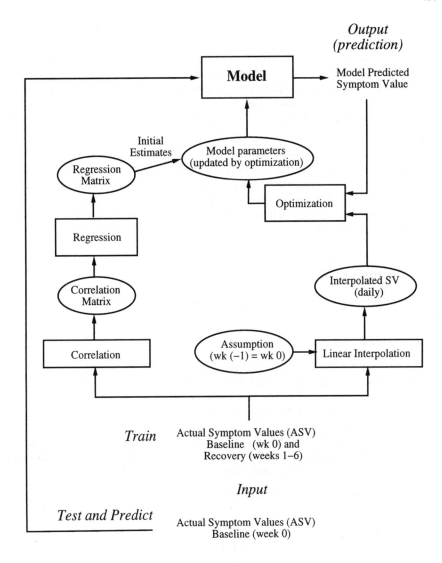

Figure 3: Overview of Training Process. Parameters were initialized with a regression matrix which was calculated from actual symptom values (ASV) by correlation and regression analyses. The model used these initial parameters to predict symptom values (model symptom values, MSV) of each patient from baseline. The optimization process iteratively modified parameters to minimize the discrepancy between MSV and ASV.

training data for these added data (week -1 to week 0), were set to the pre-treatment (baseline) values This was done by extending the ASV by one week (from week 0 to week -1); training data for the derivatives were set to zero. It was assumed that the symptom factor values before the beginning of treatment were constant and equal to the baseline. A linear interpolation was used to extend the data. The extension was necessary because the model had to use the data to learn the premise that the symptom factor changes did not occur without treatment.

Initial estimates of parameters were calculated from actual symptom values (ASV) by correlation and regression analyses. The model used these initial parameters to predict symptom values (model symptom values, MSV) of each patient from baseline. The optimization process used gradient descent through time to iteratively modify parameters and produce an optimized model (Luciano, 1996). The gradient of the objective function was calculated from each patient in turn. Parameters were updated at the end of each cycle to obtain a good fit to patients within a treatment group.

2.4   Measures of Model Dynamics

Two derived measures were used in analyzing the results obtained from the recovery model.

2.4.1   Strength of Response

The calculation for the accumulated interaction strength of symptoms utilizes the fact that the symptom factors were normalized by shifting and scaling the data to have mean values equal to 0.0 and variance values equal to 1.0, and that the maximum values of the step function and sigmoid function are 1.0. This measure is a rough approximation for the center range of the model. Measures of interactions among symptoms were derived from Equation 1 by ignoring indirect symptom influence (for instance, influence of factor j on factor i via factor k). Variables and parameters that appear in these equations are defined in Table 2.

Symptom interaction influence is given by:

$$
\begin{aligned}
W_{ij} &= +\frac{2}{T^2} \int \int w_{ij}(x_j - B_j) d^2 t \\
&\simeq -w_{ij} B_j
\end{aligned}
\tag{4}
$$

Treatment intervention influence is given by:

$$
U_i = +\frac{2}{T^2} \int \int \{w_{ii}(x_i - B_i) - u_i s(t) - v_i h(t)\} d^2 t
$$

$$\simeq \ -w_{ii}B_i - u_i - v_i(1 - \frac{\Delta t}{T})^2 \tag{5}$$

where T is the entire treatment period (six weeks), Δt is the overall latency, W_{ij} is the measure of total influence of symptom factor j on symptom factor i when x_i is small, and U_i is the measure of total influence of the treatment intervention on the symptom factor i when x_i is small.

2.4.2 Symptom Response Time

To compare the patterns of response to treatments we needed to construct the temporal structure of a patient's response. This meant that we needed a way to determine when each symptom responded to treatment. Based on the optimized model's prediction of a symptom's response trajectory, a measurement was made of the time it takes for the modeled symptom's intensity to decrease halfway from its initial intensity to its intensity after six weeks of treatment. This measurement is called the *half reduction time* (hrt). The hrt value is a prediction by the model after it has been trained on patient data, initialized with the baseline symptom values of a single patient, and allowed to evolve in accordance with the parameterized differential equations. Note that the half reduction time is not defined when a symptom is not present or does not improve.

3 Results

This section presents the results obtained for two treatment-specific recovery models. Each patient's week zero data were used as the initial conditions for a patient-specific run of the treatment-specific parameterized model to see the patient-specific predicted evolution of the symptom factors.

3.1 Validation

The statistics for the goodness of fit of these models to the data is presented in Table 3. Data from five of the six weeks studied were used in the calculation of the F statistics; the first week was used for the initial value of the differential equation. The high level of statistical significance obtained ($p < 1 \times 10^{-5}$) indicated that it was worthwhile to use this model to study recovery patterns. This supposition was confirmed (Luciano, 1996) despite our initial skepticism to question the apparent goodness of fit because of the following three reasons: (1) the assumption of data independence is violated (because the target data were time series data and therefore not independent); (2) the data were not partitioned into disjoint training and test sets; and (3) about half of the raw data was eliminated because the half reduction time was not defined in the actual data or the model predicted symptom trajectory.

Table 3: F-statistic results (79 parameters). Statistics were calculated between actual data linearly interpolated and predicted data by the model. r is Pearson's correlation coefficient; r^2 is the proportion of variance; F is an F-statistic; and p is the probability for the null hypothesis to hold. For the calculation of the F-statistic, degrees of freedom were $(N_1, N_2) = (252, 79)$ where N_1 is the number of predicted weekly data and N_2 is the number of free parameters. L_0 is the sum of squares of difference between the actual data after linear interpolation and the predicted data accumulated on a daily basis.

Cognitive Behavioral Therapy					
System	F	p	r^2	r	L_0
Second Order	5.36	$< 1 \times 10^{-5}$	0.664	0.815	17.5
Desipramine					
System	F	p	r^2	r	L_0
Second Order	1.90	0.00016	0.412	0.642	24.7

3.2 Recovery Pattern Differences by Treatment

Recovery pattern differences between cognitive behavioral therapy and desipramine can be summarized as follows: Differences were found in the order in which symptoms improved and in the timing of individual symptom improvement. The overall latency (response time over all patients and symptoms) was found to be longer in the DMI treatment group than in CBT treatment group. Direct effects were different as were interaction effects; DMI interaction effects were much stronger while the span of symptom response times were shorter. Analyses of the parameters and derived measures that resulted from this modeling effort are reported in detail in (Luciano, 1996) and will appear in future publications.

4 Discussion

This pilot study, while limited in its validity by a small sample, served to show the usefulness of these methods for extracting data about complicated relationships. As a next step, independent variables with higher temporal resolution need to be utilized. Many time series analysis algorithms require fifty weeks of data prior to the time of prediction. Typically, this amount of time series data is not available. If these methods prove useful, they may serve to encourage more frequent data to be gathered. Six weeks of weekly treatment data prohibits the use of many other potentially valuable methods because they have too few time points. In addition to more temporal data, other variables may prove to be better predictors for outcome. Finally, a truly robust model would include a specific noise model, which would again require significantly more data.

The current study has many technical limitations. First, this model does not distinguish transient from permanent treatment effects, since data subsequent to the termination of treatment were not available for either study. Second, the current method only partly distinguishes the *order* of the recovery from *causal sequence* of the recovery. For example, assume factors A, B, and C improved in this order. We cannot tell by looking at the sequence whether A or B independently or jointly caused the C to improve. They are distinguished only in the cases where a correlation method can distinguish them.

5 Conclusion

Our analyses demonstrates that mathematical models of clinical depression recovery from treatment-specific recovery data can be used to replicate and predict patient recovery patterns. Use of these modeling techniques enabled us to compare differences in the predicted recovery patterns of patients who responded to cognitive behavioral therapy against predicted recovery patterns of patients who responded to desipramine (Luciano, 1996).

We conclude that neural network modeling techniques are useful in clinical depression research and should also be useful in other areas of psychiatric research. Elaboration and further analyses of the work presented herein is found in Luciano (1996).

6 Future Directions

The starting point for clinical research on depression is usually the already–depressed person. Because we do not conduct studies that monitor the moods of persons in an attempt to determine the cause of depression, we are limited to (a) employing indirect evidence (based on other data such as animal models or pharmacological studies) or (b) working backwards studying the changes that occur in the transition from the depressed state to the non-depressed state. From what we can observe in a patient's response to specific treatments, we can attempt to hypothesize mechanisms underlying the disease. Observations made of the patients can be tested against behavior predicted by the model. The information obtained can then be used to improve the model and our understanding of the mechanisms underlying the illness.

Additional progress can also be made using newly available techniques. It is now possible to model specific neural circuits implicated in disease. Imaging data with fine temporal and spatial resolution are available using technology such as functional magnetic resonance imaging (fMRI). It is clear that future research should involve mathematical analyses at least as sophisticated as presented here, in order to understand complex and intricate relationships among data from these multiple sources. In addition, a systematic method for integration of multiple sources of disparate data, as well as mechanisms for identifying and tracking novel aspects in the data must also be considered. In other words, as more information about the biological underpinnings of depression and other psychiatric disorders is acquired, it will become increasingly important to develop integrative models that link different levels of neural organization.

7 Acknowledgments

This work was performed in collaboration with Michiro Negishi at the Department of Cognitive and Neural Systems, Boston University, and Daniel Bullock at the Department of Cognitive and Neural Systems, Boston University.

The data analyzed were obtained from previous clinical research studies of depression conducted at the Depression Research Facility, McLean Hospital in Belmont, Massachusetts by Dr. Jacqueline A. Samson, Dr. Joseph J. Schildkraut, Dr. Alan Schatzberg, and Dr. John J. Mooney.

References

Bryson, A. E. & Ho, Y.-C. (1975). *Applied Optimal Control.* Hemisphere Publishing Company, New York.

Hull, J. W., Clarkin, J. F., & Alexopoulos, G. S. (1993). Time series analysis of intervention effects, fluoxetine therapy as a case illustration. *Journal of Nervous and Mental Disease*, **181**, 48–53.

Katz, M., Koslow, S., Maas, J., Frazer, A., Bowden, C., Casper, R., Croughan, J., Kocsis, J., & Redmond Jr., E. (1987). The timing, specificity, and clinical predictors of tricyclic drug effects in depression. *Psychological Medicine*, **17**, 297–309.

Luciano, J. S. (1996). *Neural Network Modeling of Unipolar Depression: Patterns of Recovery and Prediction of Outcome.* PhD thesis, Boston University.

Quitkin, F. M., Rabkin, J. D., Stewart, J. M. J. W., McGrath, P. J., & Harrison, W. (1987). Use of pattern analysis to identify true drug response: A replication. *Arch Gen Psychiatry*, **44**, 259–264.

Quitkin, F. M., Rabkin, J. G., Ross, D., & Stewart, J. W. (1984). Identification of true drug response to antidepressants. *Arch General Psychiatry*, **41**, 782–786.

Quitkin, F. M., Stewart, J. W., McGrath, P. J., Tricamo, E., Rabkin, J. G., Ocepek-Welikson, K., Nunes, E., Harrison, W., & Klein, D. F. (1993). Columbia atypical depression. *British Journal of Psychiatry*, **163(suppl. 21)**, 30–34.